J. F. T. BUGENTAL *The Search for Authenticity*

AN EXISTENTIAL-ANALYTIC APPROACH TO PSYCHOTHERAPY

Enlarged Edition IRVINGTON PUBLISHERS, INC.

Copyright © 1981 by Irvington Publishers, Inc.
Copyright © 1965 by Holt, Rinehart and Winston, Inc.
All rights reserved.
No part of this book may be reproduced in any manner whatever, including information storage or retrieval, in whole or in part (except for brief quotations in critical articles or reviews), without written permission from the publisher. For information, write to Irvington Publishers, Inc., 551 Fifth Avenue, New York, New York 10017.

Chapters 2, 4, 6, 7, 8, and 21 include material first presented at the Fifth Post-Doctoral Institute, Arizona State University, © 1963 by Holt, Rinehart and Winston, Inc.

Acknowledgment is made to the following publishers for permission to print excerpts from the material cited below:

Grove Press, Inc., for excerpts from *Endgame* by Samuel Beckett (translated from the French by the author, copyright © 1958 by Grove Press, Inc., published by Grove Press, Inc.) and from *Krapp's Last Tape and Other Dramatic Pieces* by Samuel Beckett, copyright © 1958, 1959, 1960 by Grove Press, Inc., published by Grove Press, Inc.).

Harcourt, Brace & World, Inc., for an excerpt from "The Hollow Men" by T.S. Eliot (from *Collected Poems 1909-1962*; Copyright 1936 by Harcourt, Brace & World; © 1963 and 1964 by T.S. Eliot).

Random House, Inc., for an excerpt from "An *I* Can Never Be Great Man" by Stephen Spender (from *Collected Poems*; Copyright © 1955 by Stephen Spender).

Library of Congress Cataloging in Publication Data

Bugental, James F T
  The search for authenticity.

  Bibliography: p.
  Includes indexes.
  1. Psychotherapy. 2. Existential
I. Title.   psychology.
RC480.5.B78 1980   616.8'916   79-21163
ISBN 0-8290-0108-5

Printed in the United States of America

for Mary Edith

Preface to the enlarged edition

"I hope that implicit throughout the pages of this book will be my conviction, 'Man is a constantly evolving process, about whom we can never say the final word—these are my best estimates as of today.'" That was written in 1964 to preface this book (p. x)[1]. And now I reaffirm that thought—these are my best estimates as of today—except for one word: Today I write it, "A *person* is a constantly evolving process. . . ." Our culture and I as part of it currently are evolving to give explicit recognition to half of humankind too long unseen in implicit inclusion. "Men, women, and children continually evolve," to rescue children from the obscurity of only tacit presence in our thinking. This human evolution is the fascinating, frustrating, challenging, amusing, ever old and ever new subject matter of humanistic and existential psychology and psychotherapy.

In Chapter 24, written a decade-and-a-half after the prior section, I describe my own evolution during this period. As part of that evolution, in Chapter 24 (unlike the earlier portion of the book), I use "his or her" and "human" in lieu of sex-linked terms. Overall the direction has been that of discovering ways of simplifying, of finding that formerly disparate elements can be resolved into related aspects of more unitary perceptions. This movement provides esthetic gratification as well hope for the broader utility of the concepts; yet I view it with some caution. I want to explain that caution now because it is important to what will follow.

Complementarity vs. Competition in Subjective Experience

Our unthinking notion is that there is a "most true" way of perceiving any matter and that ultimately we hope to arrive at that most true view. We accept that some issues are difficult to grasp and that we need successive approximations until we get to that final comprehension (a word meaning both to understand and to hold). This way of thinking results in competition always being implicit when two or more ways of seeing something are present at the same time. Which is right? Which is most true? What's the answer? These are the questions we ask. I think that in the realm of subjective experience this is a wasteful and even counter-productive approach (that is, not *the right* way of seeing things!).

Questions as how to conceive and describe psychotherapy or how to think about the further possibilities of human potential are tremendously complex and extensive. Any person considering such issues brings to the task a unique personal history and thus a unique readiness to understand. For some, great detail will best fit their needs; for others, a quick overview. For some, careful spelling out of procedures will most advance understanding; for others, painstaking attention to conceptual foundations is needed.

At the time I was writing the earlier edition of this book, I was celebrating having at last some feeling of mastery of my craft after many years of preparation, and I wanted to share that attainment with others. Thus I took care to work things out in abundant detail—for my own further understanding as well as to communicate. I frequently analyzed concepts and experiences into their constituents, and I named the multiple portions thus laid bare so that pointing and discussion would be aided. Today I am at a different point in my professional and scientific evolution (not better, different). Today, as I indicated above, I find an excitement in discerning connections and identities that formerly were not seen or not valued.

The reader must take from this buffet of conceptualizations according to her/his own appetite. I am pleased to be able to add to the earlier offering, but I hope that both portions are worthy of respect for their own purposes.

I have elaborated the foregoing because I intend to speak fully from my present perspective without rationalizing consistency with earlier pages and because I want to point out a destructive tendency which we all so easily slip into and which limits our understanding and our ability to use diverse contributions. Chapter 24, then, is one descriptive overlay upon experience, an overlay that may be used to complement the more detailed overlay of the earlier chapters.

Therapy Procedure and Therapeutic Perspective

Rereading the descriptions of how the therapist works, the values and cautions he/she needs to keep in mind, the signs to be watched, and the patterns to be developed, I marvel at the wealth of detail in the earlier pages. "Of course, of course, that is all very useful (and rather well said, eh?). Yes, yes, those are good things to keep in mind, and the next time I teach a group of therapists, I must be sure to recall that it's all recorded here." Yet somehow I'm just a bit impatient—dare I say, bored?—with the earnest pedagogue who so carefully details all those good and useful matters.

And then I realize: I'm at a very different point in my working career. It is not that I take issue with many of the points the younger Jim makes (Well, now really, that 19-to-1 ratio for client talk to therapist talk [p. 115] is pretty embarrassing, isn't it?). It's just a matter of emphasis, of attitude, of practice, and experience. The younger Jim was writing the lessons he had learned from rough experience and trying—then as now—to make it a little less rough for younger colleagues. He cherished finally arriving at a coherent foundation for his work. Recording and sharing it was important to refining it, growing in it, *and outgrowing it*.

Now a different Jim reads the lessons, values them, and looks beyond them. They are like the scales and exercises the musician must master in order to get to the true music of her/his calling. As with the musician so with the therapist; artistry must grow from the soil of thorough mastery of the fundamentals and from years of apprenticeship. I want nothing I say here to question the absolute necessity of the therapist learning his/her craft, solidly grounding her/his work in considered and disciplined attitudes and methods. Only on such a foundation can the further step be taken of going *through and* beyond procedure to spontaneous and whole presence in the relationship with the client. That sort of presence grows out of having so incorporated the fundamentals that they are intrinsically part of one's being in the relationshop. And the relationship is the essential medium in which true psychotherapy can occur. Thus, therapy procedure is on the route to a truly therapeutic perspective. The perspective is not the therapy itself, but it illuminates it. Chapter 24, accordingly, speaks mostly of perspective; earlier chapters elaborate procedure.

Acknowledgements

It is an existential challenge to me to try to recognize all who, in one way or another, have contributed to my experience and thinking and thus to this extension of *The Search for Authenticity*. Certainly my clients (no longer "patients") have continued to be chief among my instructors, and I am genuinely pleased to have this means to say publicly my appreciation for them, individually and collectively. Similarly I have been enriched by students and supervisees who have been responsive, challenging, and informative.

Among those whom I want especially to recognize individually are Alvin A. Lasko, John L. Levy, Ramonda K. Bridges, Bette Harrell, Roger N. Walsh, Barbara Kessler, Patrick Thunberg, Daniel Sydiaha, and most particularly, my wife, colleague, and buddy, Elizabeth Keber Bugental.

Santa Rosa, California

J. F. T. B.

PREFACE

My work is primarily that of conducting long-term, intensive psychotherapy with people of more than average education and better than average socio-economic position. Many of these people are not "sick" or "emotionally disturbed" in the traditional, psychiatric sense. They are instead concerned that their lives are less meaningful or less vital than they sense is potential to them. They come to therapy to find help in attaining greater realization of their being as individuals. I am deeply engrossed in and find constant stimulation from this work. This book is my attempt to conceptualize what my colleagues who are my "patients" are teaching me about what it means to achieve the potential of a human being.

I find in thinking about the human situation that the existential perspective most illuminates my own day-to-day experience, including my work with these people. The attempt to open my awareness to the tremendous range and variety of human life has brought to me appreciations that no literature in itself can reproduce. Psychotherapists, and perhaps psychologists-psychotherapists in particular, are prone to overvalue the written and the public communication. For me it has been only as I have been able to let go in some measure to what my patients were unconsciously teaching me about living and personality and psychotherapy that I have been able to achieve a more encompassing grasp upon what has been constantly presented to me throughout my own life. Let me make explicit, too, that a personal psychotherapeutic experience has very much contributed to this difficult but essential letting-go process.

To Whom the Book Is Addressed

This book is written for several groups of readers. I am writing for practicing psychotherapists, but by no means only for them. While the experienced therapist may be able to carry forward my observations beyond the points at which my deficiencies in conception and articulation leave them, I hope that many others will be stimulated to such thinking. For the experienced therapist, some of the things I will say may be familiar, but a great many therapists have not had the opportunity to think through some of these matters from the humanistic-existential viewpoint. I hope they will find these perspectives refreshing and challenging.

It is my hope that this book can speak meaningfully to the great numbers of people who are engaged in working with others in the countless important and varied helping roles that are vital to our lives today: to social workers, clergymen, probation and parole officers, teachers, physicians and nurses, attorneys and judges—to any who will listen, to any who have caught a glimpse or more of the further potentials in themselves and those with whom they work. To them I write in the hope that they will find in my words encouragement to their own venturings in thinking and experiencing about human beings.

I am quite sure that I want to write to students in the fields concerned with human beings—especially to psychotherapists-to-be, but not only to them. I think I want especially to strike sparks in students with a humanistic orientation who now feel lost in mechanomorphic psychology or medicine or social work. (That word "mechanomorphic" [Waters, 1948] is a good one to characterize those views of human beings that reduce subjects to objects, that would devitalize human experience and extol the model of the machine.) To those students, I would like to bring some hope that all psychology (or all psychotherapy) is not mechanomorphic and to arouse in them a judicious bit of rebellion.

Finally, I hope I can write so that the intelligent nonprofessional may read with pleasure and stimulation. I want to encourage these laymen to think anew about what it means to be a person. In the long run, it is the big block of uncommitted voters that swings the election—not the professional politicians nor the committed party members. In the long run it is the open-minded nonprofessional who will swing the choices on man's further evolution. I am completely serious when I say I think we are in a time of such choice right now. Man's genuine further evolution or his destruction or overwhelming regression will very likely be decided in the next fifty to seventy-five years. I am concerned that too much mechanomorphic thinking—in psychology and sociology and medicine, to be sure, but also in business and advertising, and in government and politics, and even in religion and philosophy—too much of this depersonalized, inhuman thinking may get accepted as *the way* to think about human problems and human decisions. I want to add my voice to those who are calling on men to awaken to a destiny greater than that of being Mark I computers. I want to talk to some professional people and some nonprofessional people about the far horizons of the human frontier.

Plan of Presentation

Having spelled out to whom I am writing, let me say a few words about how this book is arranged. Basically the book describes what I do as an existential-analytic psychotherapist and what I think about when I am doing it. I will try to be as explicit and detailed as is realistic about what procedures seem to me to be productive in helping people who thirst for something more than they have found thus far in their lives. For the professional psychotherapist and for the student who intends to become a psychotherapist this will have its own value. I certainly do not expect them to agree with me at all points or to adopt my procedures intact. I hope they will be challenged to rethink their own views and perhaps to challenge me in turn. But for the nonpsychotherapist reader, this discussion of therapeutic procedure is helpful to my communication with him also. I can best bring to him what I hope he will receive if I say very concretely what I do and why I do it, if I help him to sit with me in the therapeutic hour and observe at first hand what the experiences are that stimulate me to the thinking and speculating and feeling I do.

Beyond the discussions of therapeutic technique, the other major areas will, I hope, be of interest to both therapist and non-therapist readers, although each will take from it according to his own readiness and interests. I have tried to provide both a general and a relatively simple introduction to the existentialist orientation as I use it and a first statement of a more fully developed metapsychology of the human condition. The latter is still incomplete; although it is at a point where it can facilitate clinical thinking and actions. To help with the process of communicating it, I have used the pattern of first stating the view in metaphoric and oversimplified fashion, returning to give it a more formal but still oversimplified statement, and then later restating it a third time in more fullness. Finally, I have tried to show some of the many open areas in which further development may occur.

Manner of Presentation

I ought to say a word about the style in which I choose to write. I am increasingly impressed with the dangerously pathogenic trend toward the mechanization of man. It seems to me that more and more we treat ourselves and others as interchangeable units, that identity and individuality get washed out in the process of acculturization. Too many books and articles about psychotherapy are written as though the authors have made discoveries that are true for all people and all psychotherapy. Certainly I have discovered this tendency again and again in what I have written. Nevertheless, I do not think doing so is existentially valid.

I have tried to write this book as a personal statement. I use the first person frequently, especially when dealing with concrete experiences and with areas of personal speculation. I hope you who read will read in a first-person fashion also. I am convinced that no one can take what I write here and apply it without transmutation of some kind. I hope that implicit throughout the pages of this book will be my conviction, "Man is a constantly evolving process, about whom we never say the final word—these are my best estimates as of today." I and you must both recognize our constant evolution and each take responsibility in this encounter. Though you may choose thus to discard some of my cherished ideas, you will have met me most genuinely if you retain your own identity in the reading. I hope thereby to speak to you, my reader, most authentically.

Throughout the book, I have tried to communicate on two levels at once: to convey ideas and concepts on the one hand, and to evoke feelings, attitudes, and emotional perspectives on the other. The reader who would understand me fully must be open-minded in these dimensions. If this book is, as I hope it is, a voyage to the new world of human experience, an exploration however tentative and incomplete, then I am convinced we will need the compass of our feelings as surely as we will need the charts of our reasoning if we are to make a true landfall on the human frontier.

Los Angeles, California   J. F. T. B.
November 1964

ACKNOWLEDGMENTS

This book is a distillation of so many experiences that it brings me to something of a crisis to attempt to set down the names of those who have particularly contributed to my writing. The reference list at the back of the book makes a beginning, but a very formal and impersonal one. Here I want to express more directly my indebtednesses. Alvin A. Lasko, Thomas C. Greening, and Gerry Haigh, my colleagues at Psychological Service Associates, have been generous with their personal and professional support, have read and helpfully commented on portions of the manuscript, and have permitted their own lives to be disrupted by my needs while writing. To George A. Kelly, Abraham H. Maslow, Rollo May, and Carl R. Rogers, go my sincere thanks for intellectual stimulation and for personal encouragement. Jerome L. Saperstein and George Frumkes taught me much about psychoanalytic theory and procedure, and I am genuinely grateful.

Some sections of the book represent revisions of earlier presentations. In particular I want to thank the following.

The *Journal of Humanistic Psychology* (and its editor Anthony Sutich) for permission to reproduce a portion of Chapter One that first appeared in the Spring, 1964, issue of that journal (Volume 4, Number 1, pages 19–26).

The *Journal of Existentialism* for permission to reproduce portions of Chapter Four that appeared in the Fall, 1964, issue of that journal.

Psychiatry for permission to reproduce a portion of Chapter Five that first appeared in the February, 1964, issue of that journal (Volume 27, pages 73–77).

Psychotherapy: Theory, Research and Practice for permission to reproduce portions of Chapter Ten that first appeared in that publication.

The Review of Existential Psychology and Psychiatry for permission to reproduce portions of Chapter Eleven that first appeared in Volume 2 (1962), Number 3 of that journal (pages 241–248).

The American Psychological Association and the *Journal of Consulting Psychology* for permission to reproduce portions of Chapter 21 that first appeared in that journal (1964, Volume 28, pages 272–277).

A very special word of thanks goes to Arthur Shedlin, who read the entire manuscript with a sympathetic but critical eye and who gave me much support and assistance in many phases of the preparation of the manuscript. Phyllis Wittenberg supervised the endless task of typing and retyping, correcting and then typing again, with equally unlimited skill and good humor.

Mary Edith Bugental, my wife, has read the manuscript with a discerning awareness to supplement her ever-present emotional support with suggestions that brought greater clarity and fewer mechanical and structural defects.

A PERSONAL WORD TO MY PATIENTS

I have had many teachers. Some were long dead before I was born, but I have learned from their writings. Some others are living and, happily, will continue to teach me. Some I have known personally, and many of these have given me not only words but example, not only example but their personal warmth and companionship. To all of these I am genuinely and deeply grateful.

But when I come to write a word to you who have honored me by being my patients, I find I have a very special set of feelings. You have given me of your thoughts, your emotions, and your living experiences. More than that, you have given me of your trust and your hope. I know a guilt and regret that I could never be all that you hoped. I know a pride and happiness that for some of you I could be what you needed. And to each of you I feel a gratitude for what you have taught me out of the living stuff of your being.

In a very real way each of you—whether you personally benefited greatly or little from your work with me—each of you is my co-author in these pages. What I feel I understand most in what I have written is what you have presented to me again and again until finally I could hear.

Throughout these pages I talk about my experiences with you. I name names, but they are not your names. I talk of people but not of any one of you. I have deliberately and systematically varied information that might in any way be identifying, and I have built composite portraits and given them single names. If you recognize yourself in any aspect of one of my fictional patients, be assured

A Personal Word to My Patients

that anything else I may say about that fictional patient probably does not apply to you.

I wish I might salute you by name as I can my more academic colleagues and teachers, because I would like to express my indebtedness more explicitly. Unfortunately, our cultural values are still at that primitive stage where to name you might be to embarrass you. You and I know that your work in therapy was an expression of your courage even more than of your despair, and so I salute you anonymously.

J. F. T. Bugental

CONTENTS

Preface vii
Acknowledgments xiii
A Personal Word to My Patients xv

PART ONE THE CONDITIONS OF BEING HUMAN   1

  1 The Human Frontier   8
      Humanistic Psychology and Existentialism 9
      Humanistic Psychology 11
      The Existential-Analytic Thesis 14
  2 Man's "Thrown" Condition   21
      Other Important Concepts 26
  3 Authenticity: The Central Concern of Psychotherapy   31
      Authenticity as the Primary Existential Value 31

PART TWO THE ANALYTIC PHASE OF THE
          THERAPEUTIC WORK   47

  4 The Experience, Concept, and Procedure
    of Existential-Analytic Therapy   51
  5 The Therapeutic Relation: Essential
    Medium of Therapy   69
      Psychodiagnostics and the Quest for Certainty 73
      Iatrogenic Complications 82
      Developing the Therapeutic Alliance 85

6 The Existential Meaning of the Resistance	88
Characteristics of the Resistance 92	
7 The Analysis of the Resistance	104
Listening to the Patient 107	
The Therapist's Interventions 115	
8 The Analysis of the Transference	134
The Transference and the Therapeutic Relation	137
Analytic Procedure 143	
9 Tragedy and the Psychotherapeutic Processes	151
Meaning of Tragedy 152	
Tragedy and the Therapeutic Work 155	
10 The Existential Crisis	166
Conceptualizing the Existential Crisis 170	
Therapeutic Procedure in the Existential Crisis	173

PART THREE   THE ONTOGOGIC PHASE OF THE THERAPEUTIC WORK   183

11 What Is a Person?	189
What Is a Person? 193	
12 The I, the Me, and the Self	200
The I-Process 203	
The Self 209	
Implications of the I-Self Distinction for Actualization and the Transference 213	
13 Awareness: The Basic Process of Being	217
The Nature of Awareness 219	
14 Ontologic Aids to Expanding Awareness	235
15 Ontologic Freedom: Emancipation from the *Self*	245
The Nature of Ontologic Freedom 247	
Emancipation 254	
16 Ontologic Freedom: Actualization and Transference	263
Transcendence 277	
Conclusion 279	
17 Courage or Dread: The Existential Issue	282
The Confrontation of Existential Anxiety 283	

18 The Existential Neuroses	291
Response to the Anxiety of Fate and Death 292	
Response to the Anxiety of Guilt and Condemnation 300	
Response to the Anxiety of Emptiness and Meaninglessness 304	
Response to the Anxiety of Loneliness and Isolation 309	
19 Ontogogy: In Support of Courage: A. Freeing from the *Self* and the Response of Faith	316
Emancipation from the Self 322	
Contingency and Faith 327	
20 Ontogogy: In Support of Courage: B. The Responses of Commitment, Creativity, and Love	334
Responsibility and Commitment 334	
Autonomy and Creativity 343	
Apartness and Love 351	

PART FOUR THE HUMAN FRONTIER 359

21 The Person Who Is the Therapist	361
Gratifications in Being a Therapist 362	
Maturity of the Psychotherapist 368	
22 Psychotherapy and Emergent Man	376
23 Beyond the Human Frontier	395
Further Levels of Emergence 396	
The Inner Life of Emergent Man 397	
An Emergent Society 403	
Beyond the Human Frontier 412	

24 The Search Today

References 417
Index of Names 429
Index of Subjects 431

*The Search
for Authenticity*

PART ONE *The conditions of being human*

What is the meaning of "an existential orientation" to the psychology of personality and the practice of psychotherapy?

An existential orientation to personality and psychotherapy recognizes the human experience as the central fact of existence, examines the vicissitudes of that experience in the perspective of the basic nature of being, and orients its growth-inducing efforts toward maximum accord with the whole of life. This is a first answer to the question. Each of the three chapters of *Part One* will answer the question further (as will the whole book, for that matter).

First we will consider the emergence of the "third force" in psychology (Maslow, 1962b, p. vi). This is a new wave of humanistic concern that initially was a reaction away from mechanomorphic (Waters, 1948) views of man and that is beginning to have a more affirmative stance as well. After looking at some of the postulates and orienting perspectives of humanistic psychology, I will make a further capsule statement of the basic thesis of this book. Here the central emphasis is on one's authenticity in relation to the givenness of the conditions of life. With this overview in mind I will next set forth some of the values I personally find in the existential orientation.

Our *second* chapter has two overlapping purposes. On the one hand it will introduce certain concepts of the existential point of view to those readers who may not be familiar with them. But more importantly, in a way, I want it to summon up, if possible, for all readers an organismic awareness of our human situation. It seems increasingly manifest to me that genuine comprehension and effective utilization of the existential viewpoint is not simply an intellectual matter (at least in terms of what we usually mean by the term, "intellectual"—abstract and cognitive only). Many people seem to apprehend the existential viewpoint in a way that makes it an experienced appreciation of living. This sort of participation in the communication process between the writer and the reader is what I hope to contribute to in the second chapter. Needless to say, the reader's willingness to "come to meet" what is written is equally important.

In the *third* chapter I say in greater detail what my existential orientation to personality and psychotherapy is. This is done by examining the central concern of psychotherapy, which is authenticity. In this discussion we will consider more thoroughly the existential givens which our awareness discloses and the existential anxieties associated with these givens. At root the distresses that bring people to psychotherapy are the results of efforts to avoid existential anxiety through living in ways not in accord with the givens of life. In a sense that is very literally true, the therapist's calling is to help his patients reclaim their lives.

Part Two of this book, which picks up with *Chapter Four*, deals with the analytic phase of the therapeutic work. This phase tries to disclose and dissolve the distortions of authenticity that keep the patient in a state of non-being. *Part Three* assumes that the analytic phase has proceeded reasonably well and introduces our attention to the ways in which a therapist may aid his client toward greater authenticity of being. The final section, *Part Four*, looks searchingly at the person who is the therapist and then speculates about the further evolution of man possible as greater authenticity is more generally achieved.

Three Constraints upon Writing about Personality and Psychotherapy

Now as I come to write about what I have been thinking and learning, I find that I will do violence to that thinking and learning if I try to cast it into the usual forms of books on personality and psychotherapy. Gradually, I have come to realize that I am confronted with an existential choice; whether to be academically and scientifically "respectable" or to be as faithful to my experience as possible. I don't think I can have both. Let me explain what I mean.

I have come to recognize that the attempt to set down in as communicative a fashion as possible what it is I think and do as I work in psychotherapy is constrained in three ways:

—"factual reporting" is distortive; only "fiction" can accurately convey my meanings.

—impersonal reporting pretends to a universality and ultimateness which I am confident are not so; I am, perforce, writing a personal document.

—the very processes of thinking and writing are part of my inquiry and discovery, so that I am always moving beyond what it is I have written. Thus any statement is in some degree out-of-date as I make it.

I want to enlarge upon these constraints, for they have significances beyond those immediately evident. It appears to me that they may throw some light on our perennial difficulties in psychological science when we try to write embracing laws or formulate dependable and replicable observations about human behavior and experience.

In brief what I speculate is this: Our observations are the very phenomena they observe. If I say, "John seems to have a need for taking a dominant role," I am not describing John, only; I am describing the "seeming," my observation. When I speak of writing a "personal document," I am amplifying one implication of this hypothesis.

THE NECESSITY OF WRITING "FICTION"

We have the unexamined assumption that technical and scientific writing is an objective reporting of public facts. However this may be in the physical sciences, or even in some parts of psychological science, it most definitely is not the case in describing psychotherapy. A report on a psychotherapeutic contact that gave a verbatim protocol of everything said, included detailed observational notes on all facial expressions, gestures, and body postures—in short, a color, sound, motion picture of the contact—would still fail to convey to the observer or reader the real nature or meanings of that contact. Such a color, sound, motion picture would indeed be something of a projective technique that different psychotherapists could interpret with quite contrasting understandings. If I am to describe what I do as a psychotherapist, I must go beyond such factual, and necessarily superficial, reporting.

Of course, it is usual to recognize that such a simple description of externals is inadequate. Most writing about psychotherapy goes beyond that level without hesitation. What is much more frequent is a kind of unrecognized fiction. The author writes of subjective processes in himself and his patient as though they were as manifest as the action on a chess board, as though he (the therapist) made each observation and intervention from a current comprehension and perspective, while these actually are more the products of hindsight and speculation. Certainly, as a therapist, I do not find that I ordinarily have such comprehension nor do I hear from other therapists who speak with me candidly that they are so blessed.

At the time of any therapeutic interview I have certain general and other, more specific, perspectives and ideas in mind (I will describe these in detail in later pages). However, the actual business of that interview would be grossly interfered with were I consciously to order my participation in terms of these preconceptions. It is, rather, my responsibility to be present in the contact in such a way that I am flexibly serving the patient's and my own purposes without undue deliberation or contrivance. As a result, what actually occurs in the interview is only in part available to objective recording or self-aware detailing. Only through taking up the novelist's skill can I hope to convey to a reader what that contact meant for me and the patient. In writing about the interview retrospectively I must recall what I can, must infer from my general orientation, and must generalize from any context. Only in this way may I approximate anything like an adequate account of what transpired. The result, of course, is that the account is not the sort of "objective" statement customarily thought to be required in science. But the result also, to the degree I am candid and perceptive, is a more valid rendering of that contact in terms of its human meanings than any other method can provide.

Let us try to illustrate this point by rather exaggerated examples. Recently I saw a new patient for intake. The impression he made on me began when I met him in the waiting room and accompanied him up the hall to my office. Let me describe that meeting.

> The patient is approximately five feet ten inches tall and weighs about 165 pounds. He is dressed in a dark pullover sweater, grey slacks, and tan moccasins. His handclasp is moderately strong, and his hand is moist . . .

Now let me describe it a second time.

> The patient jumped a little as though surprised in a guilty action when I opened the waiting room door. He bobbed to his feet in a rush of greeting which somehow managed to convey a combined feeling of his eagerness to be liked and his conviction that that liking could only come if he put on a convincing show. His clothes were cautious beatnik. His hand shake was wet and seemed to be half a yielding to social convention and half a daring himself to touch me. Going down the hall ahead of me, he hummed to himself as though frightenedly shouting his nonchalance . . .

THE NECESSITY OF WRITING A PERSONAL DOCUMENT

What I have just said will make it clear that this book is, for the most part, to be regarded as a personal document. It is comprised of statements of who I am as well as of what I think. By no means do I hold that these statements are "the" definitive statements, and I am quite convinced that other equally valid, but quite contrasting, statements can be made by other writers in the field.

To write a personal document about psychotherapy is to recognize the actual situation; namely, psychotherapy is more art than science. This means that I cannot set down specifications which another psychotherapist can take over intact and practice effectively and successfully. Indeed, I would not be able to write specifications which I, myself, would use tomorrow with effectiveness. My intent, rather, must be so to present my thinking about procedures that they become raw material, or food, for another therapist to ingest, excrete some parts, retain and assimilate others which he builds into his own being. Thus he implements his work with his patients. Although this statement of the state of affairs is especially accurate for the existential position, I am reasonably convinced it is true for all writing about psychotherapy. I know I would personally much mistrust the therapist who was a completely faithful exponent or disciple of any other psychotherapist. The uniqueness of the encounter between the therapist and patient is such that it cannot be pre-prescribed, pre-dictated by any authority, any system, or any formalized plan.

THE NECESSITY OF MAKING AN INCOMPLETE STATEMENT

In setting forth these constraints upon writing about personality and psychotherapy I have already made it evident that the very processes of thinking and writing are tools to expanding one's awareness. This means that any statement made must inevitably be the statement of what *was* thought rather than of current thinking. In trying to prepare these chapters, I find again and again that my thinking moves on beyond the point at which I have clearly formulated my ideas. Thus the attempt to describe the nature of the transference, for example, opens up new possibilities for the understanding of transference and its handling.

This seems a clear example of the operation of indeterminacy, which is inherent in trying to understand and describe significant human experience. One can commit a kind of intellectual suicide if one tries to write a definitive and ultimate statement about personality or psychotherapy. He then may either endlessly pursue a degree of completion which he will never achieve, or make a statement to which he cannot give full allegiance and find himself forever stuck with trying to defend that which his awareness strains to move beyond. I intend neither of these extremes for myself.

It is pertinent to interject here the observation that once we recognize the process nature of human experience and the infinite potentialities of human thinking and discovery, we give up hope of an orderly and completed system of thinking. But having given that up, we are begun upon an intellectual adventure which has within it high excitement and genuine creative potential. Many of us will find the ambiguity and inexorable incompleteness of this approach to be threatening. Certainly I experience these feelings myself. But I know too that once we change the conception of the enterprise in which we are engaged to that of exploration in an infinite system, once we give up the hope of making the ultimate and definitive discovery and recognize that our transaction with our experience of the out-there is a creative, artistic one, there is more to be gained than we have lost.

1—*The human frontier*

The term, "frontier," describing that region which divides the known from the unknown, graphically describes the locus of our concern in this book. Indeed, the implicit subtitle of much that we will discuss will be "Reports from the human frontier."

There was a period when I thought seriously about becoming a historian. If I had, I know surely the area in which I would have specialized. The story of the discovery, exploration, and development of the Western Hemisphere is for me one of the most enthralling and inspiring imaginable. There is an excitement in realizing that for millenia man had lived unknowingly in what was essentially close proximity to a whole other world and yet imagined he knew all there was to be known. Then the miraculous occurs: another world is discovered. The first great discovery is not fully appreciated. Other discoveries seem to make clear what has been found, although actually they but touch the edge of it. The Northwest Passage, the fountain of youth, the first inland excursions, the settling of colonies, the beginnings of a new concept of the human experience growing out of the illimitable frontier as the backdrop to all else!

I am drawing a parallel between what happened in the geographic world in the sixteenth and seventeenth centuries and what is happening in the psychologic world in the twentieth. I am quite convinced that so far as genuinely discovering or disclosing the meaning of the human experience and exploring and developing human potential we are in the very early stages. Continuing our parallel, we are at about the first quarter of the seventeenth century. Some footholds have been established in Central and South America. Now the first colonies that will endure are being planted on the continent, that will show the most remarkable development in the years to come. One can draw many parallels between the historic developments and the evolution of the behavioral sciences, but the significant parallel has to do with the attitudes of men about themselves and their world. The "new world" of the sixteenth and seventeenth centuries was not the Western Hemisphere. The real new world was the entire earth. Europe itself, and eventually all continents, was changed by the impact of the raw fact of the Americas. That impact extended to forms of government, concepts of commerce, the social class structure, religious beliefs—to all that had made the old world what it was and what it would never be again. Today, I believe, we are on the brink of just such another period of universal change, this time in our concept of the human experience.

The essential thing I want to say is in reality to express a faith and a hope. We do not know very much yet about what it means to be a human being. We do not appreciate in any depth what the potentials of human imagination, creativity, and variation may be. We are more governed by superstition than fact, more limited by tradition than recognition, more inhibited by our own fears than by external constraints in exploring the whole world of our being. I believe we have made but the barest beginnings on exploring this new hemisphere, this human frontier. And I want to share with those who have a mind to hear it, some of my excitement and wonder from these journeys on the human frontier.

Humanistic Psychology and Existentialism

In the more than two decades since World War II began, educated thinking in America about man and his condition has undergone tremendous changes. Twenty-five years ago, psychology, psychiatry, psychotherapy, and related disciplines were barely emerging into a wholistic conception of the human being. By and large the dominant influences in these fields were reductionistic, mechanistic, and part-function centered. In the intervening time, these influences seem to me to have reached and passed their floodtides. The orientation is, to be sure, still very much employed and productive, but a newer, more inclusive perspective on the human experience is growing rapidly and appears to be the ascendant one. This emerging orientation has been called variously, "the third force" in psychology (after psychoanalysis and behaviorism), "neo-phenomenology," and "humanistic psychology."

Humanistic psychology has become a rallying point for those who have been dissatisfied with what they felt were the stifling constraints of the behaviorists or the institutionalized dogma of classical psychoanalysis (Bugental, 1962e, 1963b; Maslow, 1962b; Rogers, 1963). In many ways the third force is most clear about what it opposes and least in harmony about what it supports. Within its ranks one may discern such varied figures as Abraham Maslow, Rollo May, Carl Rogers, Erich Fromm, Ernest Schachtel, Charlotte Buhler, Clark Moustakas, Dorothy Lee, Hubert Bonner, Sidney Jourard, and E. J. Shoben. Clearly, this is not a company from which one may expect an easy unanimity about many key issues.

Nevertheless there is emerging some consensus about the general subject matter and operating assumptions which guide the thinking of those who hold that man is more than a more clever rat, a temperamental computer, or a mellowed college sophomore. Client-centered therapists, Horneyian analysts, self-psychology theorists, interpreters of Zen Buddhism, neo-Gestaltists, and existentialists are beginning to find some degree of commonality while yet retaining the independence of their own perspectives.

For me, the truest existentialism is humanistic and the soundest humanism is existential. The two are not the same, but the area of their overlap is rich in potential for greater understanding of human experience and for greater effectiveness in the effort to enrich that experience. Perhaps I can best make evident the soil of humanistic psychology in which my own thinking about the existential approach to personality and psychotherapy is rooted by setting out what have seemed to me to be the fundamental assumptions and points of orientation of humanistic psychology (Bugental, 1963c).

Humanistic Psychology

The following pages will make a beginning of an affirmative statement of the nature of the humanistic orientation in psychology. I will do this by setting forth five postulates of humanistic psychology that seem to represent common elements in the perspectives of most writers identifying with this field. I will also make some defining statements about the humanistic orientation in psychology. These defining statements will be process descriptions as opposed to the substantive or content descriptions provided by the postulates. In setting forth these postulates and these characteristics of the humanistic orientation, I am well aware of their very tentative nature. We are only now beginning to discover the commonalities in the diverse spokesmen of the humanistic perspective. It is probable and highly desirable that the list of postulates that follows will be criticised, revised, and supplemented many times.

BASIC POSTULATES

MAN, AS MAN, SUPERSEDES THE SUM OF HIS PARTS

When we speak of "man" in humanistic psychology, we do so with the intent of characterizing a person rather than an "organism." Humanistic psychology is concerned with man at his most human or, to say it differently, with that which most distinguishes man as a unique species.

Our first postulate states the keystone position that man must be recognized as something other than an additive product of various part-functions. Part-function knowledge is important scientific knowledge, but it is not knowledge of man as man. It is knowledge of the functioning of parts of an organism.

MAN HAS HIS BEING IN A HUMAN CONTEXT

We postulate second that the unique nature of man is expressed through his always being in relationship with his fellows. Humanistic psychology is always concerned with man in his interpersonal potential. This is not to say that humanistic psychology may not deal with such issues as man's aloneness, but it will be evident that even in so designating it, "aloneness," we are speaking of man in his human context. The psychology of part-functions is a psychology that mechanically and incompletely handles this relatedness (actual or potential) of the human experience.

MAN IS AWARE

A central fact of human experience is that man is aware. Awareness is postulated to be continuous and at many levels. By so viewing it, we recognize that all aspects of his experience are not equally available to man but that, whatever the degree of consciousness, awareness is an essential part of man's being. The continuous nature of awareness is deemed essential to an understanding of human experience. Man does not move from discrete episode to discrete episode, a fact overlooked by experiments of the behavioristic orientation when they treat their subjects as though they had no prior awareness before coming into the experimental situation. Our postulation also provides for unconsciousness as a level of awareness of which there is not direct apprehension but in which awareness is nevertheless present. This is not the same as the Freudian concept of the unconscious, but it is probably more valid within the humanistic orientation.

MAN HAS CHOICE

There is no desire here to resume the hoary debate regarding free will versus determinism. Phenomenologically, choice is a given of experience. As man is aware, he is aware that his choices make a difference in the flow of his awareness, that he is not a bystander but a participant in experience. From this fact flows man's potential to transcend his creatureliness (Fromm, 1959), which is also to say that from this postulation we derive man's capability of change.

MAN IS INTENTIONAL

In his choices, man demonstrates his intent. This does not mean "striving," but it does mean orientation. Man intends through having purpose, through valuing, and through creating and recognizing meaning. Man's intentionality is the basis on which he builds his identity, and it distinguishes him from other species.

The characteristics of man's intentionality need to be specified: man intends both conservation and change. Mechanistic views of man frequently deal only with drive-reduction and homeostatic conceptions. Humanistic psychology recognizes that man seeks rest but concurrently seeks variety and disequilibrium. Thus we may say that man intends multiply, complexly, and even paradoxically.

Orientation

In the following statements I will specify some of the characteristics of the humanistic orientation in psychology, trying to identify those characteristics that are especially distinguishing of this point of view.

Humanistic psychology cares about man.

Humanistic psychology disavows the sort of scientific detachment pretended to or achieved at great cost by other orientations. Humanistic psychology recognizes that man cannot help but be invested in his study of his own condition. Accepting this as a given, humanistic psychology founds itself on man's concern about man and is an expression of that concern.

Humanistic psychology values meaning more than procedure.

Although humanistic psychology must find its own methods and must validate those methods as providing dependable knowledge about the human condition, humanistic psychology would be untrue to itself were it to become preoccupied with methodology to the loss of concern with the meaningfulness to the human condition of the issues with which it deals.

Humanistic psychology looks for human rather than nonhuman validation.

It is a basic tenet of the humanistic position that only that validation which is borne out by human experience can ultimately be counted significant. Humanistic psychology does not disavow the use of statistical methods or of experimental tests. However, it does insist that these are but means and that the ultimate criterion must be that of human experience.

Humanistic psychology accepts the relativism of all knowledge.

Humanistic psychology postulates a universe of infinite possibility. Thus it recognizes that all knowledge is relative and subject to change. This tenet does much to free humanistic psychology to use the imaginative and creative potential of its orientation.

Humanistic psychology relies heavily upon the phenomenological orientation.

What has been said above about the importance of meaning and about human validation will have indicated the centrality of the phenomenological orientation to the humanistic approach. The ultimate focus of our concern is the experience of the human being.

Humanistic psychology does not deny the contributions of other views but tries to supplement them and give them a setting within a broader conception of the human experience.

The Existential-Analytic Thesis[1]

We are ready now to examine the central thesis that will be presented in this book. As this is an existential point of view in a humanistic setting, our concern will be to find those ways of conceptualizing the human experience that will facilitate our efforts to release and facilitate human potential. As of now, this is how I see this matter.

I will postulate that the primary value in human life is to live in accord with (indeed, as a part of) the way things really are. Of course, that is a hazardous thing to say, for who can claim to know how things really are? The answer is, nobody and everybody. Nobody can prove he knows for sure, and everybody acts on the assumption that he knows. Probably, almost surely, there is no one "way things really are," there are only various ways of seeing our situation. I will be setting forth a way that has proven useful to me as a psychotherapist. The reader will test the degree to which these ideas fit his way of seeing things and use what is helpful, discarding the rest.

Now, just as I have postulated a primary value, I will point to a primary human process: awareness. Through awareness we dis-

---
[1] Although I will make citations to the literature, this book is not in any sense an adequate survey or abstracting of the vast amount of material on existentialism and existential psychotherapy. Burton and Lunde (1961), Lyons (1959, 1961), and Van Dusen (1959) have prepared extensive bibliographies on these topics.

cover ourselves and our world. Through awareness we can estimate our relation to world. It seems to me useful to think of that relationship as having these four characteristics:

We are limited in our awareness of ourselves and of world.
We can act in ways that affect our awareness of ourselves and of world.
We have choice about which actions to take and not to take.
While each of us is in one sense alone, in another we are all related.

When a person is aware of himself and world and lives in accord with these conditions of being alive, he is a harmonious part of all being. When, however, he distorts some of the conditions of his being, he loses that very being in the process. Unfortunately, various things happen that lead us to make such distortions. So psychotherapy becomes a way of trying to get back into life. Non-being is not just distorted being, it is literally non-being. That part of one's potential which is not in accord with life is dead.

Psychotherapy seeks to bring to the person's living awareness consciousness of the non-being aspects of his potential. These aspects, which we call his resistances, are held in their distorted (dead) condition by the person because he fears being overwhelmed by existential anxiety. This is the terrible irony: existential anxiety is itself the threat of non-being inherent in the givens of life. The attempt to escape those givens inevitably produces non-being!

When psychotherapy goes effectively through the analytic phase and thus aids the person in resolving his resistances and reclaiming his life, there is often a need for a constructive phase to supplement the therapeutic work. This constructive phase I am here calling "ontogogic" therapy. Just as the resistances on the negative side prevented the realization of human potential, so on the positive (ontogogic) side confrontation of the ontologic givens of living can facilitate the actualization of that potential.

Throughout the whole of this thesis the fundamental concern is with authenticity of being. The distortions of being that give rise to the need for psychotherapy are inauthenticities. The celebrations of being that ontogogic therapy seeks to facilitate are the products of authenticity. The influence that makes the change possible is the response of awareness to the authentic in life.

Existential-Analytic Psychotherapy and Psychoanalysis

The question may well be asked why have I chosen to use the term "analytic" in entitling this perspective when in many ways I am setting my viewpoint in contrast to that of psychoanalysis. The answer lies in my conviction that no body of clinical observation approaches the psychoanalytic in its consistency, depth, and coherence. I feel that any approach to psychotherapy at this point in our evolution must give recognition to the priority of psychoanalysis. Let it be quite clear that I am speaking about actual psychotherapeutic work rather than psychoanalytic metapsychology.

It is difficult to say just what aspects are the distinguishing attributes of psychoanalysis. Freud himself made various pronouncements at various times. Among the classically significant cornerstones of psychoanalytic theory would be the theory of the unconscious; the tripartite personality of id, ego, and superego; the postulation of basic instincts of life and death; the description of the dynamic processes in human functioning; the concept of the libidinal stream and its vicissitudes; the discovery of the resistance; the delineation of transference. In the orientation to existential analytic psychotherapy set forth in this book I explicitly disavow the tripartite personality structure of id, ego, and superego; the basic instincts postulation; and the libidinal stream concept. I find eminently meaningful the clinical aspects of the discoveries of the resistance and the transference. It seems to me that any psychotherapist who has worked intensively with patients over periods of years cannot but agree that these two phenomena are of repeated and central importance. Similarly, the dynamisms of personality functioning are again and again clinically validated. In regard to these borrowings from psychoanalytic theory, it should be noted that I particularly emphasize the clinical aspects rather than the conceptual and theoretical. This point will become more evident in later descriptions of these matters.

When it comes to the unconscious, my position is more equivocal. There can be little doubt that the concept of the unconscious usefully describes clinical phenomena readily evident. Yet my own observations increasingly suggest that the unconscious may be an artifact of our cultural orientation and training and of the basis on which we conduct our interviews. This point will also be dealt with more extensively in later pages.

THE VALUES OF THE EXISTENTIAL POSITION

Although in some ways they seem self-evident, it will be useful to set forth the values I personally find in the existential position that lead me to make it the guiding philosophy of my work.

It feels right.

In simplest, most candid terms the existential perspective simply feels right. As I read what others have written about the existential perspective, as I employ it in my own work and thinking, there is a sense of closure and even, at times, of elegance. I find I don't have to "cross my fingers" in order to accept the postulates of the existential viewpoint. Always when trying to test out the "goodness of fit" of other theoretical positions, there was the sense of the areas that could not be dealt with or the assumptions that were too tenuous. Perhaps another way of saying that it feels right is to say that so far as I can judge, the existential perspective accords with my own and with my patients' experiences.

It puts a humanistically meaningful end to the reductionist chain of motives.

Whether one accepts as basic the sexual drive, or inferiority feelings, or the need for consistency of the self, or the reduction of tension states, all personality theories have the defect that each observed condition is reduced to others which in turn are susceptible of reduction to yet others. There never seemed to be an adequately defensible, basic motivation short of some physiological state. Reduction of man to "organism" overthrows any true psychology and gives a false precedence to physiology. Man is more than and other than an organism only. While in a sense the concept of motivation is not an existential and phenomenological concept, accepting the givenness of the human condition as a basis from which to derive dynamic patterns provides a psychological and humanistic starting point for conceptualization.

It is not pathology centered.

The existential point of view speaks of man's condition in a fashion that transcends the dichotomy of pathology and health. Increasingly today we are recognizing that this dichotomy, while having once served a humane purpose, confounds our thinking and restricts our inventiveness (Szasz, 1960, 1961). The existential perspective seems to me to offer an embracing panorama in which those patterns we have typically characterized as pathologic as well as those we would deem creative, actualizing, or healthy find their places but do not constitute the most important route of access or the only basis of observation.

It recognizes the primary significance of awareness.

The existentialist has recourse always to the phenomenological world for his data and for the verification of his postulates. The psychotherapist is daily confronted with the primacy, among all human functions, of awareness. The phenomenological root makes possible the solid grounding of existential thought in real human experience.

Man-in-the-world is the primary datum.

The existential perspective takes man in his world as its primary datum, rather than some part-function of an organism, such as an instinct or a conditioned response. Very much as did Kurt Lewin (1935) with his concept of the "life space," existentialism recognizes the person as more than a mechanism enclosed in a skin. Man-in-the-world is the basic object of existential concern.

It is pragmatically useful.

Perhaps a way of saying all the foregoing is that the existential orientation "works," as far as I am concerned. It works at two essential levels for me. First, it helps me to solve conceptual problems. When I am puzzled by my patients or with myself in terms of understanding the interrelations of various aspects of what is happening in our lives, the existential perspective often proves the Rosetta Stone bringing harmony and meaningfulness to what otherwise seemed conflictful and chaotic. Similarly, many times the existential viewpoint will illuminate particular practical problems in living, those both of my patients and of myself. It offers a broad and fundamental context in which to examine such problems and with that greater perspective often the problem can be restructured and the possible choices become more evident. Note that this is not the same as saying that this view offers solutions. The existential viewpoint seldom can be called upon for solutions to problems, but it may provide a way of examining the situation which permits the person in that situation to work out solutions.

Such was the case with the professional man who refused advancements for which he was well qualified and whose rationalizations for doing so did not satisfy him or me. In time, we found how genuinely he feared making choices. Similarly there was a housewife who never could get free from her chores to play with her children even though she protested how much she wanted to do just that. As she finally recognized how much she feared the deaths of herself and her children, she could enjoy life with them.

It is an open system, presently and ultimately.

The existential orientation is a way of looking at the human experience. Strictly speaking it is not a system of postulates derived from that "looking at." The concepts offered in this book, for example, are formulations of my awareness, but they express my experience rather than *the* existential theory. Many existentially oriented theories are possible. Such a viewpoint, by its very nature, is always open for further formulations. The limits of any particular formulation are just that, of that formulation, not of the existential viewpoint. This experience of infinite possibilities is at once frightening and exhilarating. The sense that the choice is not a searching among myriad wrongs for a single right but a selection from among many different potentialities for that to which one will give actuality, changes the writer's experience from that of being tested by life to that of being a creative participant in life.

It is available to each person to use in his own way.

From what has just been said it will be apparent that existential thinking cannot offer a source of security to someone as a way of getting final answers to experience. At the same time it offers maximum facilitation to the creativity of each person, for it is a perspective that each observer will use in his own way. It is inconceivable that one can be a complete disciple of anyone else and still be an existentialist.

Existentialism recognizes the contributions of the humanities and religion.

In the existential perspective, the humanities, religion, and science are recognizable as expressions of man's concern to make meaningful his own being in the world. Each is seen to contribute in its own way, and no one can supplant the role of the others. Some psychologists have needed to belittle the contributions of the humanities or of religion, feeling that only one form of understanding (that of "objective science") was valid. Such an attitude can only operate to restrict the perspective on the human situation. Not only can important contributions to our awareness be gained from each of these approaches, but they can be profitably employed to "cross-fertilize" each other. The greatest creative efforts of literal millenia have been directed toward the conception and elucidation of the human condition. Psychology needs to keep its ties to literature, philosophy, and theology.

It restores our divinity.

Perhaps I can best summarize what existential psychology means to me by using this phrase: "It restores our divinity." I am not content to see man as mechanism or robot or even as organism. Man must partake in whatever he means by the concept of God. Allen Wheelis, in his essay, "To Be a God" (1963), expresses the same thought. Too many of our views in psychology and psychotherapy have reduced man. Reduction of man to organism—whether of the level of the conditioned response or the neurologic substratum generally—confuses parallel descriptions with explanatory potency. Existentialism restores man to his central place in man's own experience and grants us the possibility of realizing our fondest and most extreme imaginings about the human condition, if only we will have the courage and perseverance to see them through.

2 — Man's "thrown" condition

You and your family have been on a pleasant ocean cruise. Unexpectedly there is a typhoon, and the ship sinks. You manage to bring your family in a lifeboat to a tiny, uncharted island. In the midst of the immensity of the ocean, with few tools or supplies, you set up your castaways' camp. You, a city man, a professional man, a product of civilization's most interdependent form of living, must keep your family alive indefinitely with little to aid you beyond your own wits and determination.

What happens as days pass into months and years? As the hope of rescue becomes more a tribal myth than a realistic expectancy? As the first critical times of near disaster teach both the know-how needed to stay alive and the sober recognition of how vulnerable you are? What happens as finally the realization comes that this is all: this is where and how you will live out your life, and where you will die? What happens as you accept how little you know in the midst of so much you do not know?

This is a picture of man's plight; of your plight and of mine. I am on a little island of the clearly known, which is in the sea of the generally known, which is in the ocean of the barely known or but guessed at, which itself swims in the midst of the immensity of the totally unknown. Yet from the farthest galaxy may stream, even at this moment, influences so potent that the whole course of my life can be altered.

I want to evoke, not only a rational understanding, but an organismic awareness, of how each of us is surrounded by the immensity of that which is little knowable and greatly unknowable. This is the world; this is our life; this is our situation. Existentialists like the term "thrown": the thrown condition, the thrown plight of man. This is what is meant by being thrown into this moment.

Contingency and Anxiety

I have described my plight as that of living on a tiny island of the known in the midst of the vast ocean of the unknown. Here, my family and I are subject in varying degrees to influences from all the universe. I construct a shelter, farm for food, plan my life on my little island. I work within the realm of what is known, but I cannot know what storms will brew in distant parts of the sea, what tidal waves may be thrown up by volcanoes beyond my ken, though those tidal waves and those storms may ultimately reach us, disrupt our farm, destroy our shelter, and even end our lives. Even those storms I can see on the horizon will not be turned aside by my wishing and will test the strength of my building.

EXISTENTIAL ANXIETY

Leaving the metaphor, I am saying that each man lives in the midst of contingency, that even the knownness of day-to-day living is, in a sense, but a phantasy, a wish more than an actuality. I do not know, I cannot know enough to be safe, to be secure, to predict with complete confidence from one moment to the next.

Contingency means that what will become actual is contingent upon many influences, many variables, so many that they may well be infinite in number. The fact of contingency means that I never can predict with complete assurance. The experience of contingency means that I live with anxiety.

To be completely confident would be to be without anxiety. To the degree that I am not confident I must face anxiety. Anxiety is my recognition that I do not know all that I need to know to protect that which I love and to forestall that which I fear.

It will be clear that I am speaking of a particular kind of anxiety: this we can term natural or existential anxiety. The word "natural" is useful because it says this is of our very nature. This anxiety arises from the natural circumstance of man. We will examine this natural anxiety further later on.

CHOICE, FREEDOM, AND RESPONSIBILITY

We are accustomed to think of anxiety as undesirable, as pathological. Existential anxiety is not to be so regarded. It is the appropriate response to the situation in which man finds himself. There is an old story of a drunk listening to an orator recite Rudyard Kipling's poem "If." The lines rolled out, "If you can keep your head when all about you are losing theirs . . ." Then as the orator paused, the drunk filled in, "Then, buddy, you don't know the score." An appropriate response is not always the most classically desirable.

Yet it is this very situation of contingency, of never knowing enough to be completely sure, that is an essential part of our most cherished, our most God-like gift, that of freedom. There is no freedom when one knows all the determinants of a situation; that which you can predict with perfect accuracy gives you no choice in the matter. Freedom is the freedom to choose. Freedom and choice are synonyms psychologically. It is clear that we cannot know all the determinants of any given event. It needs to be equally clear that our subjective experience of choice, of action, may become a determinant, not *the* determinant but *a* determinant, and sometimes a crucial determinant. Thus is born our responsibility.

Responsibility is the experience of being a determinant of what happens. Responsibility is the affirmation of one's being as the *doer* in contrast to the acceptance of the role of the *object* done-to. We fear responsibility as we feel its weight, yet are not able to insure the outcomes of that which we do. Practicing clinicians will recognize how often patients seek to disavow responsibility, how greatly they fear it. Guilt is closely linked with responsibility, as I will discuss in further detail later. Our patients are well aware of that linkage. They are less aware that responsibility is bonded also to opportunity and self-esteem.

To return to my analogy of the island: knowing that I cannot predict what tidal waves, what storms will sweep my island, I must choose how to build my shelter, whether to put it into a cave or to construct it of palm fronds on a hill. I must weigh the advantages and disadvantages of one against those of the other. It is my responsibility. No almanac of guaranteed weather conditions will be delivered to my door.

Existential vs. Neurotic Anxiety

Thus far I have been describing the existential situation in which I find myself, man's human situation. I have not made reference to the distortions that may be introduced by my reaction to this situation. Now it is time to distinguish between existential or natural anxiety and neurotic anxiety.

So long as I recognize and fully accept my contingent situation, so long as I accept the responsibility for choice but recognize the potentiality of tragedy, I will not know neurotic anxiety. But when the load of choice, when the weight of responsibility, when the fear of tragedy strike too deeply, then I am tempted to distort the picture, to dim somehow the realization that seems too awful to bear. I may seek ways (Bugental, 1962f) which seem to reduce contingency or apparently lessen my responsibility, and thus "hedge" my choices: I may build an image on my island and worship that image, bring it gifts, and call upon it to be a god to me to quell the distant storm before it reaches my island. I may examine the stars and read portents in them or study the ocean currents and learn their meaning and tell myself that I no longer have anything to fear from earthquakes and tidal waves for I have ways of foretelling them and can take appropriate measures before they come. I may decide that I am, myself, a supernatural being, above the torments of fate, and that I will practice elaborate incantations or steep myself in learning so that I will not be subject to the vicissitudes of chance. Whatever the form,[1] I am trying to reduce my existential anxiety, I am trying to forestall the possibility of tragedy. Whatever the form, if I persuade myself that I have escaped from the province of contingency, that I have achieved certainty, that I am beyond the reach of tragedy, then I am distorting reality. When I so distort the existential reality of my life, I breed neurotic anxiety.

---

[1] It should be recognized that within this narrow perspective science, magic, religion, and superstition are all similar in their aim: to reduce uncontrolled contingency. They may, of course, differ widely in their methods and effectivenesses.

Let me interject an aside here in order that an important, implicit aspect may be made explicit. If, on my island, I study ocean currents and become skilled at reading the evidences they bring to me, I may alter the probabilities of disaster visiting us. Nothing that has just been said about the impossibility of escaping the operations of possibility should be read as a counsel of futility or fatalism. Quite the contrary, if I am wise I will do much that will significantly reduce my vulnerability. Such a response to natural or existential anxiety is a constructive one. It is only when I try to convince myself that I have won a certainty which denies the existential reality that I become prey to neurotic anxiety.

Neurotic anxiety is the distress occasioned by our yielding up of our authentic being-in-the-world to illusory hopes of being secure, of avoiding tragedy. It is always accompanied by some reduction in our total being, and for that reason it is inevitably a cancerous growth in our lives. As we try to maintain security with such an illusion, we are less real in our living and so our anxiety is renewed, thus requiring greater defensive efforts. Neurotic anxiety tends, thus, to be ever-increasing anxiety.

Tragedy. In what I have just said I have introduced a new term, tragedy. It is a word unfamiliar to much of American psychology, a word we are more accustomed to in association with literature, but it is a word that needs to be reincorporated into our psychological thinking. Tragedy is not something that is exclusively in the domain of the poets. Indeed, it is our own repression of existential reality that has obscured our recognition of this basic human experience. Tragedy is a part of living. That which we fear, that which we attempt to forestall, can, will, and does happen at times. In another chapter I will describe at greater length the nature of tragedy, but here let us recognize that tragedy lies all about us. Tragedy must be incorporated into our recognition of reality. Our attempt to distort that reality to eliminate tragedy is very much at the root of our experience of neurotic anxiety.

Existential joy. Just as we must recognize the potentiality of tragedy, so we may open ourselves to the realization of joy. That which we cherish, love, and hope for is potentially also ours if only we are authentic in our being-in-the-world. Each one of us has known the moment of exaltation in which we are at one with the world and conscious of our being with a kind of illumination that carries a deep conviction with it. Immersion in great music, the ecstasy of rich love, the moment of creative inspiration, the engrossed participation in some satisfying activity (when we say we "forget ourselves" and yet feel we are more truly ourselves than at any other time)—all these and many other occasions offer the opportunity of knowing existential joy. Neurotic anxiety destroys the potential for such times. Authentic being makes them possible, even probable.

COURAGE AND ACTUALIZATION

Still there is, because of the recognition of tragedy, a tendency to regard existentialist thinking as gloomy and pessimistic. I do not see it this way. I think it can provide a sound basis for true optimism, the optimism of reality confronted and incorporated. Paul Tillich (1952), in *The Courage to Be,* has dwelt at length on the nature of existential courage. Courage consists in a confronting of our limitedness within the unlimitedness of being. Courage consists in the exercising of our choice and the taking of our responsibility while recognizing that contingency can overthrow our decision and reverse our best efforts. Courage finds its finest expression in the choice to be.

The choice to be means that each of us is born alive but not born into being. Being requires a self-aware act of faith. Being requires a world-aware moment of actualization. By this I mean that our choices administer life to some possibilities while condemning others to oblivion. When our choices are to live, to be, when we give actuality to that which is potential within us, then we express our courage.

Other Important Concepts

There are a number of concepts that are important to the understanding of the existential orientation. Definitions for these concepts are not standardized, and various writers employ them differently.[2]

---
[2] The reader's attention is called to *A Concise Dictionary of Existentialism* (Winn, 1960), which, while by no means an adequate survey of definitions, is a good starting point.

I will offer below conceptions of a variety of terms. These will be the ways in which I will use these terms in this volume. Other concepts will be presented and defined in context in later chapters.

EXISTENCE AND BEING

Existence is. The only possible synonym for the word existence would be "is-ness." Existence is not to be explained. It is the basic given of all experience. By existence, as we are using it here, we do not mean life, nor yet awareness. *Being* needs to be broken into its two syllables to convey its most significant meaning: *be-ing*. The process of be-ing is the process of life. Accordingly, I will use "be-ing" as a name for the process of self-aware existing. In this fashion, we would then recognize that probably man alone is capable of being. This view is consonant with May's, who says, "Man is the being who can be conscious of, and therefore responsible for, his existence" (May, 1958, p. 41).

NON-BE-ING

Non-being and nothingness are interwoven and nearly synonymous concepts. Nothingness is the antithesis of being and of existence. Non-being must be recognized, however, as integral to the concept of being. Each—being and non-being—gives meaning to the other. Some writers seem to use "non-being" to designate a diminished awareness or reduced actualization of a person's potentialities. Certainly there is much to commend this, but I think it creates confusions. In this book we will use "non-being" as an antithesis of "being," in parallel to "nothingness" as the antithesis of "existence." The terms "authenticity" and "inauthenticity" will be used for the more functional designations (see later).

Death. Death is the opposite of life. Phenomenologically, we know nothing of death. The only knowledge we have of it is physical-science information which has little utility for existential and psychotherapeutic thinking. The *anticipation* of death, on the other hand, is a crucial existential and psychotherapeutic matter. Death as the definitive non-being becomes apparently synonymous with nothingness, but it needs to be recognized that this is speculative rather than documentable.

MEANINGLESSNESS AND CREATIVITY

I find myself assailed, persuaded, seduced, and promised from all sides by values that compete for my allegiance. Much of the freight carried by all forms of communication (education, theology, advertising, simple conversations) is in terms of extolling the virtues of some values or pointing out the deficiencies of others. Man is much concerned with values, expends much effort on them, will torture and kill or suffer and die for them.

The absurd. Faced with the maelstrom of competing values and finding none ultimately demonstrable, some take a nihilistic stance and proclaim all values vain and meaningless. Ultimately, these people say, life—the world—is absurd; there is no meaning. There is an existential anxiety of meaninglessness which must be confronted and incorporated if we are to be authentic. Those who proclaim the absurd flee from meaninglessness rather than confront it. Thereby, they miss the existential fulfillment of creativity.

Nothingness. The existential fact that no ultimate value is given or "built in" to our being or that the world permits us to create meaning is the base on which all meaning rests. The artist standing before an empty canvas rejoices in that emptiness, that nothingness which welcomes his enlivening touch. To fill in colors on a predrawn outline according to someone else's charting is not truly creative. Only the transformation of nothingness into somethingness may be termed *creativity*.

ALONENESS AND ENCOUNTER

Each of us is ultimately alone; yet each of us is ultimately in relation to others. This paradox describes man's situation. Viewed from the standpoint of the individual in the midst of his life, we must recognize that only the individual can have ultimate responsibility for his choices and their outcomes. Existential aloneness is a recognition that full and complete communication from one person to another can never be attained. This situation gives rise to the emotion of loneliness.

Loneliness is the feeling of having to confront *being* with only one's own awareness to illuminate existence. We can understand the nature of aloneness even more completely if we recall what has just been said about how impossible it is to demonstrate that there are ultimate values to guide one. If, for example, any particular value were to be demonstrated as universally accepted as the ultimate, then one would not be confronted with the terrible responsibility of decision in the same way that the absence of such a value makes necessary. Erich Fromm (1941) has traced the way in which the evolution of man's culture has given rise to the phenomenon of individuality. He may as well have called it "aloneness." As man comes to recognize himself as an individual, apart from other individuals, to identify himself as a unique being, he experiences loneliness. When a man saw himself as part of a corporate body, as, for example, a serf of a particular lord or as a part of the Roman Catholic Church, then he did not know existential loneliness in the same way. To be sure, it is probable that in all ages men have confronted their essential aloneness, but preceding ages, through church, state, and family, provided institutional bulwarks against the full experience of loneliness.

I introduced this section by speaking of the paradox that man is existentially alone and yet existentially in relation. Later we will recognize that man is symbiotic, depending for his essential humanness on relations with others. It is equally true that man finds his being inextricably interwoven with others. Existential literature uses a variety of terms to describe the relationships among men. Among these are: encounter, confirmation, engagement, and dialogue.

The general term *encounter* may be thought of as subsuming the other terms. It is intended to convey the self-and-other awareness—the experiencing of two or more people in their relationship to each other. Genuine encounter is the coming together of people who recognize the be-ing-ness of themselves and each other. Buber (1958) has contrasted the "I-it" relationship with the "I-thou" relationship. When I meet you and regard you as an object rather than as another subject, I give you status of a thing rather than a be-ing. This is an "I-it" relationship. It is not a genuine encounter. When I meet you and recognize you as another be-ing, this is an "I-thou" relationship and is an encounter. This process of recognition of the other as a be-ing in his own world is what is known as *confirmation*.

The words *engagement* and *dialogue* are used in many instances to refer to a further degree of interrelation than that implied by simple encounter or confirmation. Confirmation, we have said, means the recognition of the be-ing-ness of the other. Engagement and dialogue subsume this recognition, but go beyond it to portray an *involvement* in one another. *Dialogue* may be thought of as the attempt to communicate meanings of experience between two individuals (Moustakas, 1962). It presumes a willingness to risk one's understandings of one's life with the other. *Engagement*, I find, most usefully may be thought of as a further step, in which one lets the other matter in his be-ing-ness.

Conclusion

In this chapter some of the basic concepts characteristic of existential thinking have been introduced. At this point I have not tried to order them in systematic fashion, reserving that task for later. Instead, it is important to the reader who is new to these concepts that he gain more than an intellectual appreciation of the concepts only. Thus, they have been set in a connotative and imaginative framework. This is more than a heuristic need. It is a recognition that existential thinking calls for a kind of organismic appreciation of our human situation and that without this total grasp the most closely reasoned logic can carry one quite astray.

The reader may find it helpful if I synopsize briefly some of the more important concepts from the foregoing material, particularly the four major dimensions revealed to us by awareness and the attendant existential anxieties which characterize these dimensions. I will simply list these here and return to them again in the next chapter as we make a more thoroughgoing study of them.

Awareness discloses to each person (a) that he is finite, (b) that he has the potential to take action, (c) that he has some choice of what action he will take, and (d) that he is at once separate from, yet related to, his fellows. From these flow, respectively, the existential anxieties (a) of fate and death, (b) of guilt and condemnation, (c) of meaninglessness and emptiness, and (d) of loneliness and isolation.

3 — Authenticity: The central concern of psychotherapy

I have now set forth a first appreciation of the existential view of man's situation. This view makes evident the circumstances in which a person may experience distresses from which he may seek relief by turning to psychotherapy. In this chapter we will discuss in broad perspective the central concern of existential psychotherapy, the mission that existential-analytic psychotherapy tries to make it possible for the patient to perform. In the simplest terms, the main undertaking of psychotherapy is that of aiding the patient in his efforts, (a) to discard the distortions of awareness which arose to forestall existential anxiety, and (b) to accept the responsibilities and opportunities of authentic being in the world. The central concern in both phases is with authenticity. Accordingly, I will enlarge in this chapter upon the meanings and significances of this important concept and experience.

In the following pages I will develop a conceptual framework that may aid the therapist in thinking about his work and its purposes. It is not intended that this framework should be taught to the patient in the same manner. It is not a language for phrasing communications and interpretations explicitly; although it may often be implicit in what the therapist does say to his patient.

Authenticity as the Primary Existential Value

A person is authentic in that degree to which his being in the world is unqualifiedly in accord with the givenness of his own nature and of the world. Authenticity is the primary good or value of the existential viewpoint.

The value of authenticity is postulated rather than argued. It is self-evident, at least to most existentialists. Logic will support this primary value in several ways, probably most tellingly by the demonstration that one's ability to secure gratifications and avoid harms is greater in proportion to one's perception of reality, and high reality perception is closely associated with authenticity. However, this sort of argumentation is *post hoc*. The pragmatic advantages of authenticity are consequents not demonstrants. When we are in the world but in conflict with the world, we are in that measure alienated from our living. Later on, I will talk about "suchness" and hold that the fullest realization of ourselves comes about when we recognize the suchness, the givenness, the "is-ness" of Being which includes ourselves and world.

Accordingly, it is not as a functional value that we hold that being-in-the-world in accord with world is a good thing. It is rather as a recognition of ultimate suchness or as an expression of our participation in reality that we make this postulation. The functional value then derives from the more global statement. Of course, this line of reasoning brings us to the problem of defining "reality." This I cannot do objectively. I can only talk in terms of reality as I am able to apprehend it. Each reader must determine for himself the extent to which his grasp of reality accords with that implicit in what I am saying. To recognize that reality is multifaceted and is a constant construction of the individual in his relationship with world at any given moment is not the same as to deny reality exists or to hold that we may not use our individual perceptions of reality as bases for communication.

When our being-in-the-world is in accord with the nature of ourselves in the world we are authentic. *Authenticity* is the term I will use to characterize both an hypothesized ultimate state of at-oneness with the cosmos and the immense continuum leading toward that ultimate ideal.

What we call in everyday language "maladjustment," "mental illness," and "emotional distress" are examples or instances of inauthenticity. There are other examples not usually so recognized; much of what we would think of as "adaptation" or "adjustment" or "conformity" certainly has an important component of inauthenticity. To carry the point even further, we need to recognize that there is much that is inauthentic in such concepts as "success," "popularity," "trying hard," and so on.

THE NATURE OF AUTHENTICITY

Authenticity is a term used to characterize a way of being in the world in which one's being is in harmony with the being of the world itself. To say it differently, we are authentic to that degree to which we are at one with the whole of being (world); we are inauthentic to the extent that we are in conflict with the givenness of being. Clearly, I am here seeking to characterize an ideal or ultimate condition of authenticity with the recognition that we are always somewhat less than fully authentic. Also implicit in my description of authenticity, and of much more conceptual significance, is the recognition that authenticity amounts to the resolution of the subject–object split, the self–world dichotomy. As one approaches the stage of letting go to the suchness of Being without striving against it, one is attaining to full authenticity.

The postulation of authenticity, as here described, is subject to confusion from either of two bases—themselves quite contradictory. On the one hand, this view of authenticity may be mistaken for a rephrasing of the idea of adaptation or adjustment and thus a counsel of resignation or conformity. On the other hand, it may appear mystical and other-worldly. Let us clarify each of these aspects in turn.

"Adaptation" and "adjustment" have come to be odious words for many psychotherapists. It is so very evident that our patients are distressed as much because of the culturally transmitted distortions of being (Bugental, 1962d) as of those more idiosyncratically developed. To aid the patient to a "passive" acceptance of social values and avoidance of conflict may well be to assist him in making rigid a character disorder that extinguishes his very humanity and assures an end to his creativity. Clearly such an objective is totally inconsistent with the concept of existential authenticity.

The world of daily happenings is set in a larger world of human experience. The world to which one might "adapt" is within the world of authentic being. Adjustment has come to mean acceptance of the values of competitive striving, accumulation of material "goods," secrecy and separateness. Authenticity refers to a level of experience in which such values are recognized for the limited and distorted expressions of experience that they are.

Partly because of this devaluing of familiar criteria of daily life, partly because the language of authenticity has much in common (and not altogether inappropriately) with the language of mysticism and religion, it is sometimes assumed that authenticity is solely metaphysical or "spiritual" (whether that term be used with appreciation or derogation). This too misses the mark widely. As I pointed out in the previous paragraph, the familiar world is set within the broader ontologic world. Authenticity does not call for one to abandon the familiar world, rather to recognize he is very much in that world indeed, while yet recognizing that the familiar world is an incomplete arena for the human experience. The familiar world is really inescapable even if one sought to evade it, but it needs to be seen in perspective. Perhaps this is the meaning of the frequently used phrase, "He was *in* but not *of* the world."

Authenticity, then, does not consist of the rejection of the familiar world. It does not call for one to deny values, activities, associates, or any other aspect of his life. Authenticity, indeed, may be approached more through alive participation in all of these. It is, rather, the perspective or the awareness with which one participates that is crucial.

Now I must add a qualification to what has just been said. I have spoken so far about the general implications of authenticity for most of us in our daily living. It must be recognized, however, that there is an apparent contradiction, in that when a person attains to a measure of authenticity that is greater than usual, his participation in the daily world inevitably begins to change. This is as true for those who have never heard the word "authenticity" or thought on these matters, as it is for those who by reason of personal growth (for example, through therapy) develop in this direction. The term "transcendence" is used to characterize the moving past the subject-object (self-world) split. At such stages one gradually lets go of many of the attributes of the daily world as their meanings are absorbed into the broader perspective of the ontic world.

This *letting go* is a difficult process to characterize, but it is very important to an adequate understanding of authenticity. Letting go is to be contrasted sharply with rejection. Letting go does not mean a denial of even such values as striving, competition, and so on—values frequently depreciated as one first catches a glimpse of the wider perspective of being. Rather, letting-go involves first a letting be, an acceptance of all things human, and then a finding of more encompassing ways of being in relation to all such things. The too frequent mistake of the person eager for authenticity is to strive subtly and unconsciously for authenticity by renouncing that in which he is still embedded. The very denial (rejection) portrays the continuing involvement with the daily values.

So far I have been giving much attention to what authenticity is not. What then is authenticity? This is a difficult question to answer. To do so it is necessary to postulate the nature of "the world back of the world," the ontic world of authentic being. Clearly any writer's view of that world is only a statement of his own perspective at that time. Yet it is important to make that statement, while yet retaining awareness that it is limited and in no small part a projection of the perceiver. With this recognition, I will offer my best perception as of now.

Fundamental to all else in the human experience is awareness.[1] At least phenomenologically, world arises out of human awareness. It grows and evolves with experience. Learning importantly affects what one may become aware of and what will escape awareness. Emotional needs have similar effects.

The Givens of Awareness

If I am open to the stream of my awareness I find, of course, that it is varied and multifaceted and that some aspects have more immediacy or intimacy than others. The former I tend to distinguish as having to do with "me" or "myself," while the latter appear "out there." And yet the line between these aspects is a vague one, and there is a constant intermingling. It is true that all awareness "just is," is of a piece, is dissected only at some cost. But it is equally true that—at least as we in our culture experience awareness—it is in-

---
[1] To me, this seems so self-evident that I cannot but wonder how any science of human behavior can be conceived which negates this primacy. Strict behaviorism's denial of consciousness seems irrevocably a fundamental fallacy.

evitably construed to have distinguishable characteristics. What are these?

FINITENESS

Certainly one inescapable aspect of the stream of awareness as I experience it is the recognition that it is but a part of a broader stream of potential awareness. As though I stood on a rocky point watching a portion of a broad river plunge over a falls to be lost in mist below, I can discern something of the past which leads up to this moment, can catch a glimpse of the probable immediate next moments, but am ever and again reminded that there are immense stretches behind and ahead—as well as on either side—of which I know little or nothing but which interrelate with and affect the little segment of the now which I can see.

Thus I am aware but, being aware, know that there is much more of which I might be aware and that that unknown more certainly can and does affect that of which I am aware. So man discovers a first ontologic given of his awareness: that it is finite, limited, incomplete.

This discovery of the limitedness of our awareness provides the corollary recognition that we live in *contingency*. This means that because we do not know all, we do not know enough to ensure the outcomes we desire. Standing on our rocky promontory we cannot know at what moment we may discover the river is running dry, is coming to flood stage, is filling with debris, or threatens to overflow its banks and sweep us away with it.

Clearly then our awareness, in its limitedness, discloses to us our being as subject to influences we cannot anticipate. Thus is born the sense of being subject to *fate*, which in its ultimate form is the anticipation of *death*. Said differently, we become aware that we cannot know all the influences that go into the determination of a particular event and its outcomes, and yet we know that we may be affected by that event and its outcomes in any measure from the most trivial to the most final. This is the existential anxiety of fate and death.

In the foregoing section, we have studied one aspect of human awareness and developed from our study certain constructs which we will have occasion to refer to repeatedly. Let me set these out schematically so that the pattern will be more evident:

> Ontologic given: finiteness
> Subjective experience: contingency
> Ultimate existential anxiety: threat of death
> Continuing existential anxiety: sense of fate

POTENTIAL TO ACT

So far our image has been that of a passive awareness gazing out from a rocky eminence above the river which our pun and metaphor make the stream of awareness. But, of course, we are not passive. We move about and affect the world "out there" as well as changing the point from which we look. Thus we can bring about differences in our awareness. We can change the points from which we look at the river so that we see more upstream or down or to either side. We can dam the river or build a diversionary canal. This is the second important aspect of human awareness and givenness. We have the potential to take actions.

The actions we take are not random, however. We discover that we experience concern about the actions we take as they affect the awareness we have. Thus we discover that we have *responsibility*. Responsibility expresses our involvement in world and heals the breach that contingency creates, restoring us to relatedness to the world of which we are aware.

There are important psychological consequences of this experience of responsibility and its basis, our potential for taking action. These are the two forms of existential anxiety: guilt and condemnation. *Guilt is the sense* of the incompleteness of our realization of our potential. Guilt is the awareness that the actions we take express so much less than our full being. But guilt is also the appreciation that what we do matters. *Condemnation* is the ultimate threat, the potential of overwhelming guilt.

It needs to be made clear that existential guilt, in itself, is not disabling, is not a shameful thing. Existential guilt is the recognition that we do, indeed, have responsibility. It matters how we employ our potential to take action. We are not hapless bits of fluff totally at the mercy of the winds of contingency. We have weight and substance. To be sure, we are still within the bounds of the finiteness of our awareness, and so we cannot perfectly exercise our potential for action. We never fully bring it into coordination with that of which we are aware. Thus there is existential guilt as an inevitable part of the human experience.

Let us once again recapitulate the constructs we have been developing:

    Ontologic given: potential for action
    Subjective experience: responsibility
    Ultimate existential anxiety: threat of condemnation
    Continuing existential anxiety: sense of guilt

CHOICE

Recognizing that we can take action and that the actions we take make a difference in the stream of our awareness, we experience concern and feel the weight of responsibility. While yet knowing this concern and responsibility, we know too our finiteness and the ever-present potentialities of contingency. Thus our actions must be chosen in a way that expresses our concern in the midst of contingency. This is the third aspect of awareness: the experience of having choice.

The full significance of choice as part of the human experience may be gained more readily by contrasting it with what would be the case if we were instinct-governed or if a single, overriding value could be conclusively demonstrated (for our purposes, these would amount to the same thing). A governing instinct or value would make our concern about our actions a hapless one and reduce us to inert objects buffeted by the instinct or value on one side and contingency on the other. Clearly, we are not alone objects of fate and instinct, we have some say in how we will take action, and thus we have the subjective experience of *autonomy*. To be sure, as in all aspects of awareness, our autonomy is limited, but it is nonetheless a part of awareness.

In this limitedness of our autonomy, as in our limitedness of awareness and action, resides the existential anxiety that is part of the human experience. We know our limitedness and seek for some surety, some sign "out there" and, finding none, are confronted by a sense of the *emptiness* of the "out there" and the threat of ultimate *meaninglessness*.

In summary, we may list:
Ontologic given: choice
Subjective experience: autonomy (limited)
Ultimate existential anxiety: threat of meaninglessness
Continuing existential anxiety: sense of emptiness

SEPARATENESS

One of the most emotionally significant aspects of our awareness is that there are others who in some measure share our experience and yet in some measure are separate from us. It is evident that we share much in awareness and yet not all, that we can influence each other's awarenesses but not completely. This is the fourth ontologic given: that we are separate from yet related to others. (Perhaps significantly, there is no single term that can express this basic fact of our experience.)

The subjective aspect of this given is, of course, the feeling of being a part of humankind yet apart from every other human being. Again, a pun is a better communication of the two facets at once, and we may speak of *"a-part-ness"* as the experience of knowing our simultaneous being like yet different from others. The deep satisfactions of intimacy with another and the continuing frustration of being always caught within the envelopes of our individualities are involved here.

From these experiences flow the sense of *loneliness* that is continuingly with us and the ultimate threat of complete *isolation*. Day to day we know our limited awareness and our captivity within it while others around us are each in his own perspective. We bridge the gaps between us but always incompletely. As a consequence the anxiety of complete isolation is terrifying and genuine.

This fourth aspect of awareness has included:
Ontologic given: separate-but-related-ness
Subjective experience: "a-part-ness"
Ultimate existential anxiety: threat of complete isolation
Continuing existential anxiety: sense of loneliness.

SUMMARY

Our study of the nature of awareness has provided us with four aspects that may be identified for heuristic purposes. These are spelled out solely to aid our understanding and not in the belief that each is independent of the others or that this is necessarily the one correct way of analyzing awareness. Awareness is a phenomenological whole and may be analyzed into various components according to the needs of the situation. The present analysis has much value in conceptualizing and conducting existential-analytic psychotherapy. Others might do as well; certainly others would do better for other purposes.

In the study of the aspects of awareness which I have made above, the reader will have recognized certain similarities to the profound observations of Paul Tillich (1952), and indeed I have in the present context used Tillich's perspective to further my own efforts to develop schemata useful to the therapeutic enterprise. Tillich, primarily oriented to the theological perspective, recognized three forms of existential anxiety: fate and death, guilt and condemnation, and meaninglessness and emptiness. Clinically, it has seemed desirable to add a fourth aspect having to do with man's relations with his fellows (which Tillich deals with under each of the other three). This amendment is not thought of as an "improvement" on Tillich since he was writing in quite a different context. Rather, it is therapeutically useful in facilitating the therapist's thinking about his work and his patients' experiences.

We will return to this study of man's existential situation in Part Three.

We have now a first basis for understanding the nature of authentic awareness. It is awareness that fully confronts the existential anxieties of being and affirms its own being by incorporating those anxieties while yet avoiding their distortion. Man lives in contingency. He can and does take action that affects his awareness and experience. He takes such action without ultimate guide posts of universal values or built-in instincts. And man is in constant relation with his fellows while yet being separate from them.

Of course, man does not ever fully accept the givens and their attendant anxieties. Instead he feels compelled at times to deny some parts of his condition and to try to nullify their effects. When he does so, he distorts his situation and becomes prey to neurotic anxiety and inauthenticity. The analytic phase of the therapeutic task is concerned with this denial and with the recovery of authenticity.

It is necessary to genuine communication between the writer and the reader for us now to "shift gears." To this point, in this chapter, I have been talking at a level of abstraction appropriate to the transmission of conceptual materials. These are important in their own right, but they are necessarily incomplete. In a way the reader would be entitled to say now, "So the patient finds it uncomfortable to be subject to fate, to carry the responsibility of his choices, and so on. But surely that doesn't account for the grave and persistent disruptions of his life from which he suffers." In other words, what is needed now is a communication of the human experience of anxiety and the flight to symptoms to escape authenticity. This I will try to convey in the remainder of the chapter.

The Therapeutic Undertaking

THE NEUROTIC PROCESS

Neurosis consists in the denial or distortion of authenticity. To the extent that we let fear or expediency pervert our perceptions of and responses to what is real in our lives, to that extent are we neurotic.

What is reality? Reality, existentially, is being thrown into a world we cannot comprehend with the task of creating ourselves even as we discover ourselves and our world. Reality is being faced with never understanding enough while yet having to choose and act on the basis of such incomplete understanding. Reality is endlessly coming up against the walls of our aloneness.

In our transactions with life, we try to create a certainty where certainty does not exist; we try to invoke probability where there is only possibility; we try to disavow responsibility while we carry it always with us. We seek to comprehend (understand) the incomprehensible, that which comprehends (embraces) us. This is not a counsel of futility or of fatalism. It is quite the contrary. The history of man is the history of converting more and more of the incomprehensible into the comprehensible; the city of man is one of edifices of the known carved from the raw materials of the unknown. Yet we dwell always on the edge of the frontier, at the last outpost before the blank places on the map. Each advance in our knowledge wins for us also an awareness of increased realms of the unknown.

In the face of this awful (awe-full) unknown-ness, we are anxious. We fear that the world drops off into nothingness, we imagine strange and terrible creatures lying in wait for the unwary venturer. Anxiety is our birthright, our condition, our natural accompaniment to being.

But anxiety can and does become intolerable. So we turn to the circumstance that gave rise to it, our limitedness. We must rid ourselves of this frightful burden, and we place it on the world. We limit the world. We constrict world and ourselves to knowable proportions.

THE PSYCHOTHERAPEUTIC TASK

Psychotherapy is not a healing process. It is a philosophic venture. It is not the treatment of an illness. It is a daring to confront self-and-world. It is not a learning to adjust; it is a facing of infinite un-adjustability.

The therapeutic relationship is not the agent of but the medium in which therapeutic change occurs. The agent is self-and-world confrontation. What makes possible the changes in the patient's being-in-the-world is his discarding of some of the constrictions he has put on himself-and-his-world sufficiently to recognize their limiting and hurtful effects. With such recognition, the patient may choose less destructive ways of being-in-the-world, with a resulting increase in authenticity. In order to discard these constrictions, the patient must experience the anxiety (whether neurotic or existential) the constrictions were erected to dispel. Generally, this is insupportable, unless there is some other way of sustaining himself in the world during the transition. This the therapeutic relationship can often provide.

Of course, the therapist does more than provide this sustaining relationship. He may be importantly involved in making possible the patient's confrontation of himself in the world. However, the wording of the previous sentence is advised. The therapist cannot so confront the patient. Only the person himself can do this. This lonely venture is the therapeutic agent.

Basically (in the sense of functional source), the resistance is the shield the patient erects to forestall the feared confrontation with the reality of his being in the world. (Thus, the therapist who thinks of the resistance as a warding off of his own efforts misses the point and confuses the patient.) The therapist's task is to help the patient rediscover the conflict within himself that gave rise to the resistance and other defensive and constrictive maneuvers.

In speaking of the conflict within the patient, it is important to recognize that concurrent with the constrictive, self-and-world–diminishing process I have thus far been depicting, there is a process which is the patient's seeking to actualize himself in the world, which is the growth tendency striving to overthrow constriction and emerge into reality. It is the constant dialectic process of these two forces that is the dynamic of the personality. Freud in "Why War?" (1953) and Brown in *Life Against Death* (1959) discuss related views of this same dialectic process.

The therapist's perspective must be that which sees his patient as an encumbered person who yet struggles against the limitations imposed by his encumbrances. It is in this perspective that the therapist will recognize the opposition of the two processes through which the patient at once contends for and flees from his life. The making conscious of these two processes and of the conflict between them is the mission of therapy.

The Forfeiting of Authenticity

Each of us is like a person who pays blackmail to keep a feared reality from becoming manifest. So paying, we maintain a semblance of peace at increasingly heavy cost to our resources. By our very nature, we seek to actualize ourselves in the world. It follows that the threat from which we pull away, against which we erect our constricting distortions of reality, is the threat of non-being, of the non-actuality of ourselves. The paying of blackmail, then, is the trading-off of some of our actuality-of-being-in-the-world to hold off non-being. But, of course, to the extent that we so trade our actuality, we are in that measure non-actual. This is the joker in the transaction. This is the existential meaning of the race-old legend of selling one's soul to the devil (stories that usually included the devil's gift somehow betraying the buyer). When we seek to evade the anxieties of being authentic, we lose our being and incur renewed, neurotic anxiety.

We may cast this whole process into a paraphrase that will illustrate the "Waking Nightmare of Neurosis."

> I am thrown into world without instruction. Each action I take or do not take is fraught with possibility. Possibility extends on all sides through all dimensions from life to death, from good to evil, from fulfilling to negating. And I do not know. I do not know enough; I do not know what may happen; I cannot be sure of any consequences. And so I am afraid. I cannot ask, for none can tell me. I cannot study, for none can teach. What I have done and what I have not done weigh on me. What I will yet do or will not do threaten me. And yet I will be; and being, I will do and not do. And doing, I will be the doer and responsible for having done. And not doing, I will be the not-doer and responsible for not having done.

This is Man's autobiography. But yet, he writes another chapter. This chapter shows the impact of anxiety.

> I am afraid. I cannot endure not knowing. It is too much to be responsible for what I cannot control. I am so alone, so unprotected.

Then, man may write still another chapter:

> The world is really not so unknowable. If I but keep my eyes from seeing too much, my ears from hearing too much, my mind from thinking too much, it becomes quite reasonable. I can even persuade myself I see all there is. If I but worship this deity, adhere to this virtue, suffer that pain, insist on that plan, world becomes quite manageable. If I but hush the voice of possibility both within and about me, the fear grows quieter, I am no longer afraid, so much (Bugental, 1962f).

Many, if not all, therapeutic systems can have favorable results because they provide the medium, the therapeutic relation, that encourages the confronting and discarding of self-and-world distortions that are no longer functionally required. However, many therapists (and therapeutic systems) seem to stop there, others seem content to act like parents "writing an excuse" to a teacher for the patient so he can (apparently) avoid contingency–responsibility–

tragedy: "Please excuse Mr. Smith from contingency. He had bad parents."

We cannot comprehend ourselves-and-world. But this at once provides no excuse from responsibility in the world and yet prevents that responsibility being devastating. Could we know fully (comprehend) we would have no choice, no being. Were we not responsible, we would be meaningless, fluff on a vagrant breeze. The beauty and the terror of our plight is to be responsible without being able to know enough to discharge our responsibility perfectly (Maslow, 1962a).

We seek to increase our authenticity (therapy seeks to free the patient of the ways he forestalls his own authenticity). I say "increase" because authenticity is not a perfect state to be achieved but a quantitative dimension along which we can move. When I spoke of paying blackmail, I meant trading off authenticity for seeming security.

What are the attributes of being authentic?

1. Being as fully aware as I can be at the moment.
2. Choosing what possibility I will invest with my life, with actuality, at the moment.
3. Taking responsibility for the choice I have made while yet recognizing the imperfection of my awareness and the fact that my choice gave this alternative actuality and not some other. Recognizing therein that tragedy is always potential and that neither my limitations of awareness, nor my good intentions, nor my suffering, nor my virtue, nor any other extrinsic circumstance, can change that fact.

Our patients (and we) seek to be excused from this awful actuality. We want to play "not for keeps," to have it "not count," to say "slips go over."

We fear the Godlike weight of giving life and administering death to possibilities. We want to hide under the bed clothes from the shadowy Could-have-been and the relentless Is.

> For of all sad words of tongue or pen,
> The saddest are these: 'It might have been!'

And I am the one who decided it would not be.

PART TWO *The analytic phase of the therapeutic work*

When we find our lives on the brink of being swept into nonbeing—whether literal and physical or implicit and psychological—we are impelled to desperate steps to preserve what we can. Faced with the potential loss of all, we may sacrifice much to save something. Among the extreme measures to which we may have recourse in this circumstance is the yielding up of some of our very being, some of our aliveness. We make a grim trade with fate in the hope of holding on to some parts of our being. No metaphor or exaggerated language is intended in these statements. Quite literally, we realize only some fraction of what is latent in our lives. We cripple ourselves psychologically, just as Chinese aristocratic parents once broke the feet of their female infants or other peoples mutilated themselves for what they thought good reasons. We choose, knowingly or not, that some aspects of our potentials for living will not come to actuality, in order, we believe, to preserve the possibility of actualizing other aspects. Thus we become maimed creatures in our very being.

These are harsh words, but the facts are even more harsh. Our tendency is to nod and pass on when we see the devastation our fears wreak in our own and others' lives. This, in itself, is an example of the sort of distortion of awareness with which we are here concerned.

We are maimed by the distortions of awareness that we use to reduce what seems overwhelming existential anxiety. We try to change our experience of what is actual, but we only cripple our perceptions. These security-seeking maneuvers act like what Huxley called a "reducing valve" (1954a, b) to bring apparent or perceived reality to less threatening dimensions. In the process our realization of ourselves becomes so much less than is potential. These distortions, we discover in the therapeutic hour, are the very resistances our patients show in their presentations of themselves. Thus psychotherapy is concerned with the frontier of the human engagement with life.

Part One traced out the background of an existential position with regard to personality and psychotherapy. Now we are ready to examine in detail the process through which the distortions of awareness and being are reduced and the person is aided to new freshness of living. This is the work of the analytic phase.

Chapter 4 introduces the actual work of the therapeutic hour. In describing this work, I am as concerned to convey the subjective experience as to detail the conceptual structure which serves that experience. In my view the process is not properly a "therapy" or a curative one involving the "treatment of a patient by a doctor." Rather it is a philosophic venturing. Moreover, existential-analytic psychotherapy—at least at this stage of its development—is not successfully employed with all who seek psychological help; therefore I will examine the circumstances that make its use most likely to be effective. Then we will study the three phases of thorough-going therapy that may be undertaken by a person seeking to emerge as fully as possible into realization of his potential for being. Finally we will look into some procedural steps that have been found consonant with the conceptual position here advanced.

Chapter 5 recognizes in the therapeutic relationship the essential medium in which the therapeutic confrontation may occur. No single model of the relationship is generally adequate to depict what is recommended, but by using several it will be possible to "triangulate" so as to convey the kind of working together that seems most productive. Since everything the therapist does can have significant impact on the patient, I will pick out some undesirable and some desirable influences the therapist may have.

From all that has been said so far it should be evident how very centrally important are those distortions of awareness and being which constitute the resistances. *Chapter 6* studies the resistance in detail in order to make very evident its existential meaning and to establish a conceptual foundation for the actual work of the analytic phase. *Chapter 7* deals directly with the therapeutic work of analyzing the resistance. By far the most thoroughly developed technology for this purpose is that of modern psychoanalysis. Without necessary allegiance to Freudian metapsychology, one may gratefully use the clinical wisdom and skill that has been thus evolved. Within the broad spectrum of the resistances, one extremely important and wide segment is made up of those distortions of awareness and being which get built into the person's relations with others. These are called the "transferences." The study of the transference and of the method of its analysis is the concern of *Chapter 8*.

Chapter 9 deals with the existential tragedy. Tragedy is not a familiar topic in psychological thought, but the general suppression of the recognition of the tragedy has been an important factor contributing to an increased sense of meaninglessness in living. The therapist needs to recognize that tragedy is always potential, that tragedy has had some importance in nearly every life, and that tragedy is importantly bound in with guilt and despair as well as with joy and fulfillment. This chapter offers suggestions for studying the impact of tragedy upon the patient's life and for helping him to meet and accept that impact.

Chapter 10 is concerned with the existential crisis. Most patients who have a thoroughgoing therapeutic experience come at some point to a juncture that represents a choice as to the whole meaning of their lives. Here one must weigh his very being and make a choice as to how he will be in the world thereafter. Nearly everyone goes through his life on a basis compounded of parental example and teaching, cultural influences, and half-thought-through self-examination. Thoroughgoing psychotherapy raises to consciousness an embracing perspective on one's own being, and this brings about a crisis. In this crisis the therapist's acute sensitivity and greatest skill are called for, as well as his most genuine dedication to freedom and choice.

Part Three will pick up the more inclusive perspective on man's efforts to emerge into fuller being. In the present section's concern with the analytic phase we are inevitably preoccupied with what Maslow has well termed "deficiency motivation" (1962b). Part Three will inquire into what he calls "being motivation." This is a newer frontier for psychology and a realm of genuinely unmapped ranges of possibility for man.

Part Four, after taking a long, hard look at the psychotherapist's own dynamics, concludes with some speculations about a more liberated kind of society and individual experience.

4 — The experience, concept, and procedure of existential-analytic therapy

Susan just called to tell me she got a job she hoped for and yet didn't think she had a chance of getting. I'm delighted. I'm delighted for Susan and her getting the job. I'm even more delighted for Susan and her therapy. And what delights me for her therapy is that Susan called me to tell me about the job.

You see, Susan in the therapeutic hour talks chiefly in a monotone except when she weeps in a whimpering way like someone hurt too much. Susan has been hurt too much. She's been hurt in her ability to trust, to believe someone is concerned about her experience. She knows people can be interested in her as an object, but she is sure they don't believe she's an experiencing person. When she talks to me during her sessions she is very careful to be distant, factual, impersonal, and to disclaim from time to time any expectation of any but a scientific concern from me. To be sure, that's the opening move of a gambit designed to get me to make protestations of concern (which I don't do), but even were I to go along with this gambit Susan wouldn't believe me and would be even more frightened and mistrustful because she would feel that she—weak as she feels herself to be—was manipulating me.

And Susan knows all about manipulating people; that's part of why she feels so lonely and frightened. Susan looks and acts like a sexy woman, and she almost always has two men with whom she's involved: one of whom she's sure, so she's discarding him, and one of whom she's not sure, so she's winning him. As soon as he's won, he'll have demonstrated he's weaker than Susan, and so he'll have to be discarded in turn while she seeks a new man. She can't stand to be without a man, but she can't find a man strong enough to take care of her. For Susan knows that the sexy woman is just a disguise that she wears and that inside she's really just a terribly frightened little girl who wants to be enfolded and protected and comforted by a real man. Now obviously any man who would be fooled by the little girl dressed up (or undressed) as a sexy woman isn't a real man. On the other hand, any man who sees through the disguise wouldn't want the terrified little girl, so . . . (And Susan will make sure that she's too demanding as she tests each man.)

So now Susan is trying to test me. She keeps things distant and formal in the therapy hour but throws out little bits of bait to see how I'll react: "I'm afraid I might want to take off my clothes here . . . I had a fantasy about you when I masturbated, but I'm afraid to tell you. . . . You must be terribly bored with me and my miseries. . . . I don't think I'm making any progress at all in therapy. . . ." Mostly I just listen. Sometimes I point out the sad little girl putting on the heavy disguise to try to get some comfort. Sometimes I point out how impersonal and shallow is the image of herself which she presents. Occasionally I will express sympathy or concern when she gives me a brief glimpse of the little girl. Always, to the last of these, Susan responds in a rejecting or seductive way, either denying that I could genuinely feel any concern for her or protesting that my concern only frightens her or trying hastily to cover the little girl with the sexy woman.

But today Susan called to tell me she got the job. And today is a milestone in Susan's therapy, though we didn't even have an interview today. For today Susan let herself see that I had concern for her as a person and not just for her disguises and miseries.

This is an incident in the course of existential-analytic psychotherapy. It's a milestone incident, as I said. There have been many weary sessions when Susan and I despaired of ever seeing any milestones. Sometimes when she expressed her misgivings about therapy I knew they were genuine and not attempts to maneuver me into reassuring her. At such times, I would tell her I too questioned whether we were getting anywhere. Sometimes admitting despair is as therapeutic as anything else one can do in such circumstances (Farber, 1958, 1962).

The incidents of therapy are so diverse and so subtle to characterize that it is certain that any description will fall short of fully conveying what occurs. In the pages and chapters that follow, I will be trying to disclose an underlying order in what would, superficially, often appear chaotic and pointless. To do so, I will often pare away much that is also true and important in order to highlight the particular aspect with which our discussion is concerned at that point. So now, at the outset, I want to try to convey the unorganized truths of the therapeutic work. I want to dispel any illusion of clinical simplicity and neatness. Psychotherapy is a part of life, and life is varied, haphazard, complex, disorderly, and inconclusive as well as being clear-cut, unified, harmonious, and meaningful.

Gordon, a "P.K." (preacher's kid), suddenly sits up on the couch and lets go of a stream of profanity and obscenity. As he talks he gets more and more excited and more and more pleased. He practically glows as he fashions a particularly repellent combination of excretory and pious images. As abruptly as he sat up, he drops back down and lies there silently smirking with all the smugness of a schoolboy who has just run the hundred yard dash on his hands and beaten all opponents.

Katie listens to my apology for starting the hour late in furious silence, then stands, marches to and out the door without a word. Three hours later, she calls me for another appointment. She is dead drunk.

Genny can hardly speak, she is so tense with fright at her own anger. Trying to help her break through, I tell her to "Throw the pillow at the far wall, overturn the coffee table, do something physical." She throws the pillow, dumps the coffee table and all its contents, smashes an ashtray, empties my wastebasket in the center of the room, kicks off her shoes and throws them at the wall, pounds with her fists on the overstuffed chair, and screams and screams and screams. Then she collapses in great racking sobs.

Dick is late again. I tell him for the hundredth or thousandth time that he's frightened of facing himself. He doesn't say anything. He doesn't say anything through the hour; nor do I. Neither of us speaks as he leaves. Two days later the same thing. A third time we do this. I express my exasperation.

Dick smiles with pleasure and begins talking. He isn't late again.

Funny, sad, frightening, hopeful, surprising, disappointing, encouraging, boring, inspiring, frustrating, and on and on—these are the experiences of psychotherapy. I have felt hot tears in my eyes as I watched someone summon his courage to meet a demon that has long tyrannized within him, and thus win back his life. I have found my heart pounding with fear for the impending violence as long-stored rage broke through. I have been tense with sexual excitement as an accomplished siren worked her wiles of movement and voice. I have been rocked back in astonishment as a new insight opened vistas of awareness to my patient and me that surpassed any familiar landscape. I have been shamed and guilty as I have seen how my carelessness and insufficient thought have complicated life and brought added suffering to someone who trusted me. I have been furious with the calculated taunts of a masterful provoker working me over. All this and yet more beyond any cataloging.

This is intensive psychotherapy, a process of immersion in the churning broth that is the human condition. No human experience is outside its realm. No single description can do it justice. In the following pages I will try to supplement the impression thus far conveyed by examining in turn four kinds of matters: the concept of "therapy" as a treatment process, some criteria of suitability for existential-analytic psychotherapy, the three main phases of a thoroughgoing existential-analytic course, and some of the matters of procedure I have found helpful in conducting my practice.

The Concept of Psychotherapy

Thomas Szasz (1960, 1961) has strikingly demonstrated the fallacy of what he terms the "myth of mental illness." I will not rehearse what he has done so well. However I do want to point out how unrealistic an "illness" concept is to the existential-analytic therapist's task.[1]

---

[1] As an aside let us note that it is anachronistic for me to continue to use terms such as "therapy," "symptom," "patient." However, I am less concerned with being purist at this point than with transmitting my meanings as well as I can.

The illness concept implies a state of health that is native to the person, from which he has been taken by the intrusion of disease or accident (Marzolf, 1947). The healer is charged to expel the intruding agency so that the native health can re-express itself. It is often pointed out that the doctor and his medicines do not themselves "heal" or mend; rather they remove what interferes with the natural, the inborn healing process.

It should be apparent that such a postulated innate healing process has little place in it for the patient's consciousness, intent, or will. It is exquisitely mechanistic and finds its clearest representations in medical examinations conducted in silence, prescriptions written in Latin, and the curious pun that "AMA" means both "American Medical Association" and "against medical advice," as when a patient's will is exercised against the doctor's admonitions (Spiegel, 1954).

The existential-analytic recognition of the state of affairs is radically in contrast with that of the illness model. We recognize that a "state of health" is an almost meaningless concept and certainly nothing from which our patients have momentarily fallen away. It is all too clear that emotional health, whatever that may mean, is something our patients may never have had. Moreover, as we look around us at ourselves, at those we know well, and at those we read and hear about, it is readily apparent that a normative (statistical) account of "health" makes a mockery of that term.

What is evident when we step back from our preconceptions of habit and language is that the business of being a person, a human being, is enormously complex and endlessly varied. Most of us were taught much more about how to manipulate certain relatively infrequently used mathematical functions than about how to make certain crucial life decisions.

We have come to recognize that our patients' "symptoms" are as much expressions of what we ordinarily call "health" as of "illness," without fully appreciating that thereby we are basically refuting the assumption of a normality underlying those symptoms.

In my view, the person, whom I will a bit longer refer to as my "patient," is coming to me for help because the ways he has accumulated through the years for trying to deal with his living have proven inadequate to give him what he wants and protect him from what he does not want; because he has at least dimly sensed that he is not so much living his life as being lived by his fears (May, 1953b).

You will notice that I use the vague phrase "ways he has accumulated." It might be easier to say "learned" but I'm reluctant to do so because the learning theorists seem so intent upon going full force into the same cul-de-sac that mechanistic medicine went into and is now struggling to get free of. I certainly mean "learning," but not the blind, subhuman learning some mean by that term.

Suitability for Existential-Analytic Psychotherapy

The ideal patient for existential-analytic psychotherapy, it seems to me, would have the following characteristics:

An intense feeling of dissatisfaction with the way his life was going at the human level, with some genuine anxiety to spur his seekings in therapy

A fantasy or ideal of greater validity and scope in living, with some genuine hope to inspire his seekings in therapy

Age, life situation (family, vocation, and so on), and finances adequate to permit and support an extensive and intensive commitment to the labors of therapy

Psychological mindedness—that is, the "set" to appreciate subjective processes and their relations, and genuine curiosity in their exploration

Many other qualities could be added to the list (intelligence, verbal facility, and so forth), but already these specifications suffer from the defects common to most studies of this kind (Ben-Avi, 1960; Knapp *et al.*, 1960; Waldhorn 1960); the patient who meets all the criteria would not need to be a patient and, indeed, would probably be further along the way to authenticity than the therapist.

The important point, however, is that not all persons who come for help are suitable candidates for existential-analytic psychotherapy. Extreme inadequacy in any one of the four criteria listed above is usually a contraindication. Essentially, what I am saying here is that an inability to make a full commitment to the therapeutic enterprise may come from any of several sources, but whatever its source, is a nearly crucial consideration. It is generally the case that intensive psychotherapy, such as is the concern of this book, requires a minimum of two years of work, with at least two and preferably three or four contacts a week for that period. By and large, I have not seen thoroughgoing therapeutic results achieved in under 250 contacts. Even that figure is minimal. Much more typical, I think, would be a figure of 350 to 500 contacts. Clearly then, the patient must be prepared to devote a major portion of his time (and frequently of his income) to the therapeutic undertaking. By no means to be underrated here is the importance of the impact of such a commitment on others in the patient's life. The patient's family, hopefully, will have a willingness to support—or at least not to oppose militantly—the patient's therapy emotionally and frequently in terms of money and time.

Psychological Mindedness. It will be worthwhile to spend a few minutes on this concept of "psychological mindedness." It can be defined in various ways, but my own impression is that it is a cognitive-emotional "set" of the awareness which probably has some constitutional element (as in talent for mathematics or the graphic arts or mechanics) and an even larger experiential element. It is certainly something that in many people seems to appear or increase during therapy; although it is equally true that some seem "psychologically blind" and show little or no increase in this characteristic.

For my own purposes I include within the concept of "psychological mindedness" several attributes often distinguished from it: an orientation to one's own and others' behavior and experience that is open, questioning, and sensitive to process as well as to content; an emotional participation in human experience that finds expression in empathy and the ability to form a relationship. Let us be clear that it is not implied in the foregoing that the psychologically minded person is particularly articulate or informed about psychological matters or that he forms good relationships in the sense of their being healthy, pleasant, or constructive. In the latter regard, all that is intended is a contrast with the person who is so isolated that in one sense he does not seem to have left any real recognition of the person-ness of himself or others. Such a person lives as an object in a world of objects and seems in some fundamental way "out of reach." (I am, of course, describing a schizophrenic withdrawal, except that this pattern can be found in persons otherwise apparently functional, indeed sometimes quite "successful" in some aspects of our culture.)

THE CONCEPT OF "INTENSIVE PSYCHOTHERAPY"

One way of further distinguishing the place of existential-analytic psychotherapy is to call it "intensive" psychotherapy. This is what Wolberg (1954, pp. 53–87) calls "reconstructive" therapy. Whichever term is employed, what is intended is to differentiate a therapy that is designed to aid the person in a major way from a therapy that seeks only to alleviate distress of symptoms, to offer support through a difficult period, or to re-educate constricting but circumscribed attitudes. Intensive therapy, on the other hand, is therapy that seeks to aid the person to reorganize his life, to reshape his personality, to redirect his destiny. I want to list three characteristics of intensive therapy that, it will be recognized, distinguish it as a unique experience (with a very few exceptions) in our culture for anyone in his whole lifetime.

First, intensive psychotherapy deals at length with previously unrecognized thoughts and feelings of the patient, which he now recognizes with a sense of personal authorship and relevance. Here I am characterizing the preconscious and unconscious materials that through psychotherapy are brought to consciousness. The important aspect I want to point to here, however, is that these now appear in consciousness with a clear sense of personal identification, so that the patient is not learning a new language as some have mistakenly thought, nor accepting an occult or bizarre account of his experience. Genuine intensive psychotherapy helps the patient discover that which in a sense he has always known within himself but of which he has never let himself be genuinely aware.

> Linda prided herself on her golf game and took part regularly in her club's tournaments. She usually won a runner-up recognition, but she never was a top winner. Not infrequently she lost out because on just one or two holes her game would "fall apart" and she would do much worse than usual. In Linda's therapy, we never dealt interpretatively with her golf, although she would talk about it with pride or exasperation from time to time. We did work on her relations with her sister. Increasingly Linda found herself flooded with guilt as she came to recognize how she had outmaneuvered her sister

to win her father's interest and attention and as Linda felt anew her envy and anger at the sister's brightness in school, which Linda could never hope to equal. Then one day Linda was talking at the beginning of an hour in a casual way before settling down to the regular therapeutic work. She was telling with a mixture of exasperation and resignation how once again, "There I was two strokes to the good, and what do you think I did on the sixteenth hole? What do you think I did?" Her voice rose in incredulity. "I took an eight! An eight! For crying out loud! Helen just had to bogey to win the match and third place!" I kept silent. Linda took a breath preparatory to another expostulation when suddenly her whole manner changed. Her face had a look of shock, almost of fright. "I took an eight, and I did it on purpose!" She hardly was talking to me but was saying the impossible thing aloud to herself. Now she looked up, her face a study in bewildered recognition, "I did it on purpose. I've done it on purpose time after time." The tears were starting, and I found my own eyes swimming. "I had to do it. I couldn't win. I mustn't win. It's like with my sister. I've got to think how she'll feel. I can't stand hurting her anymore. It's crazy, but I've known this all the time. Except I didn't somehow. But when I came up to the sixteenth, I knew it. I mean I really did. And yet, I didn't. Oh, God, I'm so confused and frightened and yet somehow I feel relieved too...."

Only the person who has experienced this in his own life and in his own inner world can appreciate the very clear-cut difference between that which might be told one about himself and that which is discovered within one's self. Unfortunately critics of depth psychotherapy have not always understood this point and have been much confused by regarding the metapsychology of a particular school (such as psychoanalysis) as something with which the patient is indoctrinated. Nothing can be further from the truth in genuine intensive psychotherapy (including psychoanalysis). There the therapist seldom uses the glossary of his systematic metapsychology; rather, patient and therapist together create their own glossary of idiosyncratic and personalized reference words to identify the unique, personal, internal discoveries of the patient.

The *second* characteristic of intensive psychotherapy is one often stated but perhaps too shallowly appreciated. In intensive psychotherapy patient and therapist move beyond the usual constraints of propriety and rationality. Characteristically we think of psychotherapy of any degree of intensity as freed from the need for usual considerations of politeness and properness. Discussion of "forbidden impulses," of anger and sexuality, is frequently an accepted part of therapy. What needs to be recognized is that genuine depth psychotherapy does not simply set aside for the moment usual social standards; rather, it endeavors to work back of the sources of such standards. What is meant here is that these learned constraints have their effects as ways of coping with the environment. They may lead to rewards or avoid hurts. Intensive psychotherapy attempts to deal more directly with the needs for such rewards and the fears of such hurts. Thus there is not simply a setting aside of the constraints but a dissolution of them, which means that the patient will fundamentally discard them. To be sure, if the patient then acts without a concern for propriety or rationality, this is antitherapeutic. Being in or having been in psychotherapy is not a license to act impulsively. The key point here is that psychotherapy which is intensive and effective dissolves much of the binding significance of social prohibitions of propriety and rationality. The patient may seem to continue to use accepted social forms, but if he has successfully worked through the sources of his use of these, he is freed from their automatic constraining implications and uses these accepted forms solely as ways of expressing and facilitating his being. Perhaps this point can be summarized by saying that successful intensive psychotherapy results in the "shoulds" being displaced by choice.

Thirdly, and related to the second point, intensive psychotherapy explores thoughts, impulses, and feelings that cannot be acted upon fully. What is pointed to here is the fact that there is a whole realm of the subjective life which literally is beyond the span of the externally possible. This is so for two reasons: one, because much of it may partake of the character of fantasy or hypothesis for speculation, and two, because certain aspects would terminate the possibility of further therapeutic work. Thus, the commission of violent acts upon oneself and others, the disruptions of relationships and employment, are apt to end the possibility of therapy running its full course. Intensive psychotherapy must deal with the reality of such thoughts, impulses, and feelings and deal with them for what they are: parts of the internal sphere of reality. Intensive psychotherapy treats these impulses as real but recognizes it is a psychic reality that they have.

Three Phases of Thoroughgoing Therapy

There is no single term that adequately points to the total process of uncovering, releasing, and facilitating human potential in the manner here conceived. Psychotherapy, properly speaking, can only refer to the first of three phases involved in this sequence. Psychotherapy may be thought of as concerned with the removal of limitations on functioning with the intent of freeing the person for more satisfying psychological life. As we have seen, for most of our patients there is no hypothetical "normal" from which they have lapsed due to injury. Rather, full use of their potential is something they have never achieved. It is partly for this reason that we recognize a second phase, here given the name "ontogogy," which is concerned with aiding a person to actualize or make real more of his potential once the grosser handicapping effects of his emotional disruption have been overcome. Finally, I will speculate about a further phase of human development that is infrequently attained but which needs to be brought into relation with the first two. This level, which may be called "transcendence," is one at which the person would move through and beyond many of the limitations on awareness and experience that are generally taken for granted and would then realize new oneness with all being. This statement is necessarily vague for several reasons: I am able to conceive this phase only in its broadest outline; the recognition that such a level is potential is relatively recent in secular western thought; and the manner of its attainment and the forms it would take are by definition so individual and creative as to preclude generalization.

Recognition of the third (transcendent) phase of human potential is, however, essential to the whole orientation to existential-analytic psychotherapy. Only through this recognition can we put in full perspective the significances of the first two phases. Because each person has within him the potential for transcendent being, we may look to the tasks of psychotherapy and ontogogy with greater appreciation of their significance to the full gamut of human possibility.

The analytic phase (psychotherapy) undertakes to display to the person's adult awareness those self-defeating patterns of being in the world that he has acquired in his efforts to avoid being overwhelmed by anxiety or that he has learned from the culture (and which thus represent group efforts to forestall anxiety). The analogy may be made to coaching a person who wants to put himself in good physical condition: the first step may be to help him discover destructive patterns of eating, exercise, rest, and so on. These are encumbrances to healthy being that impede any constructive efforts. In the analytic phase, however, much more is accomplished than simply ridding the person of impediments to his growth. Inevitably as the patient experiences the freeing from neurotic patterns, he finds new vitality and purpose that project him toward more fulfilling experiences. Again using the physical analogy: as habits of physical being become less destructive and weight becomes more suitable, eating is better balanced and an appropriate work–rest cycle is established, the person feels new energy and readiness to undertake physical activities formerly shunned.

The ontogogic phase picks up appropriately when this release of energy and appetite for living occurs. Indeed, the two phases overlap greatly. For some this positive development comes about quite spontaneously, and there is no evident need of further professional help. But for many in our culture and under the conditions of our life that so often perpetuate or reinforce neurotic patterns, much can be gained from having a companion and counselor in the task of meeting the existential challenges of life and developing ways of maintaining and further nourishing the actualization of one's potential.

Let me close this brief synopsis of the three phases of thoroughgoing therapy by indicating in a rough-hand way something of my conception of the total enterprise. The analytic task may be likened to the overcoming of the fears and superstitions that prevented sailors of the fifteenth and earlier centuries from venturing far out to sea. The ontogogic phase takes up with the discovery of the Western Hemisphere and carries us barely as far as the founding of the principal colonies. The great work of discovery, exploration, and development of the potential before us is, I am convinced, barely begun. It is a challenging, exciting, and yet sobering and humbling prospect. I will discuss it further in later chapters, and especially in the last.

THE TASK OF THE ANALYTIC PHASE

The analytic phase of the therapeutic work is centered on the disclosure and resolution of the resistance. By resistance is meant the ways in which the patient seeks to avoid existential anxiety. The two foregoing sentences contain the essence of existential-analytic psychotherapy, and those sentences represent a major discovery about the human experience with profound significance for the whole of the psychotherapeutic enterprise.

It was Freud (1933) who first recognized the resistance and gave it a position of central importance in his psychotherapy. But Freud, lacking a genuine existential orientation, did not appreciate the enormous significance in human life of the phenomenon he had discovered. "We call all the forces which oppose the work of cure the patient's 'resistances,' " he wrote in *The Question of Lay Analysis*. This is far too limited a view, and such a view made necessary the extensive elaborations of Freudian metapsychology to account for the vicissitudes of the work of resolving the resistance.

Existential theory is deeply indebted to Freud's pioneer discoveries, but it discloses the true meaning of the resistance to be far more fundamental than is represented only in a process acting counter to therapy. The resistance is made up of those ways in which the patient seeks to avoid existential anxiety, the anxiety of being, of living. Inevitably this means that the existential anxiety is overlaid with neurotic anxieties which represent the various efforts to avoid the underlying dread of being, and thus the work of analysis must uncover layer after layer of symptoms and anxieties to get "down" to the existential anxiety. But, at root, this is the meaning of the resistance: it is resistance to authentic being in the world.

The significance of this recognition of the nature of the resistance can scarcely be overstressed. It makes evident that psychotherapy which focuses on the resistance is not an "as if" process, is not a learning process which hopefully will teach better habits for "outside" life. Psychotherapy is, rather, a centering on the patient's life itself. It is far more real or genuine or actual than any other experience the patient can have in the usual course of his life. In the therapeutic hour, patient and therapist join in disclosing the patterns of inauthenticity that are, here and now, maintaining the patient's estrangement from genuineness of being. In the therapeutic hour, the two participants are engaged in a truly vital struggle with the very processes that keep the patient in non-being. This is the raw frontier of life itself, not a substitute for or simulation of life. When therapist and patient are effective, there is no problem of "transfer of training," no question as to whether the results of therapy will be effective outside the consultation room. The patient's participation in his life is different, and the effects will be extended into all of his life.

The Transference. Each of us finds his world importantly populated by other people. We are drawn toward them and yet we may fear them. We see them as benign or malignant, as part of our being and support to our courage in meeting life, or as potential exploiters of our weakness and vulnerability, or as objects we can use to interpose between ourselves and the fearful aspects of our being. The child begins very early to form his ideas of who he is and who and what others are. Inevitably he is drawn into the mechanisms of others for forestalling their anxieties, and just as surely he establishes his own patterns for involving others to the same end. Many resistances and many of the most significant resistances are of this nature. We give the name "transferences" to those resistances that involve other people as a way of trying to avoid existential or neurotic anxiety and that are then projected onto the therapist by the patient. The analytic phase must give important attention to these transferences. Usually it is strategically wise for the nontransference resistances to be dealt with first, since during this time the projection onto the therapist can occur and the way is cleared for effective disclosure and resolution.

An Aside about the Term "Transference." This term is sometimes loosely used as though synonymous with the "therapeutic relation." This misuse seems to me to lead only to confusions. In this book, the term will be used only to refer to distortive or parataxic aspects of the therapeutic relation.

Some Matters of Procedure

In this section I want to describe some of the procedural aspects of my practice from which I draw the greater proportion of my observations. I do so in order that the circumstances under which these observations have been made will be evident and thus suggest the limitations upon their generality. Also, because this method of operating has worked out sufficiently well for me, I am encouraged to continue with it and to commend it to the consideration of any therapist-reader desiring to review his own practice. This is not to say that this is the best way. I am quite sure it is not, and that others will find for themselves their own procedural patterns which will work best for them with the kind of clientele they see. Suffice it to say that in over fifteen years of a practice which has been evolving toward the viewpoint I am describing here, these procedures have evolved concurrently and, I trust, congruently.

My average patient is in his mid-thirties, has some college education, is married or has been. He is in a professional, technical, or managerial position, or is preparing for such a position. Typically I see him three times a week, for two to four years. Presenting problems on intake most frequently are character disorders and psychoneuroses. I see about equal numbers of men and women.

I prefer to begin my work with a new patient with a schedule of four interviews a week so that the therapeutic experience can have an appreciable impact on his life and his maximal involvement with the undertaking is likely. My reasoning is that a resistance that a great many of my patients have is the desire to bring their ailments for repair and then to call back for them after a decent interval. Few of them really contemplate the total confrontation that is essential to the concerns for which they consult me.[2]

I am not always successful at intake in getting people whom I think suitable candidates for existential-analytic therapy to see

---

[2] I have fantasied at times that I would like to enter their lives even more importantly, so that their nearly total attention might be riveted on what we are undertaking. Thus, I have thought that it would be desirable if we had a residence where our patients could live when they first come to us. They might go to work or school for certain hours each day but they would come back to this residence, where they would have a variety of reminders of the kind of life confrontation that is involved.

their needs in the way I am here portraying, but I am gaining in my effectiveness as I gain in my own acceptance of the reality of what I have been describing. My own neurotic residues have encouraged me at times to underplay the significance of what the patient and I must do if he is to reclaim his life. My own resistances and inauthenticities have been importantly involved in making me hesitant to challenge the patient in the fundamental way that is important if truly he is going to come into greater authenticity in his living. Increasingly, I am able to say to a prospective patient with genuineness that unless he is prepared to make psychotherapy the most important thing in his life for a period of several years, he would probably be more satisfied to work with someone else. What I am saying when I say this is that he must put the fact of his being alive in the forefront of his awareness in a fashion which he has never done before. The result is, of course, that I get a select patient sample.

Use of the Couch. Generally I ask my patients to use the couch (Kelman, 1954). I have several reasons for this. First, I think in all candor that I am more comfortable being free to grimace and scratch, doodle and otherwise relax while the patients talk. I am more comfortable and more able to give good attention to them. I think Freud's observation here was a very realistic one and should not be used to belittle him, as is sometimes done. Anyone who has done much intensive psychotherapy is well aware that patients are tremendously concerned to pick up any minimal clues they can. They will misinterpret any datum in the effort to get them. They do get a great many clues from the way my chair squeaks, when I shift my position, when I write, and when I do not write. I am well content to reduce these clues by having them use the couch.

The second important reason is that I regard our usual conversational skills as composed as much of the resistive in the patient's make-up as of the vital. I think he is a prisoner of his usual conversational skills, and as he looks at me and talks in an everyday fashion, he is handicapped in the business of psychotherapy. Asking him to do a unique thing in his life: to lie on a couch faced away from me and to talk without any expectation of regular replies, is important in helping him to free himself from the grip of those usual conversational skills, as resistances.

Third, I think that the kinds of conditioning and learnings the patient has associated with lying on his back without anyone in sight are more apt to be those of reverie and self-aware confrontation of the issues in his life than are those conditionings associated with sitting up and talking to someone. I wish sometimes that I could have my patients talk to me while shaving, while going to the toilet, while driving a car. I think for many of us the most important existential contemplation or meditation is done when we are performing routine, primitive functions. Lying on one's back on a couch may be the nearest convenient approximation.

It goes without saying that my patients leave the couch at times, sit in any of the several different chairs in my office, pace about. However, at least in the earlier stages, I am inclined to look for meaning in these motions as actings-out of impulses that cannot at the moment be conveyed in language. Certainly toward the latter part of successful psychotherapy the patient may leave the couch and talk to me with great genuineness from a chair.

Other Procedural Matters. Later chapters will return to the procedures that have proven helpful. In the next chapter the very important topic of the therapeutic relationship will be examined in detail. Chapter 7 will discuss what I ask the patient to do and what it is that I try to do meanwhile. In that chapter I will try to explain why I think the therapist is well advised to talk minimally during most therapeutic sessions. Chapter 7, on the analysis of the resistance, and Chapter 8, on the analysis of the transference, will both describe some guides to listening to the patient and to formulating interventions.

My intent in presenting these procedural matters is dual: I want the reader to understand rather fully the conditions under which I make the observations this book reports. Also I hope to make available to the therapist in practice or in training enough details of my experience for him to select from it as he wishes. This book, however, is not an adequate coverage of psychotherapeutic procedure. It assumes that therapist-readers will already be familiar with such materials as those dealt with by Colby (1951),

Fromm-Reichman (1950), Kelman (1948), Menninger (1958), Rogers (1951), Saul (1958), Wolberg (1954), and others.

Conclusion

Intensive psychotherapy that is oriented in an existential-analytic direction is the method of choice for only a segment of all who seek psychological help. It requires a major life commitment on the part of the patient and the therapist, and, when successful, such therapy becomes one of the major experiences of the person's life. Psychotherapy may be recognized as but the first of three stages of personal evolution in the direction of increasing authenticity. Ontogogy attempts to elicit positive emergence just as therapy sought to overcome negative inhibitions. Transcendence envisions a surpassing and creative movement of the person beyond the usual confines of life.

5—*The therapeutic relation: essential medium of therapy*

Of all possible analogies, it seems to me that effective psychotherapy may be best likened to the creation of a work of art—for example, a painting—by an apt pupil under a teacher who seeks to nurture the pupil's talent even more than to make certain that the present picture is a masterpiece. One of the poorest analogies might be that of a game of chess between two experts.

The artist tries to seize upon the stuff of the world and mold it in such a way that it expresses that which the artist experiences within himself. It is very much a part of artistic creation that the product is a projection of inner living. The master artist-teacher, hopefully, is himself talented and skilled in this enterprise, but more importantly—if he is truly a gifted teacher—he is most concerned that the pupil will discover his own internal meanings and images, while he, the teacher, aids the pupil in the fragile business of translating them into shapes and colors externally visible. The master, who is all a master could be, will be filled with love and respect for the pupil's internal livingness and yet with an equal love and respect for the intrinsic qualities of the media with which the pupil works. The master will seek that intercourse of the pupil's subjective life with the materials' intrinsic nature that is most faithful to both and does least violence to either. It should be noted that in this way the master's own inner creativity may be best expressed, with equal faithfulness to himself and to his pupil and to the materials.

On the other hand, in the chess game the player's goal is to detect and negate the opponent's intent. In chess, the predetermined functions of the pieces are to be exploited within rigid limits. In chess, the act of one is always countered with the act of the other. The gambits and sequences of chess are elegant and mathematically impersonal. The personal style of a chess master is certainly evident to the initiated, but it is a cold thing and subservient to the parameters of the contest.

The psychotherapist, like the art master, ideally is filled with a loving appreciation for the uniqueness of his pupil-patient. In similar fashion, he experiences an emotional commitment to the "is-ness" of existence. To impose his own meanings on patient or world with disregard of their intrinsic qualities would violate the therapist's own internal authenticity. To aid the patient in engaging his life so that he expresses himself creatively while yet respecting the inherent properties of all existence, this is the therapist's own way of expressing his being in relation to the world.

From this introduction, it will be apparent that I do not believe that any prescription can be set down to be followed like an opening gambit in chess. Rather, I am convinced that the therapist needs a deep appreciation for the livingness of his patient and the givenness of all existence. He can usefully employ conceptual tools to grasp these more fully, but, beyond this point, the therapist must be his own being in his engagement with his patient.

Conceptualizing the Ideal Therapeutic Relationship

From all that has been said, it will be evident that the relationship which develops between the patient and the therapist may prove of critical importance to the whole enterprise. In a previous chapter the point was made that the actual therapeutic agency is the patient's own confrontation of himself and his world, but this does not gainsay the recognition that the medium in which that confrontation is most apt to occur with constructive results is the optimum therapeutic relation. Since it is difficult to specify just what makes this relation optimum, let us try to get at it along several avenues.

An Evolving Model

Various conceptions of psychotherapy have developed contrasting models of the ideal therapeutic relation. That which I am trying to delineate has most in common with the psychoanalytic and the client-centered conceptions; yet there are important points of difference from each. Such differences are most pronounced when comparison is made with the classical psychoanalytic or the early nondirective patterns. The classical analytic ideal of the therapist as a "blank screen" on which the patient projected his inner life was not only a psychological impossibility but also presented the patient with a model of inauthenticity which all too often was copied and embodied forth as that scourge of polite society, the cocktail party amateur analyst, probing everyone's motives and risking no real relationships. The early nondirective ideal has seemed to be equally a psychological impossibility: a kind of selfless mirror beaming forth unconditional positive regard for any that come before it. Again, the product (therapist or patient) tended to be a kind of inauthentic anonymity especially apt to drive spouses and children to distraction by sweetly reflecting back all feelings while yet genuinely expressing none.

It is manifest that I have presented caricatures of both the analytic and client-centered views and products.[1] However, the point is that these caricatures of the theoretical positions actually have been enacted by people, both patients and therapists. They are not complete exaggerations. Moreover, it is my conviction that the distortions were built into the initial conceptions.

Nevertheless, let me make one additional recognition. The current thinking of such analysts as Hora (1959, 1962c), Kelman (1960), May (1959a, 1961a), and many, many others would not accept the myth of the blank screen and would be very similar to that offered in this book. Similarly, the Rogers who wrote *On Becoming a Person* (1961) is fully aware of what we are here saying in a way that was not true at the time of *Counseling and Psychotherapy* (1942). In other words, I am describing a general evolution of the understanding of the psychotherapeutic relation, not a unique discovery of the existential-analytic view.

THE CONSULTANT MODEL

But let us return to that view. I have previously used comparisons with a master artist and a chess expert to try to clarify my con-

---

[1] Certainly one could, with equal humor, describe the existentially processed patient—and therapist—as always taking Hamlet-like stances, mumbling darkly, "To be AND not to be," and walking in front of trucks with transcendent but ignorant bliss shining on his features.

ception. Perhaps another comparison will fill in the picture further. The existential view sees the patient as a person busy in the midst of his own life who finds he needs a "consultant" to aid him (the patient) in making more of his living satisfying.

This term "consultant" is important in conveying much of what I want to say, yet it has disadvantages too; so it must not be carried too far. What I mean to convey with the term is this: the consultant is always in some measure external to the on-going business of the patient's life. No matter how much the patient may seek for the consultant to take over—indeed, no matter how much the therapist tries to guide or manage his patient's affairs—the existential reality is unchanged, the patient is the only responsible one in his own life. This does not obviate the very real, and often very heavy, responsibility a psychotherapist bears in his own right (see Chapter 21). Certainly as we work with our patients we can try to do much to aid them in their exercise of their autonomy, but we need always to recognize and respect that autonomy.

Let me make this point even more evident, for it is an important one. Ultimately, the existential-analytic goal of therapy is to help the patient achieve his most authentic personhood. This ideal outweighs such secondary goals as improved efficiency or comfort in living. Accordingly, the authenticity of the therapeutic relationship itself must be maintained as fully as possible. The distortion of seeming to transfer responsibility from the patient to the therapist is often attempted by the patient's fear-defense maneuvers but must not be abetted by the therapist's own countertransference (Hora, 1962d; Kaiser, 1955; Menninger, 1958).

A SHARED ENTERPRISE

The therapeutic relationship, we must recognize, is much more than the model of consultant-client conveys. It is not merely a commonsense relationship; it is not impersonal, and it is not as limited as the analogy suggests. It is essentially a relationship between two human beings, each in the midst of his own life, neither fully adequate to deal with all the contingencies he is encountering, and yet for a time endeavoring to communicate between them so that they achieve more understanding of what it is they are experiencing about one of them especially.

Implicit in what I have just said is the recognition that therapy is a shared enterprise in which the therapist gains as well as the patient. I am sure this is so. It is important to recognize this reality, to free ourselves of the idea of the patient as the one to whom things are done and the therapist as the one who does things. Maslow's term (1962a) "the synergistic relationship" is suggestive here, the relationship in which each gains from the fact of being in relationship to the other. This is not a kind of license to the therapist to use the relationship in a self-serving fashion or with blind faith that whatever fulfills his needs must somehow be useful to the patient, but it is a recognition that only as each is importantly committed to the relationship can he draw meaning from the relationship, can there be a potential for real therapeutic impact.

Everything the therapist does, of course, has its effect on his relation with the patient. As we have seen, so much else beyond what the therapist says explicitly or intends consciously contributes to its evolution. Having gained some impression of the ideal sought for, let us now examine some specific procedures and circumstances through which the therapist may unwittingly—but importantly—affect how he is experienced by the patient and what the patient may come to expect of him and of therapy. We will discuss the use of examinations of the patient, the kinds of complications in the treatment process that the therapist may introduce, and some steps that may aid a favorable relationship.

Psychodiagnostics and the Quest for Certainty

Psychology first earned its place in the clinical field through the development of procedures and skills in the psychodiagnostic assessment of patients. The work of many gifted and creative people developed this approach to an excellent degree. In what I will be saying about the use of psychodiagnostics I intend no diminishing of the contribution that has been made; instead I am going to be speaking solely from the perspective of an intensive psychotherapist of existential-analytic orientation considering the possible values of psychodiagnostics in outpatient practice. Needless to say, the physician-psychotherapist who conducts a physical examination of his patient will want to consider the implications of doing so in a manner similar to that we will employ below (Saul, 1958, p. 67).

I make no regular use of a formal psychodiagnostic study before undertaking psychotherapy with most of the patients I see. The reasons why I do not do so fall into two main categories, those that relate to me as the therapist and those that relate to my patient. I will detail these in later pages, but first I need to review some aspects of our basic existential perspective.

EXISTENTIAL-ANALYTIC ORIENTATION

Man finds himself in "a world he never made," a world of apparently infinite possibility. In this world, man is constantly confronted with choices for which he must always be less than adequately prepared. Thus man is constantly faced with uncertainty, with contingency, with the possibility that his choices may fail to bring him the results he intends. That failure may range from the simplest disappointment to a fatal misstep, from being late to a pleasant evening's recreation to being killed as he walks across his normally quiet, residential street.

This contingent plight is the constantly present and always overriding fact of our existence. Much of the time we do not think about it, and each of us joins in some measure in a universal conspiracy to suppress, repress, or displace awareness of this fact. The manner of our doing so is varied and often subtle as we use the defense mechanisms that Freud so brilliantly disclosed. But whatever the particular dynamic pattern, the common element is in some form the *quest for certainty* (Schwartz & Wolf, 1959).

Let us pause to examine this quest for certainty. By "certainty" I mean the opposite of contingency. Having survived a disastrous fire in our neighborhood and being concerned about my home, I decide to investigate the likelihood I would not be so fortunate again. I find my odds are 1000 to 1 against the likelihood that my house will burn, but I am not content and so have the brush cleared back some distance. Now the odds are 1500 to 1, I find. Still concerned, I have an automatic sprinkling system installed. Now I'm told my odds are 3500 to 1. However I try, though, I must recognize always that I cannot achieve certainty that the house will not burn. I may do much, but I can't be sure that a nuclear firestorm will not make my efforts vain. I may build my house underground, but still I can't be sure but that the earth might be drawn closer to the sun and the whole world thus be ignited.

Now these are ridiculous extremes, of course, but the point remains: there is no true certainty to be had. So it is with any issue. Nevertheless, we seek that certainty constantly. We buy insurance, seat-belts, medicines, door locks, education, and much else to try to protect ourselves against tragedy, to secure good outcomes. So long as we recognize we are dealing in probabilities, such choices can be useful. But every therapist has seen the pathology of seeking for certainty instead of better probabilities.

THERAPY AND CONTINGENCY

The task of therapy may be conceived, in an oversimplified fashion, as that of helping the patient reconfront the contingency situations from which he has fled to the seeming certainties of his symptoms and character defenses. In this process he must contend anew with the frightening impulses with which he could not deal in the past, accept—and hopefully, learn to welcome—the responsibility for choice that is his as he gives up the blind repetitions of parataxic living and reawakens his awareness to the full reality of his being-in-the-world.

EXISTENTIAL IMPLICATIONS OF TESTS

Let me now make some observations about the implicit and existential meanings of tests. Tests can only measure aspects or parts of persons. No test can measure a whole person, nor can any battery no matter how intensive and extensive. Only a whole person can grapple with the task of encountering—I do not say, comprehending—another whole person.

Each test must do some violence to that which it seeks to describe; some tests do much violence. An inadequate or inaccurate description of a person is a kind of destruction of that person, at least in many situations in which we use such descriptions to make decisions importantly affecting people.

To think that we can measure or assess human personality with 10 inkblots or 550 true-false questions is to assert we have climbed Mt. Whitney because we have mastered the hill down the street. True, they are similar tasks but only in one part or aspect.

Many psychological tests are founded on an image of man as a relatively simple animal built up additively of units such as habits, instincts, traits, and the like. Such a view of man is rapidly becoming as outmoded as the running board. The true nature of man, we are increasingly recognizing, lies precisely in the fact that could we efficiently tally all his habits, instincts, traits, and so forth, man would still be something other. Man is the process that supersedes the sum of his part-functions (see Chapter 1).

INTAKE PROCEDURE

When a new patient comes to me and I see him for intake, I typically try to become aware of any extreme distortions in emotional status that may suggest the need for procedures with which I am not equipped. These would include those people who show a potential for extreme acting-out, a possible need for hospitalization, or the likelihood of organic disease. Early in our contacts I try to secure an evaluation and opinion as to the medical suitability of this patient for outpatient service. The intake and initiation of therapy may run to five or ten interviews. In addition to the bases for ruling out therapy I have described above, it may well be that in this initial period the patient finds that he wants some other form of service or that he is not ready to undertake intensive psychotherapy with me at this time. On occasion I have used psychological tests to facilitate this decision-making process on my part or on the patient's part, but this is not my usual procedure.

DISADVANTAGES TO THE THERAPIST

Now why do I conduct my practice in this way? As I said above, the reasons fall into two categories; those relating to the therapist and those relating to the patient. Let us first examine those relating to the therapist. There are three of these. First, the aid given by the psychodiagnostic battery and work-up "costs" more in terms of conflict with the therapeutic task than it contributes to that task. Second, the introduction of psychological testing produces an interference with the therapist's ability to encounter his patient as a total human being. Third, the therapist may unwittingly make use of the test information as a resistance to confronting his own unsureness in the face of the unknown in the relationship with the patient. Let me expand on these.

THE "COST" OF TESTING

The first point has to do with the extent to which the gain from the introduction of a testing battery balances the cost. In most instances what a test battery yields can be grouped into three categories: structural information, information about dynamic processes, and information about intrapsychic contents. The structural information includes intellectual level, something about the functional relationships of the psychological systems within the personality, and indications of ego strength, superego functioning, and impulse control. All of these kinds of information are indeed interesting and suggestive where we need to treat the patient as one example of a class of people—for example, applicants for service at a clinic. There we must make administrative judgments as to which patients will be given service and by which therapists. This, of course, is a valuable social function, but the information needed to perform it is not necessarily the most useful sort of information when undertaking long-term, intensive psychotherapy.

The information in the area of defense patterns applies somewhat more directly to the therapeutic task, in that awareness of these patterns is essential to the therapist in conducting his work with the patient. Nevertheless, very often the psychological testing does not present these data in a fashion most useful in actual work with the patient. The patient himself will present these data more meaningfully in the course of the interviews. Then one can see the layering pattern that permits a more orderly process of analysis and forestalls the kind of chaos in the therapeutic work that Wilhelm Reich (1949) warned against. Similar comments may be made about the intrapsychic contents: the kinds of conflicts persistent in obsessive patterns, the important figures in the patient's earlier and present life, and so on. All this information is certainly suggestive, but it develops more naturally and more usefully in the interviews themselves, rather than at the time the therapist is undertaking his first sessions with the patient.

INTERFERENCE WITH ENCOUNTER

In some ways a more important objection is the interference occasioned in the therapist's encounter with the patient when he has a great mass of information about the patient in advance.[2] It seems essential to the existential-analytic viewpoint (and perhaps to others also) to meet the patient in the uniqueness of his being. This some-

---

[2] This interference effect can be occasioned also when one receives a patient on transfer from another psychotherapist. Then it is usually preferable to see the patient several times before having detailed transfer notes.

what esoteric-sounding term simply means that the therapist as a person needs to come freshly to the person who is to be his patient, to find him as *the individual* rather than as a class representative; to meet him with awareness uncontaminated by other information so that the therapist may know how it is the patient presents himself, what sorts of responses he elicits in others, and what it is he seeks to do in the interpersonal relationship. It is almost impossible to have this fresh outlook when talking for the first time with a patient on whom one has a wealth of information.

RESISTANCE TO THE UNKNOWN

Probably this same interference is a part of the resistance the therapist may erect to confronting that which is unknown in his relationship with his new patient as they undertake psychotherapy. It is all too easy to forget that the test findings themselves are but probability statements and, forgetting, to accord those scores a precision they do not have. As indicated above, contingency is uncomfortable; not knowing, not being sure, can be frightening. And yet this discomfort, even this fear, is an essential part of one's sensitivity in getting to know the new patient with whom one is working. If we dull the edge of it with the pseudo-security of test interpretations, then we probably dull sensitivity to some of the things that are going to be most important in the work with the patient. One gains a measure of security by losing a measure of awareness. One gains a modicum of knowledge as he sacrifices more than a modicum of being-in-the-relationship.

These three reasons for hesitating to use tests at the outset of intensive psychotherapy with a new patient suggest that the over-all cost of using tests is more than the therapist may care to pay, more than responsibly he can pay in undertaking his work with this patient. This is even more true when we look at those reasons which from the patient's standpoint argue against the use of the psychodiagnostic battery.

PATIENT'S STANDPOINT

DEPERSONALIZATION

First of all, basically, is the fact that the testing inevitably depersonalizes the relationship in some measure, whether the therapist administers the battery himself or some other psychologist does so. The effect of the battery is to make of the patient an object for study, to be understood by another, more than it is to foster his own self-understanding. Since a common element in the psychopathology of many patients is an already present tendency to depersonalize themselves, to make themselves into objects, one cannot in good conscience undertake a procedure that so massively reinforces this tendency. The patient is asked on the questionnaire to look upon himself impersonally and to describe himself objectively. The patient is asked, when looking at the inkblots, to turn over his perceptions to someone else for analysis with the manifest message that obviously he cannot understand what these perceptions of the inkblots say. He is divorced in a sense from his ego-function, while his self-concern is asked to divorce itself from his perceptions and the report on them. This depersonalizing works exactly contrary to the therapeutic purpose of helping the patient regain the sense of his own identity and of aliveness in his being.

FALSE CERTAINTY

The second reason that the psychodiagnostic battery is undesirable from the patient's standpoint relates to the quest for certainty I have already described. The use of the tests, particularly those that yield numerical scores and those that are mysterious, such as the inkblots, plays into the patient's seeking for a certainty outside himself: a quantifiable, statistically precise authority on which he can lean. The dependency element in the make-up of many patients is very important. Those things which foster that dependency, which make it seem that mysterious but powerful forces are being mobilized in the patient's behalf, work against his successful therapeutic course. This is particularly so in relation to the transference: for if the patient is asked to submit to tests and then the therapist esoterically interprets these, either telling him the results or not, a support is lent to a parataxis, to a distortion, and this is a support that will add complications to the therapeutic task.

MAKING THE PATIENT AN OBJECT

The foregoing two points on the depersonalizing effect of tests and the illusion of certainty they create set the stage and are part of the third and final point: use of a psychodiagnostic battery takes from the patient some of the responsibility he must have to tell about himself. It says in effect to the patient that there are other ways of learning about him and more important things that can be learned about him than he can or will tell of his own accord. One of the main functions of psychotherapy is that of providing the situation in which the patient is called upon to talk meaningfully about himself, to himself and to the therapist. Too often the patient tends simply to turn over information about the object that is himself to the therapist and wait passively for the performance of miracles, like a man who leaves his shoes at the shop and says he will call back for them at the end of the week. A great deal of work in therapy has to do with dealing with this resistance, this defense against taking responsibility for oneself. Employment of the psychodiagnostic battery unnecessarily adds to the probability that the patient will see himself as not fully responsible to account for himself.

SUMMARY

I have tried to say why I do not regularly include a psychodiagnostic battery as a part of the intake procedure with patients entering upon long-term, intensive psychotherapy with me. The reasons fall into two categories, those that relate to myself and those which relate to the patient. Obviously this is a heuristic rather than an actual distinction, since the two categories interweave, just as that which is of concern to the patient and to myself interweaves. The reasons I have described are, in summary, that the tests provide too little aid for the psychological cost they entail. That cost I have spelled out in terms of the interference the test results and other extraneously derived information occasion in my fresh encounter with the patient as a total person; in terms of the support to my resistance to encountering that which is unknown in my relationship with the patient; in terms of the depersonalizing effect of making my patient an object for study as opposed to a responsible person in his own life; in terms of the pseudo-certainty the tests seem to provide and the support this gives for parataxic projection upon me and upon the process of therapy of an authority which does not reside in us; and finally in terms of taking responsibility away from the patient to tell about himself to himself and to me. Clearly, most of these same considerations would contraindicate the physician-psychotherapist's conduct of a physical examination of his patient also.

VALUES IN TESTING

Nothing I have said above should be read as denying that there is a very real place for the psychodiagnostic battery in situations where administrative decisions must be made about the patient and we desire to make those decisions on an informed understanding of the nature of the patient and his problems. I think there is often, but not always, a very real use for (and on occasion I do use) psychodiagnostic instruments in counseling cases where a situational problem is presented, such as disturbed relationships in marriage or parenthood. These instruments are helpful in vocational and educational guidance situations and certainly where there is a question as to case management and disposition. The sort of information that can be derived quickly and efficiently through the use of psychodiagnostic instruments makes them well worth our reliance. When a person finds it impossible to tell me about himself and he is not able or ready to undertake intensive treatment, I have no hesitation in using the diagnostic instruments as a way of facilitating my aid to him in certain important decisions he must make.

In concluding this section, the following quotation from *Amiel's Journal* (1866) (Cantril and Bumstead, 1960, p. 14) is pertinent.

> To understand is to possess the thing understood, first by sympathy and then by intelligence. Instead, then, of first dismembering and dissecting the object to be conceived, we should begin by laying hold of it in its ensemble, then in its formation, last of all in its parts. The procedure is the same, whether we study a watch or a plant, a work of art or a character. We must study, respect, and question what we want to know, instead of massacring it. We must assimilate ourselves to things and surrender ourselves to them; we must open our minds with docility to their influence, and steep ourselves in their spirit and their distinctive form, before we offer violence to them by dissecting them.

Polybius of Megalopolis, writing in the Second Century before Christ, spoke of the error of . . .

... the notion that the contemplation of the *disjecta membra* of a once living and beautiful organism is equivalent to the direct observation of the organism itself in all the energy and beauty of life. I fancy that anyone who maintained such a position would speedily admit the ludicrous enormity of his error if the organism could be revealed to him by some magician who had reconstituted it, at a stroke, in its original perfection of form and grace of vitality. While the part may conceivably offer a hint of the whole, it cannot possibly yield an exact and certain knowledge of it (quoted by Cantril and Bumstead, 1960, pp. 18–19).

Iatrogenic Complications

There are some ways in which the therapist may actually increase the patient's alienation and self-fragmentation. These may be termed "iatrogenic complications" of the therapeutic process. They can be likened to the effects of physicians who used to bring sepsis on their hands from the surgery into the sick room in the days before antiseptic practice.

DISPLACING RESPONSIBILITY

When the therapist encourages the patient to displace responsibility for that which he experiences or does, the therapist is subtly enfeebling his patient. It is all too frequently the case that the patient from his own needs and the therapist from his cause-seeking orientation join in demonstrating how parents or spouse or others brought about some untoward incident, some undesirable pattern of behavior, or some other unwanted element in the patient's life. The therapist may feel he is siding with the patient in helping the patient to see how this way of behaving today was a result of the other person's actions. But the patient needs to learn that such causality is a limited concept which is not a sufficient answer to the problems of his experience. Certainly historic sources of response patterns can be distinguished with profit at times. This sort of insight gives the patient some sense that he is not to be blamed for developing the pattern. But that removal of blame is only in terms of the *sources* of the pattern. *The present enactment is the patient's responsibility.* The need to remove interfering blame can cause a therapist to go too far and remove from the patient the sense of choice and responsibility.

OPPOSING EGO-FUNCTIONS

A second way in which the therapist may complicate the patient's efforts toward achieving greater authenticity is through the therapist's interdicting intellectualizing, control, reasonableness, and other such patterns. Therapists may also indicate skepticism about volition, determination, resolution, hope, and prayer. All these human functions can be part of the well-being of the patient and only their misuse is interdicted by the wise therapist. Certainly intellectualizing can be used as a resistance and often is, or control can be an expression of the patient's fear of himself, which is most unhealthy, but our patients need to be able to use their intellectual resources and to exercise control. It is the *misuse* of these that is important. When a therapist, particularly in the early stages of therapy, teaches a devaluing of these human functions, he may in the later stages of the therapy regret that teaching, for he then finds his task complicated, as the patient's choices and values become centrally important.

There seems to be a kind of mythology of the naturally good man involved here, a mythology that is not truly humanistic. I prefer to envisage the situation as one in which there is no instinct toward either good or evil. The concept of instinct robs man of choice. I am convinced that when we are free of distortions we are able to see existence in such a way that we will make choices which are in harmony with life in general, because these become the choices that are most fulfilling to us as individuals. This is akin to the concept of enlightened self-interest but is not synonymous with that concept.

NONRATIONAL ASPECTS

We need also to recognize the less rational and more mystical aspects of the therapeutic relation. Primitive people often have a superstition that if another person knows one's true name then that other person can conjure with the name and have power over its owner. Thus such people have one or more public names they use more frequently than their true names in order to protect themselves against the magic in relationships. This is a vivid example of the fear of being truly known and of the belief that to be truly known is to put oneself in the power of another. We are accustomed to scoffing at these "superstitions" without recognizing that there is a great truth in them, a truth important to the therapeutic relationship. We ask our patients to let us truly know them, and it is avowedly so that we can help in their process of emergence. Their fear of being so truly known has deep roots in man's history. What is overlooked by the fearful patient is that in the therapeutic process he too will learn to know himself more. To be known more fully by another than by one's self is to be vulnerable to that other; but when self-knowledge equals or exceeds that of the other, the danger is appreciably lessened. Yet the therapist needs to respect his patient's fear of being known. The therapist needs also a dedication to use the knowledge he obtains about his patient in the patient's own interests and toward the goal of the patient's increased self-knowledge.

There is another side to this coin of being known by another. For the most part we, as therapists, fear to be truly known by our patients, and we name our fear "therapeutic discretion," "the blank screen," "detachment," "disengagement," and so on—all words that suggest that it is for the patient's good that we avoid being known. I question whether it is not more than this. I am not suggesting that we should be known by our patients in the same way or to the same degree that we seek to know them. I am saying that the relationship may suffer if we introduce too many distortions into the images of us that the patients gain.

Finally, let me point out that the therapist plays a unique role which is probably also tied in with the shaman in primitive ritual: the therapist is the one who names names. A great deal of social intercourse is conducted on the presupposition that we do not name candidly, we do not say always what is so. We talk of polite "white" lies, of "tact," "discretion," "good taste," and so on. All these words indicate that in everyday usage we avoid speaking completely explicitly; we are cautious about saying what we know or observe. But in the therapeutic situation one of the main things a therapist does is to lift aside this veil of polite deception and name names, say words. The therapist names the sexual body parts that are usually avoided in conversation; the therapist uses the forbidden four-letter words (Feldman, 1955); the therapist talks of hate toward parents and loved ones; the therapist points to covert discourtesies and offensivenesses between patient and therapist. We need to recognize how potent this tool of naming names can be. The therapist is the one who is seen as being unafraid to say the unsayable.

What I want to convey here is that there is a great deal of magic being practiced today by all of us: we are all firm believers in the mystical and magical. The therapist who by his forthrightness hopes to dispel mystery may only gather the charisma of a wizard by his evident unafraid handling of what is so clearly potent with tabu. We should note too that many of us as therapists have engaged in a reaction-formation against our own fear of naming names. We have made a display of our lack of fear, and thus have needlessly terrorized our patients or estranged ourselves from them by our need to demonstrate to them and to ourselves how unafraid we are to say the words (see Chapter 21).

Developing the Therapeutic Alliance

The familiar psychoanalytic concept of the therapeutic alliance with the ego of the patient is basically a useful one. I prefer not to think in terms of alliance with some subpart of the individual (the ego) but to think in terms of the alliance with the patient, himself, as a total person. This seems to me to be most veridical to the actual situation: two people engaged in a mutual endeavor to help one become more effective and fulfilled in his life experience. Those procedures of therapists that we described above as producing iatrogenic complications may contribute to a negative therapeutic alliance. Let me now speak about some of the tactics one can employ in developing a creative therapeutic alliance.

DEALING WITH SPEECH BLOCKS

When the patient finds himself resistant and unable to talk to the therapist, it is sometimes helpful to speak to him in a manner which assumes the alliance even though he is little aware of it at that point. For example, when a patient falls silent for some time, the therapist may say to him, "Does it help more if I am quiet or if I raise questions from time to time?" This inquiry assumes that therapist and patient are joined in mutual effort and are mutually confronted by the resistance, so that they can consult together as to what to do about it. Obviously there will be points at which the patient calls on the therapist to question him or talk as a way of resisting. In such an instance one may say to him "You're afraid of where your thoughts may take you and so want me to help you keep control."

PATIENT'S SELF-REACTIONS

It is frequently helpful to watch the patient's implicit response to his own ego-alien feelings and attitudes and to highlight them. Very often the patient has difficulty in recognizing what it is he experiences as he encounters his own feelings. Responses like the following are helpful in cementing the therapeutic relationship: "You're embarrassed by your sensual feelings toward me," as opposed to, "You're feeling sensually toward me." Obviously this would only be appropriate where embarrassment is evident. Another example: "It makes you uncomfortable when you can't find anything to say," instead of, "You seem to be blocked." Or to the patient who is showing a lot of anger because of his not doing well in expressing himself: "You're furious with yourself when you don't perform up to your standards."

AIDING DISCRIMINATION

These same responses can serve the useful purpose of demonstrating to the patient the ego-syntonic aspects of responses that are otherwise distortive or overreactive. This is a tremendously important kind of learning for the patient to make: to find out that his impulses to use his will, control, intellect, and so on are not subject to indiscriminate challenges but need to be modulated in a more constructive fashion. For example: "You need to be unusually careful about getting emotionally involved," when the patient is overcontrolling, or "You're fearful of where your emotions may carry you." An important consideration in these kinds of responses is to demonstrate acceptance of the patient's need for control or reasonableness but also to show how it is becoming overextended as a response to fears of himself. Again: "You're so afraid of your emotional hungers that you dare not permit them any expression" instead of "You're afraid to let go emotionally."

DISTINGUISHING BLAME FROM RESPONSIBILITY

Another way of helping the patient who is fearful of his impulses can reduce some of the neurotic guilt or self-blaming tendency without shifting that guilt and blame to some other figure. This involves pointing to the source of the pattern but emphasizing its present functioning: "You've been made to feel guilty for wanting love" instead of "Your parents made you guilty about your emotions." Similarly with the affect-blind patient, one may say "You were taught to fear your emotions so much you can't even let them come to awareness."

This last example is in some ways the epitome of the kind of response it is useful to make when dealing with resistances. Here the intent is to help the patient sense his own seeking for more actuality, his own desire to cooperate with the therapeutic process. So the therapist says things that ally him with the patient's healthy seeking and tries to avoid saying the things that ally him with the resistance. The aim is for the patient increasingly to feel, to be aware, that the resistance is a resistance to his own self-knowledge rather than to communication with the therapist.

Conclusion

The therapeutic relationship is the essential medium in which any genuine therapeutic growth will occur. It is not in itself sufficient to induce deep-seated growth, but it is a necessity that that relationship be as authentic and as creative as it can be. No amount of sophistication of technique, no degree of thoroughness of grounding in theory can substitute for a sound therapeutic relationship.

6 — *The existential meaning of the resistance*

"The whole of psychoanalytic theory is in fact built up on the perception of the resistance exerted by the patient when we try to make him conscious of his unconscious," wrote Freud (1936) in his *New Introductory Lectures on Psychoanalysis*. Yet as significant a place as Freud accords the resistance, existential-analytic theory regards this discovery as even more fundamental. The resistance shown by the patient in the therapeutic session—the ways in which he avoids awareness, displaces responsibility, maintains his alienation, and so on—is the very pattern through which the patient maintains his inauthentic relation to his life, is the very source and process of his non-being.

This is a recognition of tremendous theoretical and practical significance.[1] As was pointed out in Chapter 4, this perspective makes it evident that in psychotherapy we are engaged with the

---

[1] As with many fundamental insights, it is not possible to assign to any one person the title to this discovery. There can be little doubt that Freud was critically important in paving the way, but his own philosophic perspective militated against his full appreciation of the significance of his own discovery. Wilhelm Reich (1949) is most evidently a next link in the chain of discovery, and his appreciation for the architecture of the resistance and the process he called "character armoring" began to make explicit the bridge from a phenomenon of the analytic hour to a characteristic of the life stance. A follower of Reich, Helmut Kaiser, took the next big step by breaking rather completely with the Freudian metapsychology and focusing almost entirely on the genuineness (au-

very life processes of the patient. Although most therapeutic views do not deal with the matter explicitly, it is often assumed that therapy is concerned with a "projection into the interview" of the patient's characteristic ways of reacting—a kind of "sample" or instance but scarcely "the real thing." Such a view, of course, made it necessary to give much attention to "insight" as the explanation for how learnings in the therapeutic hour might carry over into "real life." But insight proved an inadequate principle, and many—including Freud himself—came to recognize that "insight alone is not enough." This recognition makes clear that something is amiss with the conception of the problem which the insight principle was supposed to solve. If patients improve without insight—and this we know occurs—and if other patients get insight but don't improve—which we also know to be true—then insight as a way of explaining the transfer of therapeutic gains to the out-of-therapy living is obviously inadequate.

To this situation, some have come with an alternative explanation: the patient, they explain, undergoes "a corrective emotional experience." This is a helpful concept. Usually coupled with it is an emphasis on the "growth-facilitating relationship"—that is, the benign effects of the therapist's acceptance and concern. Rogers (1959, 1961a) has especially well developed this line of reasoning. There can be little doubt that the therapeutic relationship can be tremendously significant in its influence, and the discussion in the previous chapter should make it evident that I feel attention to the relationship is extremely important. However, as I postulated in the earlier discussion, the therapeutic relation is (often) the essential medium in which therapy can occur, but it is not the therapeutic agent. We know, for instance, that therapeutic gains do not always

---

thenticity) with which the patient presents himself in the therapeutic hour. Implicit in Kaiser's thinking was the meaning that authenticity in the therapeutic session is crucially related to or isomorphic with life functioning. (I have not had an opportunity to see Kaiser's posthumous book [1964] and to ascertain to what extent he has given his views an existential or other theoretical setting. In personal contacts with Dr. Kaiser I received the impression he was far less concerned with the conceptual framework than with pragmatic treatment results.) The recognition of the existential meaning of the resistance here made explicit is implicit in the writings of May, Hora, Boss, and others.

occur when a good therapeutic relationship exists and that gains can occur in the absence of a good therapeutic relation.[2]

So we can accept the idea of the corrective emotional experience as the therapeutic agent, but we must ask, "What is it that gets corrected by this emotional experience?" Here the several theories tend to part company. Let me only say that in my view what is corrected is one's very way of being in the world. Thus I believe psychotherapy can operate on the most genotypic level. From such change we would expect, and we do see, changes flowing to attitudes, expectancies, self-and-other perceptions, and so on.

With this orientation to the importance of the resistance and its fundamental significance, we may study its nature and functioning in more detail.

EXAMPLES OF RESISTANCES

Let us start by examining some instances of patients being resistant.

> Ann talks to me in a listless voice, complaining of her supervisor at work, complaining of her landlord where she lives, complaining about the hours I make available to her.
>
> Ann is resisting, Ann is resisting even though she talks regularly, and indeed, if I say nothing, can run through the whole hour with scarcely a grunt from me.
>
> Now look at Ben. Ben has made tremendous progress from the socially borderline truck driver who came to me several years ago to the university student I talk with now. But listen to Ben, "I don't know why; everything went very well at school yesterday, but I looked at all those kids, and I felt old and useless and afraid I'd never get married. I just had a horrible fear that five years from now I'll be finishing my graduate work, and I'll still be alone, and ten years from now I'll be working, but I'll still be alone. What really gets me is this terrible fear." Ben is talking, and talking about feelings, but Ben is resisting.

---

[2] On the basis of some studies she is conducting at Mt. Sinai Hospital in Los Angeles, Hedda Bolgar reports in a personal communication that it seems the therapist's relation with the patient is less crucial than the patient's feeling that the therapist at least will be dependably "there." This, to the present author, further supports the view that the relationship is only the medium and not the agency of therapeutic change.

Charlotte resists in a different way. "You know last night all I could think about was our talk yesterday. I mean, you really helped me so much. I felt so much better after I talked to you. And I keep thinking, I wish I had you all the time. Why did I have to find you so late? I wish I'd known you sooner." Charlotte is resisting in her way.

Why do I say each of these people is resisting? Well, perhaps the reader can see it already. Ann resists, among other ways, by picturing herself constantly as an object maneuvered and manipulated by everyone else, particularly by those having any authority in relationship to her, her boss, her landlord, me. Ann resists by refusing to be a person in her own name, by fearing to take responsibility for her own life.

Ben's resistance is more subtle and difficult to convey simply through words. It is not in what Ben says that you can find his resistance. You have to hear Ben bring in this sort of dreary report week after week after week and into the months to realize that what Ben does is to cling to his fears, to insist on his fears. And yet these fears, as he tells me about them, were always just this morning, just last night. Never, when I challenge him, can he find the fear feeling right now. Ben's fear is his "security blanket," and Ben knows now that if he ever let go of being fearful and struck out for himself, then he would really find the fear—or so he is convinced. Ben said himself one time in a burst of recognition, "If I ever gave up my misery, I'd never be happy again!"

Charlotte nuzzles up to me and tries to get within my protecting embrace. Charlotte offers me adulation, appreciation. She would offer me her body gladly. She offers me everything except Charlotte, except a person to meet me. Charlotte can be coy or tearful, frightened or arrogant; but Charlotte cannot be Charlotte.

It will be apparent from my examples that when I talk about the resistance I am talking about something far broader than resistance to talking to me. It is a confusing error to think of the resistance as directed principally against the efforts of the therapist. The therapist needs to recognize that the resistance is much more significant than that. It is the way the patient formed his symptoms and meets his life. It is the manner in which the patient forestalls authenticity in his own being.

An important observation to consider in trying to understand the nature of the resistance is that the patient may talk readily and feelingfully, he may to the best of his ability fulfill Freud's impossible injunction to say "everything that comes into his mind," and yet the patient may still be resisting. This is because the resistance is in the patient's way of meeting life. It may be in the way his account is subtly warped to avoid life confrontation rather than in the telling itself. The therapist who thinks of the resistance as being directed toward himself or toward therapy, makes the same mistake that many patients do when their resistances are pointed out to them: They protest, "I'm trying to say whatever comes to mind, and you're finding fault with me!" Or they complain, "Well, you said to say whatever I thought about the way my dad acted, and now you're telling me I'm dodging responsibility!" In other words there is the easy confusion of the resistance as an existential life experience with the pattern or spontaneity of the patient's talk, two quite importantly different (though not unrelated) phenomena.

Similarly, the patient who is not talking freely, but who is experiencing great stress in trying to talk at all, may be less resistant than the open talker. Confrontation of one's self-defeating ways of being in the world may—when genuine and direct—leave one quite speechless for a time. Resistance at such a point would probably take the form of fluid talk.

Characteristics of the Resistance

Although I have given a general description of the nature of the resistance, it will be useful now to make a more thorough examination of certain aspects of particular importance in the analytic or therapeutic situation. From all that has been said thus far, it will be apparent that I believe genuine intensive or depth therapy depends upon the patient's being enabled to confront the reality of his life as directly as possible. Only through a full appreciation of the tremendous significance of the resistance is this goal possible for the therapist and his patient.

The five aspects of the resistance which we will recognize are: (a) the resistance arises as the patient's effort to cope with overwhelming threat, (b) the resistance is part of a fictitious world interposed between the patient and the real world, (c) the resistance is exposed in the patient's presentation of himself in the therapeutic situation, (d) the resistance is layered and sequential in organization, and (e) the resistance expresses the patient's courage as well as his fear.

THREAT AND THE RESISTANCE

Directly or indirectly, all resistance arises from the patient's efforts to cope with threat that seems to him to be overwhelming. *It is this threat that is resisted by the resistance.* Such threats may be real or imaginary, truly overwhelming or actually inconsequential, current or long past—to the external observer. What matters is that the person experiences the threat (phenomenologically) as real and overwhelming.

Resistance is the name given to those ways in which a person distorts his awareness to avoid becoming conscious of insupportable threat to his being. Resistance is, as Freud recognized, a barrier to the coming into consciousness of what seems intolerable. But what Freud did not recognize is that this barrier is a part of the person's whole way of being in his life and is not solely a phenomenon of the therapeutic hour. Moreover, since ultimately the awareness that the resistance bars from consciousness is an awareness of the person's actual condition in the world, the resistance reduces the actuality (authenticity, being) of the person in his life. Thus we identify the resistance as in fact the very inauthenticity (or, in an older language, the very illness) from which the person suffers and which may impel him to seek psychotherapeutic help.

THREAT

What is threat? Threat, existentially and phenomenologically, is a meaning experienced as implicit in a perceptual experience. The threatened person takes a particular meaning from some perception he is having. The particular meaning that arouses the threat experience is the potentiality of non-being for the perceiver. All threat, we are saying, ultimately is the threat of non-being, is the existential threat. To be sure, the threat may be distant or imminent, vaguely possible or highly probable, susceptible of easy change or immutable, and so on. Further, the threat may be seen as presaging total non-being of the person or simply the non-being of some relatively peripheral aspect of the self or as involving any amount of totality and of centrality. Each of these qualifications is reflected in the varying degrees of intensity of the threat experience.

Threat, I am postulating, is the meaning of potential non-being of one's own being, experienced as conveyed by a perception. Clearly the manner in which I define myself will have much to do with what will and will not threaten me. Thus, if I am earnestly identified with the Democratic party, a success of the Republicans will be threatening. If I believe myself an intellectual, the noisy shouts of the "anti-eggheads" are threatening, and so on.[3]

ANXIETY

Threat is a meaning attributed to a perception. Anxiety is a subjective experience accompanying that meaning which is the threat. Anxiety is an emotional state.

We distinguish existential from neurotic anxiety in several ways. Existential anxiety is anxiety that arises in response to perceptions of the ultimate givenness of the human condition and the threats of non-being implicit in those givens. Neurotic anxiety is always resolvable ultimately to existential anxiety. Neurotic anxiety comes about as defenses against existential anxiety fail and new distortions of awareness of the human condition are employed to ward off the existential anxiety.

Whether the anxiety is existential or neurotic, when the patient finds these feelings flooding his experience, he is impelled to defend against them. He may be able to meet the threatening situation in such a way as to reduce his experience of anxiety while maintaining authenticity. In this instance, no resistance would be engendered. On the other hand, he may feel unable to contend with the threat sufficiently to reduce his anxiety to tolerable proportions. He may then begin to distort the actuality of the threatening object or his own authenticity so that the perception of threat is modified and

---

[3] It is the confused appreciation of this fact that leads to the "cool" philosophy. A certain segment of the population, appreciating in a vague way that one can be "reached" (touched emotionally, threatened) by whatever one invests in emotionally, preaches and tries to practice the quasi-religion of "cool," of uninvolvement, of detachment. To the converts to this faith, a short-cut Nirvana is to be had by a kind of schizoid denial of concern. Of course, all this primitive Stoicism achieves is a

the anxiety is reduced. This process of distortion is the root and substance of the resistance.

A Case Example. Let me illustrate this process in a highly oversimplified segment of an actual person's experience.

> When Larry was small, his father, a police captain, seemed the center of the world and clearly the most important and influential person around. Larry found he could get away with things with adults and children alike when they knew whose son he was. Larry confidently planned some day to be the captain of police too. Later, as his world expanded, Larry's dream grew also and the goal became that of captaining a larger force than his father led. Through all of this, Larry was consistently using his father's position and his own vocational aspiration as a way of being different, of avoiding full responsibility for his own actions, and as a reassurance against his failures and shortcomings. When Larry didn't grow into the strapping man his father had been (although a younger brother did), when he found he had little success in positions of leadership he managed to attain, Larry went through a very confused and anxious period. He emerged from it to go to college with the goal of becoming either a psychologist or a personnel man and with a firm conviction that he had an unusual ability to size up others quickly and very accurately.

In schematic sequence we can think of Larry's experience as follows. Encountering the risks of contingency and the weight of responsibility, Larry was not ready to accept these directly. (One part of his story that we did not have time for has to do with the family emphasis on success in visible terms and the family censure of weakness or failure.) Finding himself smaller, he displaced some of his identity onto the tie to his powerful father. Probably this worked well with his encounters outside the family but less well at

---

sense of heightened meaninglessness to one's life, an uneasy guiltiness about whatever healthy emotions remain, and a head start on a truly schizophrenic withdrawal. What the "cool cat" fails to recognize is that one finds his being not by flight but by aware and courageous involvement. Some are able to move through involvement to a further participation in life that seems to the adherents of the cool philosophy like what they practice but is in fact its complete antithesis. This "cool" philosophy is discussed further in Chapter 22.

home. There he began to re-experience anxiety as the protection of the identification with his father proved insufficient. Thus he erected a second level of resistance to his anxiety: his own plan to be a police captain. With this he could handle in-family threats because someday he would be the dominant one. But then this plan was defeated by both his physique and temperament. The resurgence of anxiety was quite marked in high school and seems only to have been bound up when Larry emerged with a new resistance, his new vocational goal and self-image.

The sequence may have been something like the following.

Existential anxiety:	awareness of being finite in a contingent world
Resistance level one:	identification with father
First neurotic anxiety:	at home others also so identified
Resistance level two:	plan to become a police captain
Second neurotic anxiety:	not big enough or a good leader
Resistance level three:	natural judge of men

It should be evident that I am not describing a conscious process. The small boy did not appraise the world as contingent and himself as finite and make a conscious decision to identify with his father as a way of avoiding this existential anxiety. What did happen was that Larry found he could not make things happen the way he wanted them to but that his father seemed able to do so. It felt good to be close to the big, powerful man, to be swept up onto his shoulder, from which point he could look down on his mother, the furniture, and so much else that normally loomed over him. It was frightening and lonely when his father was away or ignored him and he was left to himself. But that fright could be made less when he wore his father's spare uniform cap or his big shoes, for then Larry would remember the smell and feel and strength and power of his father. So, unwittingly, he came to meet the frightening times of loneliness by changing his awareness of himself from Larry-the-little-boy-alone to Larry-the-captain's-son.

It needs to be clear also that the child's identification with his father, as well as his vocational goals and any other specifics of his life, are not the resistances themselves. These same identifications and goals may be used in a creative way to increase authenticity. It is the *use* made of these percepts, the distortions of the reality of experience, the warding off of uncomfortable awareness, that constitutes the resistance.

The foregoing sequence portrays the "direct" causal pattern from which the resistance arises. However, some aspects of the resistance are importantly rooted in learnings from the culture at large and from particular significant figures in the person's developmental years. Thus the child who is taught to put "what the neighbors will think" ahead of authenticity-in-being is taught a resistance and incorporates it indirectly (Bugental, 1962d).

World as the Construction of Awareness

We are so accustomed to maintaining an external, objective perspective in looking at ourselves and others that the phenomenological orientation often seems surprising or even an illustration of the perverseness of human nature. We find ourselves intrigued by the strangeness that people behave in a phenomenological rather than a behavioral or "actual" world. "Actuality" we think we know to be the external world. In point of fact, the reverse is more congruent with the human experience: that is actual which is the direct material of awareness, which is immediately experienced; while that which must be inferred must await verification by other awarenesses.[4] Perhaps another way to make this point is to call attention again to the fact that the basic human experience is the experience of awareness. Only through awareness is there knowledge of world, of self, of other people. Once the primacy of this recognition is fully appreciated, there can be little surprise that it is in this realm of awareness—the phenomenological world—that behavior is determined. The so-called objective world is always an inferred world, is always a secondary world, and obviously is always known incompletely and in some measure inaccurately.

What is "world"? As I experience world, it is made up of people, things, places, relationships, values, distances, activities, feelings, ideas, and much else. Some of these parts of world have

---
[4] The point is sometimes overlooked by the over-zealous "objective" scientist that there is no route to world or to knowledge of world except through human awareness. Even electronic instruments and statistics are but ways of impressing the awarenesses of certain human beings.

attributes such as color, weight, mass, smell, and taste. Others are true, interesting, important, frightening, ugly, and many other things. I know that some aspects represent things that I should do or should not do, that other people will agree or disagree with me about, that have always been so or are but recently discovered, that have much to do with me or little. But, if I only reflect, I must recognize that the overriding fact is that all exist for me solely through my awareness.

We are accustomed to making the assumption that world is a shared awareness of all normal people. Such is not the case. World is a construction of each person in his relation to life. That there is much overlap between my world and yours is not denied, but this is far different from saying that they are identical. It is impossible to write general descriptions of world just as it is impossible to write general translations of dream symbols, and for the same reason.[5]

The essential point for the therapist is that he must open himself to learn the world of his patient rather than assuming that they share world. In its way this is not an unfamiliar point; what is important is the recognition that the resistance plays an important part in structuring the world each of us experiences, and changes the experience of world from the creative product of person–life intercourse to a by-product of a person evading life.

Although I have said that world is the always new creation of each person, I have not said that each world is totally idiosyncratic, nor that communication between worlds is impossible, nor yet that nothing is shared between worlds. The work of analysis itself depends on the realization that two people physically in the same place, ostensibly open to the same stream of communication, both intending the greater understanding of the world of awareness of one, will share much. It is the breakdown of this sharing, the breakdown that comes about because the two perceived worlds do not coincide because the patient is bringing in his characteristic distortions of world (his resistances), that makes possible the work

---

[5] The paradox is, of course, represented by the fact that the very sentence which says it is impossible to write generalizations is itself a written generalization. Yet we must recognize that this sentence is a statement of my world which I hope will mean something similar in your world. In the same fashion, general trends in the meanings of dream symbols are familiar.

of analysis. It will be apparent at once that an intensive personal therapeutic experience thus becomes an essential part of the preparation of the therapist. This is not in the naive hope that the therapist will thus be relieved of all distortions or resistances. It is because there will be a lessening of the number and pervasiveness of his resistances and because he will have a deeper appreciation of the relativism of all awareness.

Larry, in our example above, came dangerously close to seeing his world in terms of "might makes right." Deriving from his intolerable feeling of powerlessness, he became polarized, as it were, in terms of power. In the therapeutic hour his accounts of people and situations were always implicitly or explicitly with reference to power relationships. He admired this friend because of the way he used his power for good, and he feared the increasing power of certain minority elements of the society. He seldom used the word directly, perhaps partly because it was so ubiquitous in his thinking. Money, position, relationships, and ideas were chiefly assessed in terms of their power potentials. His own efforts to grow were, of course, to grow in power: through education, through making the right contacts, through being an attractive person, and so on and on.

Yet Larry would have been very surprised to read the preceding paragraph as descriptive of himself and probably would have angrily denied it. One of his important lines of resistance was to deny the significance of power in his own life. Of all the reasons for this denial, the need to avoid confronting his basic feeling of powerlessness was one of the most important.

Larry's way of implicitly eyeing his world through the filter of power significances represents what I think Hora (1962c) means when he speaks of the "assumptions" and "inventions" that create a fictitious world in which one "conducts" his life. These assumptions are, in our present language, major resistance patterns that forestall one's authentic being in the world. Subsidiary to these major patterns are the resistance layers that are more immediately evident in the therapeutic hour. These layers, in turn, are compounded of the multitude of specific resistances, which take the form of distorted percepts, of emotional reactions, of specific denials or displacements (and all the array of "defense mechanisms" so well disclosed by psychoanalysis).

THE FICTITIOUS WORLD

Hora, who writes with unusual clarity about existential psychotherapy, puts this matter in terms slightly different from those I have been using, but does so with evident similar meaning (1962c).

> For everyday life proceeds largely in the realm of inventions; that is, everyday life is not really lived but "conducted" along routine, preconceived lines and assumptions of what "should be" and what "should not be." Mental assumptions tend to become more important than reality, and human consciousness tends to be hampered by them in its cognitive function. The process of dis-covering the authentic being consists of uncovering, *dispelling the "inventions"* which mask and cover the truth of what really is. (Emphasis Hora's.)

We have been using the general term "the resistance" to subsume what Hora calls "inventions" and "assumptions." His language has the advantage of making more evident that the resistance results in the patient being entangled in an unreal world and that this "realm of inventions" is that of much of everyday life. Implicit in this recognition is the meaning that society inevitably compounds the distortions of perception which are the very stuff of the resistance. In this way the person comes to experience additional, nonexistential threats (the "shoulds" and "should nots," Hora; Horney, 1950). The process of resistance-elaboration is thus accelerated and made more complex.

EXPOSURE OF THE RESISTANCE IN THE THERAPEUTIC SESSION

The resistance is the barrier against overwhelming threat that the person raises because he feels he cannot sustain the anxiety with which he is flooded. The resistance is displayed in the therapeutic session because the patient carries his resistance into all his life. He cannot step out of his resistance any more than he can step out of his world, for the resistance is the way he is in his world. These recognitions make it extremely evident that psychotherapy is not to be likened to a laboratory in which we simulate the "real life" situation in order to discover its principles for later applications. Nor is psychotherapy similar to a classroom in which learning is sought for subsequent, extramural employment. Psychotherapy is more like a surgery or a garage in which the work proceeds directly on the functioning organism and the corrective efforts are immediate to the disruptive influences. But even this parallel is inadequate, for in the surgery (at least as it is presently conducted) and in the garage the conscious participation of the organism worked upon is not needed and may even be considered (in the former!) a distraction (many surgeons would be happier if their surgery patients were more like automobiles in a garage). In psychotherapy, the conscious participation of the patient is not only needed, it is the one truly essential element.

Perhaps our best parallel is—as so often—the work of exploration on a new frontier. One may study maps at home endlessly without adding much information to the white places. Only actual exploration in person will tell what lies in a mountain fastness, how that desert is to be crossed, where the animal trails are in this forest. Of course, one can make informed guesses from aerial photographs, from previous experiences with other, similar terrains, but only direct encounter with the unknown can make it known.

The therapeutic session is, then, an opportunity for the patient to make a direct encounter with that which is unknown in himself and his world. In this exploration, the psychotherapist may serve as an experienced guide who has been into other somewhat similar unexplored regions, but he must not make the mistake of thinking that he thereby knows the present terrain.

Since the actual process of exploration is to be dealt with in much more detail in later pages, which describe the analysis of the resistance and the transference, I will not elaborate here further on the significance of the display of the resistance in the therapeutic hour.

"Layered" Sequence of the Resistance

Wilhelm Reich (1949) nowhere better demonstrated his genius than in his discerning appreciation of the clinical nature of the resistance. Although he predates our current concern with existentialism, he helped to pave the way for it. He has most effectively shown the layering of the resistances that constitutes the character structure and that like so much scar tissue prevents the patient from vivid engagement in his own life. Reich's observations constitute an empirical demonstration of the futility of the effort to protect one's self by distorting awareness. As we saw in the case of Larry, the distortions which first are interposed to ward off the dread contingencies so disrupt the person's aware being in the world that new (now neurotic) anxiety is engendered. Accordingly, further distortions are required to overlay the earlier effort, but then these too prove inadequate and must in turn be covered over. The result when we see the patient therapeutically is that we must "peel the onion" sequentially, must help the patient recognize and relinquish layer after layer of "assumptions" (Hora) to help him work toward living in new innocence.

COURAGE AND THE RESISTANCE

Although we have needed to attend particularly to the disruptive and distortive nature of the resistance, we must keep mindful of the more creative aspect also implicit in it. Confronted with what seemed overwhelming threat, the patient fought for his survival through the creative use of his potentiality. No resistance is a pure fabrication. Every resistance is a compromise with the givenness of experience, in which the patient has sought to preserve as much as he could of what was authentic in himself and his experience.

This perspective is essential in the existential-analytic orientation, for we seek to support the patient's seeking for authenticity even as we help him to resolve his resistances.

SUMMARY: AUTHENTICITY AND INAUTHENTICITY

The resistance, I have been saying, is the process that works against the patient's being authentic in his life. Let us return now to the matter of authenticity itself. By authenticity, I mean a central genuineness and awareness of being. Authenticity is that presence of an individual in his living in which he is fully aware in the present moment, in the present situation. Authenticity is difficult to convey in words, but experientially it is readily perceived in ourselves or in others.

In Chapter 3 I proposed that authenticity has three functional characteristics:

1. The authentic person is broadly aware of himself, his relationships, and his world in all dimensions.
2. The authentic person accepts and seems to go to meet the fact that he is constantly in the process of making choices, that decisions are the very stuff of living.
3. The authentic person takes responsibility for his decisions, including full recognition of their consequences. It is here that the terrible threat of authenticity resides.

In Chapter 2, when I described "man's thrown plight," it was evident that one can never truly know enough to make completely "safe" choices. Therein lies the potentiality of tragedy. When we face the fact that we are constantly in the process of making decisions and that inevitably we cannot know enough to guarantee the outcomes of those decisions, then we are in existential anxiety. Such anxiety we call natural; nevertheless, it can become too heavy. When the contingencies work out so that our choices have tragic consequences, we may find the load of this responsibility more than we can bear. Thus we begin to distort our reality. Then we begin to deny responsibility, to negate the fact that we have made the decisions. Then we begin to yield up our authenticity.

To Summarize. Resistance is the name that we give to the general defensive wall the patient puts between himself and the threats that he finds linked to being authentic. Resistance is antiauthenticity.

"THE TRANSFERENCE"

Now I need to say a word about the transference in relation to the resistance. The term, "transference," is used so loosely and in so many ways that I want to specify how I will be using it. By transference I will mean the patient's unconscious attempt to reestablish with the therapist a symbiotic relationship the patient earlier had with some other person important in his life. This definition will be expanded in Chapter 8, in which I will particularly deal with transference analysis. For our purposes here it is sufficient to recognize that the transference is a special form of the resistance; that is, the patient has learned to involve others in symbiotic relations which seemed to offer protection from contingency and which, as always, led to new anxieties and thus new symptom (resistance) formations.

7 — The analysis of the resistance

The resistance, as we have now come to realize, is the key to the manner in which a person meets the givens of his life. Compounded as it is of that which is his effort to preserve his being from the threat of non-being and that which is the very thief of his actuality, the resistance is the expression at once of the person's anxiety and of his courage. It is to this vital fulcrum upon which the patient's life is balanced that the therapist will direct his primary attention.

In this chapter I want to describe what I ask, implicitly or explicitly, that my patients attempt to do in the therapeutic hour and what it is that I am attempting to do concurrently. I hope in this description to make evident the procedure that currently seems to me most productive in displaying and analyzing the resistances and in thus making it possible for the patient to resolve them.

When a patient begins work I let him talk in whatever way is most spontaneous with him. For some this means a recital of symptoms and complaints, for others this means a narration of life circumstances and history, but there are always some who have great difficulty in doing what they think I want them to do or what they imagine they should do.

>Several years ago I began the treatment of Don, a third-year graduate student in clinical psychology from one of our local universities. He had great difficulty during the two intake interviews in telling me very much about himself and tended frequently to be reduced to silence and covert misery by the oppressive guilt and fear he experienced. From some things he

said, I reasoned that he had certain guilty confessions he felt a need to make. These so pressed on him for expression that he could not let himself talk because also he had in mind a kind of model of therapeutic talk which he felt compelled to achieve. What I mean is this: he had read sufficiently about analytic practice to think that he should "free associate"—say everything that came to mind. At the same time, his guilty thoughts were so frightening to him that he couldn't express them. Still, his need to perform well, to free associate well, insisted that he say the guilty things if he said anything at all. The resulting impasse could only be handled by silence and misery. Accordingly, I began asking him simple questions that had the effect of setting aside the injunction to say everything that came to mind, and in this way he could talk to me. As he gained more relief, I was able gradually to broaden the focus of my questions so that he could talk more easily and could tolerate making some selection of subject matter himself.

Now, in a nutshell, this was a picture of Don's resistance, indeed of his neurosis and life stance. A third-year graduate student and one who has done exceptionally well in his graduate studies, he was a person who needed approval, who needed to perform excellently. He was skillful in finding out what the rules of the game were and then performing according to those rules. So he knew that the rules were to free associate, to say anything that came to mind. But he was also very guilty about his masturbation, his sexual adventures with his girl friend, his hostile thoughts toward his parents, and probably other things too. This guilt pressed on him, indeed was part of what brought him to therapy. To be authentic he would need to take responsibility for all the "bad things," but the value system with which he was inculcated meant that admitting to masturbation, for example, was admitting to having done poorly, was admitting to being less than an "A student" in life.

Don came to me because he was fearful and miserable. To be authentic he ought to have told me of his fear and misery, of his sex experiences, and of his disloyal thoughts toward his parents; but in order to tell me authentically about these he would have had to take responsibility for them. This he could not do; for that, in his eyes, was the mark of failure. To be authentic he would have to say, "I have failed," but this breaks down his whole resistance façade of doing well. So Don was caught in a double bind and could not talk to me. My questions served to grant him permission to set aside the injunction to say everything that came to mind. In his responding to my questions the transference was revealed, since in one sense the highest imperative ought to have been his own need and his own sense of what would help him. Instead, the transference made my authority override his need, and so he could respond to me.[1]

What do we know about Don? Just from this much, we know that he was fearful of himself and guilty about himself, that he handled his fear and guilt by trying to meet external criteria of performance and appear excellent, and that he felt the reverse. He resisted the pain of not being what he felt he should be by denying his own responsibilities and choice and thus by reducing his awareness. We know that he used relations to others as ways of forestalling his own choice-responsibility. We know that he was at a juncture where these contrary forces were nearly equal, and he had no way of resolving them. It is no surprise, then, to learn he guiltily, frightenedly, harbored strong, suicidal thoughts.

What the Patient Is Asked to Do

At some point many patients will ask me, what ought they to be doing during the therapeutic hour, what do I want them to talk about? On occasion I will point out the dependency involved, but many times I will accept this as a valid question in which they ask guidance because I do have specialized knowledge and resources to help them. Usually I will answer in somewhat the following fashion.

> Tell me what is of concern to you, what matters to you in your life today, right now as you lie here. What is it that you want to think through? What is it in your living that you want to make different? As you talk to me about your concern let yourself be open to mention any other awarenesses that come in whether or not they seem pertinent to what we are talking about. Sometimes these other awarenesses will be memories, sometimes physical sensations, sometimes emotions.

---

[1] As an aside, we may note that there is also an "ought" which says that I am a knowledgeable person, and therefore he ought to cooperate with me because I was trying to help him. Unfortunately, I don't think that "ought" governed his behavior, but rather it was the transference "should."

Whatever they may be, let yourself mention them and then continue with what you were telling me about, or follow whatever you find is of concern to you at that point. Talk to me about what concerns you in your life.

When the patients mention "free association," as many do, I let them tell me what they think it means and encourage them to try it if they wish to. Some of my patients feel that they always free associate, others feel that they do it on occasion. I am not concerned with terminology so long as the patient is able persistently to try to tell both of us of his concerns in his life.

My intent in this kind of guideline is to treat the patient as a whole person in the midst of his living, trying to order his life in a constructive fashion. My intent is to call upon him to be aware and responsible.

Listening to the Patient

It is difficult to characterize what it is I try to do as a psychotherapist during the session with my patient. In one sense it seems to me that most descriptions of therapeutic work ignore the essential point or imply it only indirectly. The difficulty of adequately phrasing the functioning of the therapist is very real and a part of our limited glossary of terms for authentic human relating. Perhaps existential language gives us a good opportunity to attempt a new description of the therapist's role.[2]

AUTHENTICITY AS THE KEY TO THERAPEUTIC ATTENTION

Carl Rogers (1961a) has rightly emphasized the importance of "congruence" as a condition in the therapist essential to his contribution to succcessful therapy and as a goal condition for the patient. He describes his concept of congruence in the following way.

---

[2] It is to be recognized in this section that I am very particularly describing my own experience and that others may find the subjective aspects of the therapeutic process to be different. Nevertheless, I believe there is a certain common core in what many, though by no means all, experienced therapists do; this is what I am trying to characterize.

By this congruence we mean that the feelings the therapist is experiencing are available to him, available to his awareness, and he is able to live these feelings, be them, and able to communicate them if appropriate. No one fully achieves this condition, yet the more the therapist is able to listen acceptingly to what is going on within himself and the more he is able to be the complexity of his feelings, without fear, the higher degree of his congruence (p. 61).

From my perspective, I am in agreement with all aspects of this statement. There may be some difference in operational implementation of this concept when it comes to deciding when and how the therapist will express his own feelings in actual interventions with the patient. However, I want to make it very clear that this agreement with Roger's postulation is no mere casual thing; that the genuineness or congruence he prescribes as desirable in the therapist is seen as equally essential in the present orientation.

I do not find the term "congruence" a fully satisfying one. Congruence describes the interrelations of aspects of a person and their harmony. However, it seems to me too limited in perspective. It is my feeling that congruence is a part of existential authenticity, that the person who is genuinely authentic in his being-in-the-world is congruent within himself; and to the extent that one attains authentic being in his life, to that extent is he congruent. I prefer the broader conception and term because it seems to me to facilitate understanding of the therapeutic impact, the growth-facilitating potential of the condition to which Rogers points by the term congruence and to which I am pointing with the term authenticity.

AUTHENTIC PRESENCE

In listening to the patient I want to be authentically present in the situation with him, regarding this as a central here-and-now experience of my life, and becoming jealously aware of any intrusions on my presence. When I achieve a measure of such authenticity, and only to the extent that I do achieve it, I am ready to attend to the patient. This seemingly very manifest point needs emphasis since in actual practice I think it is very often overlooked. The therapist is prone to assume his own authenticity and attend only to inauthenticities in his patient. I have found increasingly that self-awareness reveals to me many ways in which I am not authentically in contact with my patient or authentically in myself in the therapeutic hour. (This matter of the authenticity in the therapist received some attention in the examination of the therapeutic relationship in Chapter 5, and will be inquired into further in Chapter 21, where we consider the person who is the therapist.) Just as any conscientious craftsman looks to the maintenance and improvement of his tools, so the psychotherapist will seek constant growth in his own authenticity, knowing that in this way he realizes more of his own potential even as he becomes more what his patients need him to be.

THERAPIST'S "SET" AS PATIENT TALKS

The therapist is most apt to be able to function effectively if he listens to his patient with a paradoxical combination of attitudes. On the one side he will seek to attend to the patient *in toto*. This means that he will listen to what the patient says and how he says it, watching how he lies on the couch and how he gesticulates. This means that he will give attention to pauses and to what is not said as well as to what is said. And yet all of this is not in an effortful way. The therapist can defeat himself by a kind of forced concentration as opposed to an open attentiveness (Hora, 1962c).

Psychologists who are experienced in psychodiagnostics are familiar with a difference between "attention" and "concentration" that is important in the therapist's set. When someone is given a series of digits orally and told to repeat them after one hearing, it is usually the case that the person who is relaxed and not effortful does better than the one who struggles to enforce the numbers on his memory. (This is the same difference Rappaport *et al.*, describe between performances on memory for digits and arithmetic; 1945, p. 179.)

The difficulty in conceiving and expressing the therapist's approach here is that it so easily can be misinterpreted as a kind of concentration, alert figuring out, or astute use of knowledge, training, and skill in a self-aware process similar, for example, to that most of us use in solving a problem in algebra. This is most definitely not what is intended. The kind of concentration and figuring involved in solving mathematical problems is antithetical to the subjective state desirable for the therapist.

The therapist needs to adopt an openness of listening that has been variously characterized as "passive receptivity," "free-floating attention," "wakeful awareness," and so on. The characterization of this attitude or set of the therapist's attention is difficult when we try to state it affirmatively. It can be somewhat better indicated by saying what is not the kind of attending here being described. It is not concentrating, nor yet is it idle wandering of one's thoughts; it is not figuring things out, nor yet sleeping or dozing; it is not listening to meaning alone, nor yet listening in terms of some mixed set of ideas.

Again attempting to state it positively, effective therapeutic attention involves open, aware availability to all that the patient presents through any modality of his being in the therapeutic hour and concurrently to all that is arising within the therapist himself during that time. Such attention is difficult, tiring, exciting, risky, demanding, fulfilling, and essential to genuine depth therapy. It is the basis of that much maligned term, intuition.

Subjective Awareness. Now we have pointed out, too, that on the other side the therapist will be attempting to be aware within himself, aware of the kinds of imagery he has, of the moods induced in him, of the fantasies that may form, of his own physical comforts and discomforts. Let us be clear, this is not a subscription to the belief, which some enunciate, that the therapist is a passive tablet upon which the patients write, and that therefore the therapist can read everything "written upon himself" as coming from the patient. This is not so for me, and I doubt that it is so for anyone. On the other hand, to the extent that the therapist can be open and aware within himself and equally aware of his patient, he can form impressions of what it is the patient is evoking in relation to the on-going business within the therapist himself. This is much less precise than one might ideally desire, but it is much more authentic, more human.

When I am most able to attend to my patient in the way that is creative, I listen to him and experience his total presentation of himself in a fashion which subjectively gives me the experience of participation with him in his telling of himself. Then it is almost as though I can feel his words flowing from my own awareness concurrently as I hear them from him. From time to time my immersion in this stream of his talk and all that goes with it will be intruded upon by awarenesses from within myself which may either be disruptions due to my inauthenticity (incongruity) or may be my sensing of the patient's incongruity or inauthenticity. This is not an intellective or rational or deductive matching of what the patient is presenting with what I deem to be the reality. It is a wholistic response of my subjective awareness to the experience of being immersed in the patient's presentation of himself.

If the foregoing description sounds mystical or vague, it is because our categories for examining subjective life are poorly developed in the "scientific" glossary, and are better developed in the literary and philosophic or metaphysical areas. What is intended in what I have said is by no means a mystical or other extraworldly experience; rather, what I think happens is that one's awareness can be brought into a measure of attention so that incongruities emerge (like discords in music) in the total presentational pattern of what the patient is saying. Needless to say, this is only possible if the therapist is as congruent or authentic as possible and if he is free of striving and distractions that would contaminate his reception of what the patient presents.

The Need to "Cure." Several writers (for example, Menninger, 1958) have warned against the need or urgency to cure. One place where this guidance is most pertinent is in relation to the attention to the patient. Such striving clearly disrupts the ability freely and openly to attend to and intuit about what is experienced. The therapist who is encumbered with too strong a need to "cure" often is the therapist with marked doubts about his own competence or about his vocation. The openness of attention and readiness to know his patient in depth essential to the therapist is disrupted by an urgency to produce reassuring changes. To be sure, we are not unconcerned that our patient benefits from his work with us, but if we are wise we know that only the patient can meaningfully alter his own life and that we serve him best if we remain steady in our task of understanding him and aiding his awareness.

THE "DOMINANT EMOTIONAL THEME"

Leon Saul (1958), in a valuable book on the technique of psychoanalysis, speaks of the "red thread" (p. 96) for which the therapist must wait and around which he must organize his interpretative efforts. His concept is a productive one, but I want to adapt it to our present purpose and so will retitle it.

The *dominant emotional theme* may be likened to a composer's use of a musical theme in a symphony. He may develop it in various ways: at times dropping it out of the score and then reintroducing it, changing its key, even changing its tempo, but returning to the basic theme again and again. In a patient's talk, if it is not interfered with too much by the therapist, a dominant emotional theme may usually be discerned. I employ the operating hypothesis that each segment of patient talk, whether an entire interview, a portion of an interview, or even several interviews, will have a dominant emotional theme to which the patient's associations are all related in some way. This is not to say that the content is unimportant. One needs to be aware of content. But it is to say that the process and the implicit emotional themes are the core around which the therapist's interventions need to be organized. Interventions, especially if they be interpretations, that are offered apart from this dominant emotional theme are most apt to be rejected, dealt with superficially, or accepted only rationally. Interventions designed to make the dominant emotional theme both conscious and explicit are in most instances essential to other therapist activity.

AN EXAMPLE

The patient is Greta who is well along in her therapeutic course. Today she is telling me about her school, where she is a graduate student. She tells me first how a particular professor seems to take delight in calling on her with challenging and difficult questions. In the past, she says, she would have been terrified by this, but now, as a result of her therapy, she rather enjoys it and meets the challenge. This leads to some thoughts of performing well in a competitive way with her brother when she was a child and the approval she won from her father. Then she tells, with obvious distress, of a sexual fantasy which she links to her father or her brother. She is weeping and struggling to get this fantasy out. Several times she starts to use overgeneralized language such as I have in the past pointed out as a resistance to describing embarrassing material genuinely. Today without my bidding she is explicit; though it is clear how frightening and painful she finds it to be so specific and detailed.

Now, what is happening here? An experienced patient is following her associations in a productive fashion. She is not concerned, as she once was, to understand every connection between her thoughts; she can allow herself to report embarrassing material; and she can determinedly report it in detail despite her discomfort. But what is the dominant emotional theme? The dominant emotional theme in this passage I believe to be, "I am doing so well in therapy." She sounds this theme first with the account of her response to the challenging questions of her professor, in which she gives explicit recognition to therapy's contribution. Next, she plays a variant on the theme by linking doing well with sibling rivalry. And finally, she brings it into the therapeutic hour by her suffering candor as she enacts her theme once more. Now, knowing no more than what I have said so far, we cannot tell why this theme is being sounded and played with these variations. It is probably too soon to interpret even this much, but we can say something that will help to prepare the way for interpretation.

> T: You seem determined not to permit yourself any evasiveness in telling me about this sexual fantasy.
> P: Well, I'm just sick and tired of the way I've dodged, and I want to face up to things now.
> T: You don't want to allow yourself the detours you once needed.
> P: That's right. I'm through being so cowardly and frightened. My sexual feelings are perfectly natural, and there's no reason to hide them.

At this point we let Greta proceed with her thoughts, and we know several things of importance. She is trying very hard to do well, and this need to do well is so strong at this point that she has split herself into a taskmaster and a slave. The challenging questions of her professor are nothing compared to the demands she is placing on herself now to perform well here. The dominant emotional theme having been recognized in each of the associations, we are able to use it as an access to the patient's associations without disrupting them, and with a kind of focusing. I will not try to synopsize more of the interview with Greta. What comes out, as may have been anticipated, is that she feels guilty because of sexual thoughts toward me, and the resistance is taking the transference pattern of trying to control what will happen in our relationship by splitting herself and demanding excellence of performance. Certainly I am not going to try to interpret all this to Greta at this point, nor would I now interpret the further significance that this is a re-enactment of the pattern that she used as a child in vanquishing her brother for her father's affections and in keeping the relationship one in which she could be sure of doing well.

THE DOMINANT EMOTIONAL THEME AND THE RESISTANCE

It is important to recognize that the dominant emotional theme is not synonymous with the resistance. In Greta's case it is at once true that she is doing well in therapy and that the excessive need to do well is part of her resistance. We were led to understand the resistance by becoming aware of the dominant emotional theme. The theme is an expression of the patient's being-in-the-world at the moment he is talking. As such, it will often have both authentic and resistive components, or it will thread through both in the patient's experiencing and portrayal of himself.

INTERPRETATIVE SEQUENCE

The therapist does well to avoid confusing the theme and the resistance, for to do so is to reap but a portion of the benefit awareness of the theme makes available. Interpretations that reflect back to the patient only the resistive aspect of the theme soon are experienced by the patient as "nagging" and disruptive. The patient is unconsciously seeking to express his seeking for authenticity also. The more effective use of the therapist's awareness of the dominant emotional theme will be that of helping the patient first become aware of that which he is trying to *express* (with Greta: "You feel more aware of how well you are progressing in therapy today," for example), then aiding his discovery of his own *response* to this theme ("You're very determined to continue to do well, aren't you?"), and then displaying the *distortive aspect* of that response ("You're trying so urgently that you seem to have no patience with your hurt or frightened feelings.").

In the examples cited we are assuming that the interaction flows along smoothly between therapist and patient. It is important that the therapist be sensitive to signs of disruption in the patient's stream of awareness and talk which might arise from the patient encountering threat, the therapist misperceiving the dominant emotional theme, or other influences. Forcing through to all three phases of using the theme vitiates the worth of the effort. It should also be noted that many times sensitive reflection by the therapist of the theme may aid the patient in taking one or both of the next two steps himself. Needless to say this is a desirable result.

The Therapist's Interventions

The phrasing of interventions is very much an area in which individual style and personal authenticity are essential. It is plain that the attempt to develop a standard pattern of intervention would be antithetical to the orientation to presence and mutual encounter which we deem fundamental to existential-analytic psychotherapy. In this section no such attempt will be made. Rather I will describe guidelines that seem to be consonant with our general approach. First I will consider the values of the therapist being sparing in his talk, then I will suggest a model for selecting points at which to intervene. Next I will offer several considerations to guide the content and phrasing of interventions, and finally describe some of the more typical defects in interventions.

THERAPIST SILENCE: A USEFUL POINT OF DEPARTURE

From what has been said it should be evident that the therapist is well advised to avoid talking a great deal in the therapeutic hour. There are many exceptions to this. At certain points he may talk a lot and may even talk more than the patient does, but over-all one can speculate in favor of a ratio of at least 19 to 1.

What this means in actual practice for me is that at the time I introduce the patient to the couch, usually around the fifth to tenth interview, I make it evident that I will not be engaging in a usual conversational exchange with him. Sometimes this comes about implicitly and requires no structuring; sometimes I say something like, "As you talk to me, I will generally not reply directly. I want to be free to listen to the 'music' as well as the 'words' of what you are saying, and I want to encourage you to inquire into your concerns in your own way." Many patients require no more explanation than this. Some need to test out the relationship by trying to involve me in usual conversational gambits, and they can often be shown the resistance involved. A few are frightened at first by the feeling of being abandoned, and I may give brief verbal responses for a time to help them meet the fear sufficiently to prepare to confront its meanings (often linked through parental threat of abandonment to the existential anxiety of isolation).

With many individual variations, then, the usual pattern of the therapeutic hour is the brief greeting as we meet, perhaps a quick comment on the weather or some other superficiality,[3] and then the patient takes the couch and begins talking where he deems appropriate and without my intervention. From time to time I may comment or question, but for the most part I am silent.

There are several reasons for this recommendation:

1. Usually the therapist can keep from contaminating the patient's perceptions best by maintaining silence (Robinson, 1950, pp. 101–105). The silence itself may be a contaminant in some cases at some times, but it tends to be more constant than almost any other kind of participation.

2. The therapist will find it advantageous not to be a participant in a usual conversational exchange with the patient. Anyone who comes for therapy has had years of developing conversational skills that are heavily colored with his resistances and transferences, with his inauthenticity. He is as much a prisoner of them as unconsciously he seeks to make the therapist. One reason for encouraging the use of the couch, as pointed out in Chapter 4, is that it tends to offset these usual conversational skills. There is a real value in having the situation somewhat unique in the patient's experience, particularly in the early stages.

3. The therapist ought not carry the responsibility of having to respond to the patient regularly. Rather, the therapist will profit from being free to pursue his own train of thought, to let his own

---

[3] Of course, the greeting and the superficial comment may each be a source of information or a part of the resistance. I do not feel, however, that the therapist needs to be so purist as inflexibly to refuse all social amenities as an invariable rule.

associations lead him for a bit. Generally the therapist needs to be aware of what it is the patient is saying, but there are times when he may not be. Generally he can appreciate what would be required for an answer at any given point, but it is another matter to move from open, attentive listening to more active responding, and the therapist should not be burdened with this necessity.

4. The silence provides a relatively neutral medium or baseline to which the therapist can return and which helps to give more emphasis to the interventions he does choose to make. The things the therapist does say gain added force from the fact he does not say very much. And since he will want to choose what he says carefully and wants it to be heard as thoroughly as possible, the therapist will value this augmentation.

The Occasion for Intervention

While the therapist listens with the open set we described in an earlier section, he will have a general orientation that guides his awareness and helps him discern when an intervention may be most useful. As I listen to my patient, I generally have in mind a model something like the following.

> This is a person in the midst of his life trying to make sense of what he experiences, trying to guide what he will do, trying to be more fulfilled and comfortable. When he is talking to me, another person, he knows at some level that I am in a very similar situation. He is talking to me because he wants to be more able to be in his life and to accomplish his purposes in it. At some level he knows I am neither all-knowing nor all-powerful. How does he talk to me? Does he talk to me in line with this reality, or is there implicit in what he says some distortion from this reality?

As I listen I hear certain repetitive ways in which distortions from the reality of our situation occur. Some of these are apparent, more nearly explicit; some are more subtle and covert. I do not respond to all that is said, but as I hear the repeated, dominant emotional theme, and as I see the manner in which this is being played out with me today, I am moved to comment to try to help my patient become more aware of some aspects of distortion.

Guides to Content of Interventions

In phrasing my intervention I try to serve a number of interwoven purposes concurrently. Let me comment on these and make evident how they guide what I say.

Help the Patient Reclaim an Alienated Portion of Himself. When the patient gave up some of his authenticity in order to try to be more safe, he became alienated from a portion of himself. This is so very evident when Ann (in the early part of Chapter 6) tells me about how unfairly she is treated. She has so clearly turned over a measure of herself to others. Perhaps I err in saying "*re*claim," for Ann in a sense never had possession of that portion. She was taught as a child to divest herself of much of her autonomy. One of my goals in phrasing my intervention is to help the patient claim that which is basically his.

Reduce Blame. One of the influences that most makes it difficult for the patient to lay claim to himself is his heavy indoctrination by our culture with the fallacy that *blame* is synonymous with *responsibility*. I think that responsibility needs to be seen by my patient eventually as synonymous with *opportunity*, rather than as synonymous with blame. So I try to deal with the cultural loading in his thinking that makes him dread blame. Let me be clear, this does not mean that I try to help him do away with *guilt*. I regard guilt as a more valid matter with which the patient must contend, but his general apprehension of blame is largely a culturally derived one and needs to be dealt with as profitless and stultifying.

Demonstrate Needful Motivation. Many times the patient is unable to see how his symptoms and his resistances are as much a product of his seeking to preserve himself as they are of his fear and guilt. It is useful to point out repeatedly to the patient the needful basis on which his resistances were formed. Particularly in the early stages, I am apt to say such things as: "You need to be vague as to how you feel about your boss." "You need to be overly generalized when you talk about sex." "You need to be unclear in your memory of your anger."

Another way in which this can be done tellingly is when a patient's emotional reaction to his experience is manifest, for example: "You are embarrassed by your sexual feelings." "You're ashamed of your anger toward your daughter." In this fashion the patient may be helped to accept the interpretation more readily. He is enabled to recognize the constructive aspects of himself as well as those of which he feels ashamed.

Increase the Feeling of Authorship of His Own Behavior. I watch for ways of phrasing and timing my interventions that make possible a heightening of the patient's feeling of being the author from whom his behavior flows. It is so often evident that the patient has lost the sense of being the originator of that which he does, so that I will sometimes come in briefly to underscore a dim recognition of his own role in bringing something about: "You can see how your fears made you trigger your wife's anger."

Change Compulsion to Choice. Neurotic behavior is compulsive behavior. My patient's inauthenticity has made of him an automaton. In phrasing my interventions, I am alert to try to help him recognize the points of choice and to recognize the points at which he has given over choice to compulsive repetition. Self-aware, responsible choosing is close to the heart of authenticity, and I want to help the patient move toward this goal. "Because you were so afraid of your anger, you couldn't risk really looking at the situation before you acted."

Describe What the Patient Is Doing, not What He Is not Doing. This rather simple guideline has much of importance to it. If the therapist is able to tune in sensitively on the dominant emotional theme and then to recognize the form the resistance is taking at any given point, he is ready to help his patient become conscious of a way in which the patient is unwittingly constricting his life. The point is that the patient is helped to recognize something in which he is already engaged. When the therapist's interventions, then, are accurate and well timed, the patient experiences *recognition*, rather than instruction. Subjectively he experiences a sense of the rightness of the interpretation, as his conscious contents correspond with what has been preconscious or unaware before the therapist spoke. It is this accord between consciousness and a formerly unrecognized pattern of living which gives the patient access to that which has been hidden but self-defeating.

This pattern of effective intervention may be contrasted with interpretations that tell the patient, in effect, "You're not being authentic." This may be accurate, and indeed the patient may accept the validity of the statement, but he is confronted with a more cognitive task that often decreases his immersion in the flow of awareness and is less facilitating to his self-discovery. The patient being told that his talk is not being authentic must then seek to identify and set aside what he is doing and try to find something that is more genuine.

> Beverly is restless and her voice has an irritable edge as she talks today. "So I kept thinking of how long Jack was going to be away, and I couldn't get to sleep. It's just like it's always been. I don't think therapy's helping me a damn bit. And you just sit there so impassive. You don't care what happens just so I pay my bills. Isn't that right?"
>
> It's clear that she's spoiling for a fight; yet there's an odd quality to her voice and manner, as though she's pushing the anger beyond its actual intensity. If I tell her what she's not doing now, it might go like this:
>
> "You're not telling me about what you were thinking when you couldn't sleep."
>
> "Oh, what does it matter; nothing ever changes anyway."
>
> The therapist begun on this course is apt to find himself feeling like, and being heard by his patient as, a nagging parent, complaining about the patient's failures. Meantime, the therapist will sense the on-going process of the patient's exploration of his concerns slipping away—the unconscious intent of the patient. However, when I tell the patient what she is doing, the results are different.
>
> "You want to get in a fight with me now."
>
> "Well, I don't think we're getting anywhere; do you?"
>
> "You'd rather fight now than risk getting anywhere."
>
> "What do you mean?"
>
> "You're uneasy about what you were telling me about when you couldn't sleep, and you try to pick a fight to get away from that uneasiness."

"Yeah, I guess so. Well, I can't see what it matters, I just was kind of unhappy and hot and restless, and I dozed and woke up and dozed and woke up and—Oh, I just remembered!" Beverly suddenly stops talking and lies very quietly and then begins to weep like a frightened little girl. After a bit, during which I am quiet too, Beverly tells of masturbating last night. She is very frightened and very filled with shame.

The significant point to this example is the fact that many times the therapist will unwittingly play into the resistances if he focuses on what the patient *is not* doing, while a clarification of what the patient *is* doing may deepen the awareness and disclose the resistance.

RESISTANCE "CHAINS"

Sensitive recognition of the resistance expression currently being employed by the patient, coupled with concise interpretation, often results in the dropping away of that resistance expression almost immediately. It is not "gone," but it is less apt to be used again as soon. Very often a second resistance layer is then encountered. At times, when patient and therapist are working well together, several such layers may be penetrated within a single session. The following example will illustrate this.

Dave has been talking for some time about his running battle with his wife. He details one frustration after another at her hands. Throughout his tone is suggestive of someone telling a diverting anecdote. At length, I intervene, "It sounds like you find it hard to take this situation seriously."

Dave counters, "Why do you say that?" His voice has noticeably sobered.

"You sounded as though you were ready to laugh any moment."

"Well, it's not funny, and I'm not going to laugh either." His voice is developing a hard edge. "I'm getting fed up with her, and I've been letting her have it a bit too. . . ." Now he begins telling for the first time of some of the ways he provokes and antagonizes his wife. His manner is almost defiant. After he has elaborated this for several minutes and as the defiance becomes more overt, I intervene again.

"You seem to expect that I'll berate you for doing these things to your wife."

"Yeah? Well, you can just keep your damn nose out of it. I told you I was sick of her making my life miserable, and so it's her turn to swallow it for a while...."

I don't wait this time, for the anger is coming to the surface rapidly. "You're ready to fight me or anyone about this you're so mad."

"Oh, hell, Doc, I'm not mad at you. It's just that I know I shouldn't be treating her that way, but . . ." Now his voice is dropping, and the anger is passing. Dave now does some of the most productive therapeutic work of the hour in examining his feelings of impotence in dealing with his wife except when he just gives way to his anger and torments her. He talks of this for some time before I speak again.

"It sounds like you have to be angry in order to ask for what you feel are your rights."

"Yeah, that's certainly true!" There is a rush of recognition in Dave's voice. "You know, that's just the way it was when I was a kid. Why my dad . . ." And Dave goes on working with memories which he has not allowed to drop away into the past but are being bitterly re-enacted daily in his marriage.

It is important to see how this whole chain of resistance expressions has to be worked through sequentially if Dave is to get to a point of dealing with the real issues in his life. Not on this day, but in time, Dave and I were able to discover how Dave's fear of responsibility for making decisions was importantly bound up with his relation with his wife. At an unconscious level, he had looked to her to be the ultimate one to shoulder such responsibility (just as his mother had done for Dave and for his father). His wife's unwillingness to fulfill this role had projected Dave into anxiety time and again.

When resistances chain this way, one cannot leap ahead along the chain without disrupting the therapeutic work. It is essential that the therapist let the patient set the pace. It is enough to help the patient recognize what it is he is doing at each point. Sometimes this must be done repeatedly; sometimes a single confrontation will serve.

For many patients these sequences of resistances tend to be rather persistent and organized in the same way in the same patient. Thus it proved to be typical that Dave moved from taking-it-too-lightly, to defiance, to anger, to guilt. We probably went along that chain twenty-five or thirty times before it began to disappear. Some other examples of persistent chains include:

>Airy offhandedness to silly laughing to flirtatiousness to heavily portrayed claims of superiority
>Inability to think of anything to say to anger to tears
>Overly earnest therapeutic work to hurt innocence to anger to guilt about fantasies

Guides to Phrasing Interventions

Let us examine some aids or guides to the phrasing of interventions.

Using the Dominant Emotional Theme

I have already talked about the importance of the dominant emotional theme. The more the therapist can phrase his interventions in language harmonious with the dominant emotional theme of the patient's associations, the more readily will the patient hear it. We know there are exceptions to this: a resistant patient can deny a simple repetition of the statement he has just made. The process of denial and repression can be very prompt and very sweeping. Nevertheless, the more one can find the wavelength on which his patient's associations are being transmitted, the more the likelihood that the interventions will be useful to the patient.

Patient's Repetitions

One way of determining when to intervene is to be alert to recognize those elements the patient is repeating in various ways. Repetitions are usually woven into the dominant emotional theme, as has been illustrated above. Further, it seems generally true that the repetition represents the "working to the surface" of material which has been less conscious. For this reason, also, it is well to avoid premature seizing upon simple repetitions before one has allowed sufficient emergence to be reasonably certain just what it is that is being reiterated.

>Ann tells me that the landlord wants to raise her rent and that she feels unfairly treated. Then she tells me that her boss let some of the other women leave on time while keeping her behind to do some overtime work.

It is clear that Ann is repeating a theme. What is that theme? She is being unfairly treated. People take advantage of her. Certainly these are accurate, at least to this point. I might say, "You're saying over and over how unfairly your world treats you." Such an intervention might aid her in inquiring further into her awareness. However, if I just wait a bit, I may understand better what she's trying to express.

Now Ann contrasts her own solitary apartment with the homes to which the other women at the office go at the close of work. There is still complaint in her voice, and she makes clear that she feels she has as many desirable qualities as the others. Still the unfairness theme. But as she continues, it is possible to use the indicator of her repetitiousness to locate the more significant element in what Ann is protesting.

"You feel you're made helpless and vulnerable unfairly by being so alone." The sob with which Ann answers reveals that this intervention has truly responded to Ann's feelings.

THE THERAPIST'S USE OF REPETITION

Just as repetition in what the patient says may signal material emerging toward consciousness, so the therapist's use of repetition may facilitate such emergence. The therapist who understands the layering of the resistances which has been described above will recognize as best he may be able that layer which is "on top" at any given point and focus his interventions on it. In this way the use of repetition follows naturally from the therapist's observations. Similarly, this procedure helps to forestall the sort of scattered or chaotic interventions that tend to keep the therapeutic interaction superficial and unproductive. In general, then, the therapist will find it helpful to phrase his resistance interpretations in a way that brings out the compulsive, repetitive aspects of the patient's thinking and experience.

Thus, with Charlotte the main thing I pointed out to her for the first several months of her therapy was, "You're so afraid of your feelings." "You're frightened by what you're feeling." "Your feelings seem so terrifying to you." At first she objected; then she became furious; then she fell silent. Today she can recognize with a sense of new-found strength when her fears are mounting, and she can deal with that mounting fear in a constructive fashion she never knew before. Many of our intellectualized, obsessive-compulsive patients literally are affect-blind and must be told over and over again that they have and respond to feelings.

VIVID LANGUAGE

The therapist does well to phrase his interventions in vivid language, watching for opportunities to build a private, metaphoric glossary with the patient. The terms that the two of them have worked out together from the patient's life experience have peculiarly poignant significance for him. Many times these are from events in his life; sometimes they are from anecdotes or jokes therapist and patient have told each other.

> Ben was a devout atheist, whose atheism was a point of pride. Ever since the day that I interpreted his repeated recital of his fears as a "telling of his Rosary," we have used this phrase again and again. We wryly observe that he is very faithful in his devotions, running through a list of fears in a blind ritualistic fashion, as though saying a prayer learned by rote. The impact of this metaphor is much greater than might be the case were I to phrase my intervention more academically.

> A very attractive, hysteric woman, much sought after by men, was tremendously shocked when I said, "You're a whore. You offer your love to anyone who will take over responsibility for decisions in your life!" (Needless to say this was at a point where we had been working together several years and our relationship was quite solid.) The interpretation was quite accurate, and its impact on the patient was of lasting value. I think its appropriateness was demonstrated when she later came to use this very metaphor herself.

INADEQUACIES IN INTERPRETATIONS

I would like to conclude by making several observations about points at which therapists are apt to have difficulty or to be unsuccessful in offering interpretations of resistance.

ARGUMENTATION IN INTERPRETATION

One such point that psychologists particularly are apt to be prey to is the attempt to document or qualify too much. We are, as psychologists, trained to value the presentation of evidence rather than personal endorsement as a basis for judgment. We tend many times when making our interpretations to try to demonstrate their accuracy by marshaling instances and unrolling deductions. Similarly, our statements are apt to be phrased in a conditional or qualified fashion. I think these habits of ours mean that many times our interpretations are flaccid and inadequate. Many of our patients need to encounter us as people willing to take a stand. Rather than piling up the evidence of what the patient has been doing in order that that evidence may speak instead of us, it is incumbent upon us many times to tell the patient flatly what we have observed. The dangers of mistaken interpretation may be less than those of flabby interpretation.[4]

Lucy had grown more and more uncommunicative in the past two weeks. Each session she professed difficulty in knowing what to say, and every topic she chose soon ran out. She had been drawing in tighter and tighter despite my efforts to show her how threatened she was. "Lucy," I told her, "Since you started to tell me how you really feel about your father you've been finding it hard to talk. You remember several weeks ago you described how he was the mainstay of the whole family, how everyone always turns to him for help. Then you told me you were so proud of him, proud that he was your father. Remember, I told you that your voice just wasn't very convincing, and you were so angry with me. Maybe you're still angry or maybe you're scared. Don't you see, it must be something like that?"

Lucy nodded, her mouth a straight line, her face impassive. "Yes, I guess so. I'm not aware of feeling that way, but you're probably right. You usually are." It was the end of the hour. She rose with her back to me and left without saying anything further.

At about twenty minutes after midnight, the phone jolted me awake. It was Lucy. "I think I need to talk to you, if you'll forgive me for disturbing you at this hour." Her voice was stiff, formal, almost prim. I started to suggest a special appointment in the morning. Instead I said, "I'll meet you at the office in thirty minutes."

When I got to the office, Lucy was there. Seated in the office, her face was a mask except for darting eyes that con-

---

[4] Heavily argued and documented interpretations often evidence a therapist who is listening to his patient with problem-solving concentration rather than open, authentic attention.

stantly moved in a hunted way and her fast short breathing. "I came from Santa Ana," she said conversationally. "I drove very fast. Almost 100 miles an hour. And I thought about just shutting my eyes and letting go of the wheel. Do you think I'm crazy? Should I go to an asylum?"

"Yes, I think you're crazy! I think you're a damn fool for driving like that. I think you're crazy with fear for your feelings about your father. That's what I think." I blasted out my anger at her.

Lucy just stared at me for what seemed an endless period. I started to think that perhaps I'd been too abrupt, responded too much in terms of my own feelings. Then I stilled these thoughts. Something was happening to Lucy's face. Suddenly it seemed to squeeze up, and the tears fairly spurted out of her eyes. "Ohhhh!" The sound was almost a curse. "That's right! That's right! He was so good and so right and so aloof and so kind and so distant and so phony and so . . . He was just everything, but he never cared a thing about any of us . . . about me!" Now she started sobbing with great hoarse sounds.

Later we were able to see how my careful, detached, well-documented interpretations had made me seem so very much like her father. When, however, I risked being wrong but frankly confronted her and showed that she mattered enough to me to bawl her out, I helped her win free of the icy control she had imposed on herself to hold back what she had been taught to regard as her shameful anger with her father.

We may note too that it probably was extremely important to have seen Lucy that night. The way she drove and the thought of suicidally letting go control of the car were evidences that she was on the verge of a violent acting out. To smash herself in the car would have served to violate the law (father's will) while yet punishing herself for her bad feelings and stilling both the tortuous conflict within her and the guilty promptings.

TIMING

A second frequent difficulty in interpretations is that the timing is not sensitively keyed to the patient's readiness to receive the interpretation. It is usually well to try to sense what is in the process of emergence in the patient's awareness.

An Example: Changing the Subject. One may discern that the patient is becoming uncomfortable with his associative material, beginning to sense that it is shallow, repetitive, or profitless. Many times the patient will not be ready spontaneously to recognize this as a resistance or as a difficulty occasioned by emotional forces. He will tend to see it, if he becomes aware of it, as a difficulty in the topic with which he has chosen to deal. Left to himself, the patient would handle the difficulty by changing to a different topic. The therapist's intervention to disclose the resistance saves the patient from a wasteful search for topics which will be more readily discussable. At such a point the therapist can pinpoint the kind of difficulty the patient is having, with the result that the resistance interpretation is experienced then as that which it most truly is, a facilitation of this patient's purpose. When the interpretation is less well timed, it may be heard as a reprimand or challenge.

Howard has been telling me of his reluctance to sign a new lease for the office which he shares with his partners. Howard has been talking with some other, younger dentists who propose a joint practice in another part of the city. He is strongly tempted to join them, having come to see the kind of dependent relationship he has with his present, older partners. At the same time, he is hesitant to seem ungrateful to the latter for the help they gave him in getting his practice started. He has talked about this dilemma for many minutes and seems to be "running dry" on the topic as he alternates between feeling that he wants to assert himself and move out with younger colleagues and feeling that he would be ungrateful to leave his present partners. He finds himself repeating these two themes with minor variations and appears restless. From past experiences I know that Howard will shortly switch the topic, probably without being fully aware of what is happening. Interpretation can help Howard at this point; so I may say, "You seem to be uncomfortable with the implications of this choice you face," or I might say, if he seems closer to awareness of his discomfort, "You'd like to get away from this uncomfortable choice between seeming to be dependent and seeming to be disloyal."

It is difficult for many patients to recognize the kinds of intrusions on their associative material occasioned by emotional processes. The spontaneous tendency frequently seems to be to regard the problem as one of having no more ideas and thus needing to change topics. It is an important therapeutic step when the patient begins to recognize the fact that he can talk indefinitely on almost any topic of genuine significance to himself.

> Charlotte says, "I've hardly begun on this snarl my husband and I keep getting into and yet already I'm running out of ideas. I can't see why, but I must be frightened in some way." Charlotte has come a long way from the days when she jumped from topic to topic. She now has an effective aid in exploring her own awareness: a signal of the presence of otherwise hidden fears.

Teaching Persistent Exploration. In the earlier stages of the analytic work, it is helpful to teach the patient a different concept of the therapeutic talk than that he usually brings with him. Thus, typically, the patient will talk about a matter until he finds difficulty or discomfort and then tend to take up a new topic to deal with in the same way. When this happens in rather clear-cut fashion, I interrupt and say something like this:

> You've just moved to a new topic for the second time today. Each time when you did so, it seemed that you'd run out of ideas or were having trouble saying clearly what you wanted to. Now I'd like to suggest that unwittingly you're serving your fear of yourself by switching topics. Think of it this way: When you're driving a highway and come to a detour sign, it's appropriate to move to a different road in order to get where you're headed. But when you're working on the road crew and come to that detour sign, it has quite another meaning. Then it means "This is where I'm headed; this is where there's work to be done." You and I are the road crew. When you have trouble or run out of ideas abruptly on something you're talking about, take time to find out more about what's going on in you. When you have trouble like that it means you're doing a good job and we've come to a place where we can help you win back more of your own awareness.

OVERINTERPRETATION

A third frequent difficulty with our interpretations is our tendency to "unload" too much on the patient at one time. The most astute observation and accurate interpretation can be rendered futile and even vitiating if we overload the interpretation with too much material at a time. The phrasing of an interpretation needs to be made with primary attention to the "perceptual feel" of the patient rather than that of the therapist. This is to say that it is important to try to have an awareness of how the patient is seeing the situation at the moment we choose to intervene. In recognizing this criterion, it will be evident that the patient is seldom attending to the same internal "display" of topics that the therapist may have developed in his mind as he listened; rather, the therapist will do well to try to find the point of overlap between his own awarenesses and those of his patient, and use this as the entering point for his intervention. This will mean that that intervention must be concise and fairly pointed.

> In the example of the intervention with Howard above, it would probably not be useful, unless we were ready for a major confrontation, to say to Howard "You're uncomfortable with this choice between assertion of your own desires and loyalty to your older partners, just as you're uncomfortable with your wanting generally and with the feeling that your wanting brings you in conflict with the kinds of values you were taught by your parents. This is like the choices you had to make when you left home and is a re-enactment of your discomfort in rebeling against your father. Every time that you've come to a choice between acting on your own desires and being loyal, you feel the same discomfort."

Now everything about this hypothetical interpretation is accurate; indeed it might be used as a major confrontation at some point. However, since this instance came early in Howard's exploration of this problem, such an amount of material "thrown" at him at once will act to dissipate his mounting emotional immersion in the choice situation he faces. The result will then be dilution rather than focusing of the question he is confronting.

Omnibus Interpretation. Even more ineffectual is the kind of omnibus interpretation that tries to teach process points concurrently with elucidation of a present resistance.

> Charlotte, when she is talking about her feelings about her sister and her competition with her sister for her father's love, finds herself becoming restless and wanting to change the topic. She is now able to recognize these symptoms of resistance and, as indicated above, say that she feels she must be fearful. If the therapist at this point makes an omnibus

interpretation it could take the following form: "You recognize that you are fearful in talking about your feelings about your sister and your father, and you get fearful this way whenever there is any hint that you may be hostile toward someone you love. You remember the other day this occurred when you were talking about your husband. Often, too, you get fearful when you find that you have thoughts that you don't approve of, such as some of your sexual thoughts or some of your angry thoughts. Another thing that seems to make you fearful is the sense of not performing up to your standards, as when you were telling me the other day about the mistakes you made in grammar at the club. . . ." The therapist might feel he was helping Charlotte to see the kinds of situations that make her fearful, but such an interpretation does far more to confuse the situation than to illuminate it.

The Unity of the Resistance

A point that needs to be clearly recognized if analysis of the resistance is to proceed effectively is that ultimately the resistance is not an additive composite but is the life stance of the person in relation to the existential givens. Thus the resistance is a unity. As we listen to the patient we become aware of this or that aspect, at one or another level of generality, sensing some facet of the total posture of the patient thus involved. But these differences are in our perceptions and interpretations, they do not truly represent different resistances.

> John talks of his conflict with his wife who protests that he is distant and cold. He tries to see things through her eyes, he says, but he can only conclude she is too demanding. He'd like to make her happier, but he just can't see what he could do. Then he finds himself "stuck" as to how to inquire into this matter further, although he is far from content with leaving it so "up in the air." After a moment's hesitation he begins talking about some reading he is doing in preparation for a new assignment at his work.
> Now, I could follow John to this new topic and doubtlessly in time the underlying dominant emotional theme would emerge that joins the two topics (difference with his wife and reading for the new work), but I have seen John go through this sequence sufficiently often for me to be ready to try to

interpret the resistance pattern involved: "You're leaving this problem with your wife up in the air."

"Well, what can I do? I can't figure anything out except that she wants too much, and I can't do anything about that."

"So you just have to drop it, eh?"

"Well, what else can I do?"

"What would happen if you didn't drop the matter, but stayed on the topic right now?"

"I'd just go on getting no place like I've been doing so far this hour."

"Would you? Well, why don't you summarize the way you see it now and then see if anything else comes to mind."

"Oh, okay, but it won't do any good."

And so John makes a summary, except that somehow he finds additional thoughts occurring and reopens the topic and goes a bit further before he again wants to leave the matter. This time it's pretty clear he is getting into uncomfortable ideas about his lack of responsiveness to his family. So I can say, "You find this idea of not being very giving to your family so uncomfortable that you'd like to change the subject."

"Well, I don't know what else I can say about it."

"How convenient!"

"Yeah," he grins self-consciously and picks up the topic. And so we move a little closer to the recognition of the fear that he experiences when he is close to another person.

John's pattern of changing the subject in his associations during the therapeutic hour is an aspect of his total life resistance pattern, which has other aspects such as being too busy to be available for close engagement with his wife and children, such as changing his employment periodically, such as having a number of friends but no intimates. John fears "getting to depend on" anyone or anything if he becomes "too involved." Ultimately, we find, John is unable to accept and incorporate the fact of being responsible for his choices and their consequences. This is tied to his fears of being abandoned, and so he has developed a pattern which we can characterize in oversimplified form as that of leaving the other (or the topic or the job or whatever) before he is left.

The important point to recognize is that the in-interview resistance (changing the subject) is the same process of John-meeting-his-life as is the ultimate existential resistance of avoidance of genuine encounter and presence. It is not a sample of the existential resistance, or a parallel to it, or even a part of it. It is the existential resistance itself as we are able to recognize it in the interview situation. As we expose it to John and he is able to set it aside in some measure, he is grappling with his very life process, with the actual influences that keep him in non-being.

From the therapist's point of view it is essential that this recognition of the unity of the resistance be taken very seriously, for its significance for the analytic work is profound. Casual inferences about the resistance and erratic interpretations may not only be ineffectual, they may do much to confuse the patient and make more difficult any eventual orderly and successful analysis.

The responsible therapist will be concerned to recognize that aspect of the resistance which is most exposed in the interview, to bring this to the patient's awareness repeatedly and poignantly, to follow the chaining of resistances back to the patient's existential life stance, and to help the patient discover the constructive being–seeking authenticity as well as the loss of his being which is portrayed in his resistance. In this fashion does the therapist authentically bring effective aid to the patient's seeking of his own authenticity.

CONCLUSION

The analysis of the resistance is the key step in existential-analytic psychotherapy. It calls for the greatest sensitivity, self-knowledge, and skill on the part of the therapist. When the therapist is effective in conducting this phase with a well-motivated and alert patient, the sense of genuine therapeutic engagement and the evidence of clear-cut therapeutic changes in the patient's life are among the most immediate and unequivocal in intensive therapeutic work.

8 — The analysis of the transference

Bruno Bettelheim, in *The Informed Heart* (1960, pp. 264–265), tells of an incident in a German extermination camp during the infamous reign of the Nazis. A group of prisoners stood naked outside the crematorium, waiting numbly for their executions. As so many thousands and even millions of prisoners went passively to their deaths, it seemed it would be with this group. However, the commandant of the camp learned that one of the prisoners, an attractive young woman, had been a dancer. He ordered her to dance for him. She did so, and in the whirling of her dance moved close to him until suddenly she seized his gun and shot him. She was instantly shot down herself.

This dancer took back to herself what so many of those exterminated relinquished: choice. This dancer became again a person, and in her personhood achieved a dignity by choosing to die in a self-affirming way. As Bettelheim says:

> Exercising the last freedom that not even the concentration camp could take away—to decide how one wishes to think and feel about the conditions of one's life—this dancer threw off her real prison. This she could do because she was willing to risk her life to achieve autonomy once more. If we do that, then if we cannot live, at least we die as men (p. 265).

Let me set in contrast to this dancer what has been happening with Betty.

Betty, in her middle forties, is still unmarried. Betty works at a lower occupational level than that for which her education prepared her; indeed, lower than she has worked previously. Betty's days are made up of her work and her small apartment and her therapy. She seldom goes out, either alone or with others. In therapy, as in her thoughts away from therapy, she repeatedly goes over and over her relations with her mother, father, brother. Sometimes she does this in terms of the way it once was at home and the fancied and real injustices she suffered then. Sometimes it is in terms of her current correspondence with each of these people and all the subtle meanings that she can find in the way they write to her, the things they say and do not say. This is Betty's life.

Betty is like one of the naked prisoners waiting outside the extermination oven. She is drained of her humanity. She is simply waiting to be marched away, because Betty cannot let herself choose, does not choose to have her life. Bettelheim tells of prisoners who lived in barracks next to the extermination ovens and denied to themselves what was happening. As a result, docilely they let themselves be killed off. Betty is like one of these. She denies what is happening in her life, how her days are being killed off.

Non-being: The Price of Escape

As we have seen in earlier pages, our efforts to escape anxiety lead to non-being. Betty only shows in exaggerated form the terrible toll taken by all of our compromises with actuality, the toll that is exacted in our very livingness. We have seen how this experience of existential anxiety can increase to a point at which we may choose to distort our real situation in the hope that we can reduce the unbearable anxiety. Having made this choice, we develop the symptoms that are the expressions of our flight from anxiety. Faced by the need to make life decisions which we know may have far-reaching and profound significance, we are constantly tempted to deny the choice, to act as though the choice were not ours or had other meanings. Again and again we find ourselves trying to slide past decisions, dreading the issue.

Betty, in our example above, daily slides past looking at what is happening in her life. She wants to be, clings to the hope of being a wife and mother, while actually the likelihood diminishes daily. Like a person who goes to the same motion picture again and again hoping that the unhappy ending will somehow change and become a happy one, she goes over and over her disappointments in her childhood and early adult years as though somehow seeking to have them come out differently and thus to regain her life. By not choosing to be in the now, she continues her non-being and loses her life.

In the therapeutic relation Betty is by turns helpless, sulky, and demanding. She protests the frequency of her contacts and their times during the day as though these were personal impositions I made on her to gratify myself. She frequently says she has nothing to say, cannot remember some key incident or dream, or finds superficial thoughts pre-empting her awareness. In all of these instances she waits passively for me to fix things up. Her verbal behavior with me tries to make of the therapy hour an unwelcome intrusion of her life which she tolerates only because this is the only way she can please me enough that I will give her what she wants. What does she want? In fact, the very life she so readily cedes away.

You will not be surprised to learn that Betty's father was a demanding, mercurial person who needed frequent demonstrations that she was appreciatively dependent on him. Whenever she seemed to take his support for granted, he would pull it away, and she could only regain it by a tantrum or by elaborate demonstrations of how lost she was without her father's backing, how helpless and inadequate she was. Autonomy and initiative were treated as proofs of disloyalty.

Betty learned to fear contingency and choice-responsibility dually. The world was an even more unpredictable place for her than for most of us because her father needed to make it so. For her the only sure way to a measure of stability was through using her emotions to influence her father. Today Betty avoids being in the world just as she was taught, and similarly she concentrates on manipulating me through her emotions.

We may say that Betty acts toward me as though I were her father and that this is a transference. It is also, of course, a resistance. Having looked at the resistance earlier, let us now try to understand the nature of transference and the distinctions we may make between resistances and transferences.

The Transference and the Therapeutic Relation

THE CONCEPT OF THE TRANSFERENCE

In my discussion I will define "transference" as the patient's unconscious attempt to re-establish an earlier, symbiotic relationship with a person important in his life. By symbiosis I refer to a collaborative way of being in the world. In the transference, the patient tries to recreate a collaboration such as he had in the past with some important person. He sees the therapist, unconsciously or consciously, as a powerful source of new contingencies that may heighten his dread. This increases the patient's need to find some way of relating to the therapist that will reduce or constrain the contingency-emitting potential the therapist is seen as having. In the past with other persons, particularly his parents, the patient has been in a similar situation, and he will try to use with the therapist that pattern of relationship which worked best with one or another of these earlier figures. The choice is made chiefly in terms of two variables: (a) the kinds of cues he gets from the therapist that make him like one of the earlier figures on a reality basis; and, (b) the kinds of internal promptings, both of distress and of hope, to which the patient is most subject at this point in the relationship.

THERAPEUTIC SIGNIFICANCE

The transference may be thought of as a seeking for re-establishment of a situation of known limits of variability in which the patient feels he has ways of coping with the therapist and preserving himself in the world. It is not simply a blind repetition of earlier patterns or a chance product of a repetition compulsion trying to work out earlier, incomplete, emotional business; rather, it is purposive in the present situation. It represents a falling away from authentic transaction with the therapist in the present. The significance for psychotherapy is clear: much can be learned about the patient's probable transferences onto the therapist from study of the important relations of his early life; and interpretation of the unreal elements in his relation to the therapist can be facilitated by showing their learned basis in the earlier relationship.

As I have conceived the transference it will be evident that the kinds of symbiotic relationships in which the pattern of relating (which I now term transference) was originally learned were always such as to breed inauthentic dialogues. Therefore, the transference is always a resistance. (It should be noted that this is not the same as saying that resistance is always transference.[1])

THE DUAL IMPLICATIONS OF THE TRANSFERENCE

The transference is a patterned way of being in the world that involved a significant other and that is reactivated in the patient's relation to the therapist. This way of conceiving the transference has the advantage of calling our attention to an aspect frequently overlooked: the transference is not just the patient's way of perceiving and responding to the therapist. It is an evocation of the sub-self of the patient that has been symbiotically related to the earlier figure. Saying it somewhat more starkly, when my patient reacts to me in a transference manner he is a different person than he is in other circumstances, just as he seeks to transform me into a different person than I am in the interview situation.

DISTINGUISHING THE RESISTANCE AND THE TRANSFERENCE

From all that has been said, it should be apparent that the fundamental datum is the experiencing person in the midst of his own life; nevertheless, there is heuristic value in recognizing two aspects of the person's distortion of his present situation, each of which we deal with in appropriate ways in the therapeutic undertaking. It will be useful to make evident the contrasting conceptions of the resistance and the transference that are helpful in actual therapeutic work. We will do this by making a number of statements in parallel about each.

RESISTANCE
"Designed" to prevent internal awareness from coming to consciousness and causing the eruption of anxiety, either existential or neurotic.

TRANSFERENCE
"Designed" to involve the therapist in ways already familiar to the patient so that the therapist will take over some part of the patient's coping with contingency and anxiety.

---

[1] Because the transference is such an immensely important part of the resistance and because its handling requires particular sensitivity and skill, I am treating the transference separately and will even, at times, refer to it as separate from the (rest of the) resistance.

Prevents authenticity.	Prevents genuine encounter.
Internally directed.	Expressed in the relationship to the therapist.
Prevents the free production of associations or reporting of awarenesses.	Prevents genuine relating to the person whom the therapist is in fact.
"Layered and peelable."	Persistent, changing only in superficial form when being displaced onto other objects.
Requires orderly analysis for dissolution.	Requires repeated exposure and working through for dissolution.

ASPECTS OF AN EFFECTIVE THERAPEUTIC RELATIONSHIP

Although I have dealt at length with the therapeutic relation in earlier chapters, it is so important to the understanding of the transference that I must carry our considerations further. Heuristically we can analyze the therapeutic relationship into three main aspects. It is important to recognize that this analysis into components is artificial, that these three aspects are not distinct but are really three ways of looking at the same process. Nevertheless, having recognized this, there is genuine value in distinguishing the aspects in order to appreciate more clearly what is involved in the relationship between the therapist and the patient.

Real Relation. The first aspect is the realistic relationship between two people. This includes the business arrangements between them as to time, fees, and so forth. It includes the reality of their intimacy, sharing, and common effort, of the mutual respect and appreciation they come to develop for each other as real persons.

Transference. The second main aspect may be thought of as composed of the transferences from past significant figures in the lives of both participants. Generally we are inclined to give more attention to and recognize more readily the transference that the patient projects upon the therapist. However, it is well to keep in mind that counter-transference projections by the therapist are also present. The projections of both vary along a continuum from those that are largely accurate to those that are completely parataxic and distorted. Much therapeutic effort must be devoted to helping the patient learn to distinguish that which is parataxic and distorted and that which is accurate in the way he sees the therapist.

"*Display.*" The third aspect of the therapeutic relationship we can think of as the "display" of the intrapsychic life of the patient. The word display is used here in a sense similar to that in which systems analysis people use that term, the laying out of all aspects of a system. The patient displays his being-in-the-world in his way of relating to the therapist and of using the therapeutic opportunity. This is not the same thing as the transference, which is the distortive carrying forward from the past of relationships to previous significant figures. The therapist is a present significant figure, and the patient is portraying in his whole manner of presenting himself and relating to the therapist a cross-section of his subjective life.

As we regard the third aspect of the therapeutic relation, it is evident why this relationship is the most important in the patient's life, for in one sense it *is* the portrayal or display of the patient's life. No other relationship can be as central, because no other relationship is so organized as to allow this total display. Psychoanalytic theory recognizes this in the concept of the transference neurosis, which is the microcosmic summation or representation of the patient's total neurosis or personality. The patient who needs to forestall this display of his inner life has a major therapeutic resistance which must be dealt with if any genuine therapeutic product is to be obtained.

The Subject–Object Split as a Transference

Many of my patients are inclined to split themselves into an observer and an observed; frequently this becomes a taskmaster and a slave.

> Donna had made good progress in the analytic phase of her therapy, for she was conscientious and intelligent. However, the point came at which this very conscientiousness was increasingly revealed as a way in which she avoided authenticity. It took the form of her saying implicitly, "If I don't watch myself and keep after myself every minute, I'll probably goof off and not do well in anything; certainly I'd give in to my fears and not progress in therapy."

As the therapist pressed on Donna's awareness the fear of herself, the splitting of herself involved in this form of conscientiousness, Donna for the first time began to consider relinquishing this pattern (resistance). One day she began to feel acutely what that letting go would mean: "I get panicky about just letting go. I feel like I'll just give up and die . . . I won't try to learn anything or do anything or accomplish anything. . . . When I think about letting go, it is like living, and I feel a great big hurt in my throat."

This is a succinct statement of the being and non-being issue. Letting go is dying—to the old way of living, of non-being. But letting go is also living—coming into new aliveness.

Why should Donna feel panic at what apparently would mean taking it easier on herself? Where does this split pattern come from and what purpose has it been serving? Too many of us, recognizing the same attitudes toward ourselves, are apt to feel that such a split is indeed necessary to ensure that the person will do the things he needs to. Such is the pervasiveness of this lack of self-trust, of this resistance to authentic wholeness of being. After all, who is it that is concerned about getting things done? And who is it that will do them if they get done? The answer, of course, is in each case the person himself. Indeed, it is the splitting into taskmaster and slave that brings about the non-doing, at least in part. When one feels basically a slave, then why not idle away the time when the taskmaster is away? The splitting is not the symptom of the failure to follow through on one's own purposes, but the cause of it.

Back of this sort of splitting within the person is almost always a parent or other significant figure who regarded the patient much as his authoritarian voice (the taskmaster) now regards his object-self (the slave). Usually the early figure was not as stringent as the patient has become over the years for a reason we shall see in a minute. That same earlier figure who so controlled the patient was usually also a source of strength or support. The earlier control provided direction and relief from the anxiety of choice, and it provided a seeming security from contingency and responsibility (if only it were faithfully obeyed). The patient, leaving behind (actually or psychologically) the earlier authority, feels the absence of the attendant security and protection from anxiety. Usually there is a concurrent falling away from the "good" habits or behavior the authority enjoined. Thus there is an attendant shame ("What if the authority could see me now?"). The patient then establishes the authoritarian voice within, the "good" things get done once more (at least in some part), and the sense of attendant protection returns (also in some part).

But why does the authoritarian voice within the patient grow even more suspicious and demanding than was the voice of the original figure? Clearly, because of two associated influences. First, the patient performing the "good" acts not from his own (intrinsic) motivation but from the "should" of the (extrinsic) earlier figure, is apt to do them less faithfully as the distance from the earlier figure increases. Thus there is increasing shame and decreasing security. Second, the authoritarian voice within the patient, "powered" by increasing shame and insecurity, increases its rantings in the effort to restore comfort. Clearly the effort is vain, for as the breakdown of the resistance (self-transference) proceeds and anxiety mounts, new distortions are brought to bear. These new distortions may take the extreme forms of masochistic self-injury, of piling on additional (compulsive) tasks as a ritual for atonement, or any of a variety of other forms. In any case, they so dissipate the energy and security remaining to the patient that he is even less apt to be able to perform the "good" acts or to trust himself and heal the subject–object breach within himself.

A POINT OF CRITICAL DIFFERENCE: THE NATURE OF MAN

Every therapist needs to examine his own conscious and explicit as well as his implicit beliefs about this matter of the basic nature of man. Many times, if he is candid with himself, the therapist will find that—at least for himself and his family—he acts in terms of a traditional and nonhumanistic view of man. Freudian psychology and much of Christian psychology have taught the view that man's impulses are bad or dangerous and have to be restrained and redirected. Striving and inhibition are key concepts—even values—in such a perspective. Control is not for artistic modulation but for protective restraint.

Some psychotherapists insist the reverse: man is basically good; only release him in every way possible and all will be well. To me, these seem the familiar mistrust ideas inverted. Such assertions have the ring of protest and, sometimes, of overdetermined blindness to the world of actuality.

It seems to me that existentially we must recognize that "good" and "bad" are not characteristics of the given world of being. Were they so, we would have less choice than I believe is our condition. If one can genuinely counsel that man is inherently good, then all we need is an improved technology for releasing man, and our real freedom is at an end. The best technology becomes the operational equivalent of the ultimate good, and man is but an object of that technology and his inborn goodness. No, I do not believe it.

Man is. Not man is good or man is bad. Within the limits of his awareness, responsible for his choices, without the guideposts of instincts or innate nature, and trying to find meaningful relation with his fellows, man is, period.

Analytic Procedure

Recognizing the Transference

Many therapists speak glibly of the transference without really recognizing how very genuinely the patient sees the therapist in a projective fashion. We are accustomed to think of this as a matter of the patient seeing the therapist "sort of like" he saw his father. This is not so. Unconsciously the patient experiences the therapist *as* his father or another earlier figure. This is to say that, unless the therapist intrudes so much on the patient's awareness that the transference has no chance to be truly projected onto the therapist, the patient will reenact and relive his relationship to the father in the relationship to the therapist. It is hard to find the words to express how literally this is so. Usually much experience and an adequate personal therapeutic experience are required for the therapist to appreciate the vividness of this projection.

In general, unless the transference is being acted out in the relationship with the therapist in such a way as to interfere with the therapeutic work, it is best to delay interpretation of it until a great deal of work has been done with the rest of the resistance. The more the patient has begun organismically to experience what it means to be authentic and has developed some awareness of when he is approaching authenticity and when he is in flight from it, the more ready he becomes for transference interpretations. By and large much important therapeutic work will be done by the patient in learning to use the therapeutic hour as a place for self-exploration and for development of emotional awareness. In this endeavor he will many times bring forth memories and self-perceptions that relate importantly to the transference. Certainly when he himself begins to make parallels between his manner of relating to the therapist and his manner of relating to important figures in his early life, the therapist will want to join him in this sort of inquiry. However, in general practice a real transference confrontation and working through is well postponed until a good deal of progress has occurred in the analysis of other aspects of the resistance.

THE RELATIONSHIP REPERTOIRE

While the patient is learning to work therapeutically and learning to explore himself in the direction of being more authentic, the therapist has abundant opportunity to develop a picture of the patient's *relationship repertoire*. This is a concept that helps in planning for transference interpretations. Each of us, from his earliest years, is engaged in trying to discover how to be a person, what it means to be an individual. Each of us draws heavily on our parents, siblings, and other significant figures in those first years for many kinds of information about ourselves and our world. One of the most important kinds of information thus acquired constitutes the dyadic definition of who we are. By "dyadic definition" I mean the definition that describes one's self in relation to others. It is not a definition of the person in isolation but in relation. This is an important point to keep in mind. The child learns that with certain others he is weaker or more helpless; that with still others he is more adequate but must be distant, and so on.

As the therapist listens to his patient he acquires a composite picture of the various relationship patterns that are available to the patient for meeting and dealing with others. The therapist needs to be able to distinguish the kinds of persons who are most apt to elicit particular patterns in the patient and to recognize those points at which the patient experiences confusion or conflict in the patterns evoked within him.

LISTENING TO THE PATIENT

Let us now examine the process of listening to the patient to pick up these clues. It is a difficult process to put into explicit language without doing violence and becoming more confusing than informing. It is handicapping to the therapist if he attempts to be too attentive to the explicit content of what the patient is saying. The therapist needs to develop what Freud called "free floating attention," which permits him to sense not only the words but "the music" of the patient's talking. It helps to listen to the total pattern, the tempo, and the phrasing with which the patient speaks. When the therapist does so, he may become aware that the patient is not really talking to him as he is in fact, but talking to him as though he were someone having a different kind of relationship to the patient. The patient's voice may be pleading or apologetic; his voice may be demanding, or querulous; his manner may convey a supplication, or it may be unusually distant and formal. Then if note is taken of the content of what the patient is saying, the therapist may understand better why it is the patient is talking to him, what it is the patient talks about, and what it is he implicitly expects, having said this.

Another type of information that is frequently useful is to see what the patient can tell of his relations to other current figures in his life. In his relationships to his spouse, to his superior at work, to inferiors, to companions in various enterprises, he is demonstrating other parts of his relationship repertoire. Similarly, when the patient enters group therapy there is a chance to observe the various relationship patterns he has available.

INTERPRETING THE TRANSFERENCE

If the therapist has been successful in interpreting the patient's other resistances, patient and therapist will have "peeled back several layers." The patient will be learning gradually to talk with greater authenticity. Inevitably in the course of this process of "peeling the onion" we come to those resistances that are acted out through the transference.

The point was made above that it is generally well to allow these to remain until the patient has developed a feeling for authenticity in the therapeutic hour. There are certain instances, of course, where this generalization does not hold good. Thus, if a patient, even quite early in his therapeutic course, begins to accuse the therapist of judgments of him and is unable to talk openly because of these fancied judgments, the therapist can aid communication by making a partial transference interpretation by way of a direct confrontation. For instance, he may say to the patient, "You feel so guilty that you're sure others are judging you as you judge yourself." Again, a patient who tries to lure the therapist into departing from the therapeutic regime by asking many questions, by behaving in a seductive fashion, or by trying to entertain, may profit from interpretations of his behavior; for example, "You are fearful that you may not have control over what is happening in this interview, and so you have to try to gain control by questioning me," or "You're fearful to let me know you, and so you try to amuse me instead of telling me about yourself."

SEQUENCE FOR INTERPRETATIONS

These are, of course, incomplete transference interpretations. The behaviors were learned in relation to earlier significant figures and are being acted out in the therapeutic situation. However, it is seldom well to make a full interpretation of the transference at this early stage. Instead it is useful to treat the behavioral aspects as resistances and help the patient work through them in that fashion.

One effect of working through the resistances in some measure first is that then the transference resistances emerge in which the patient more and more focuses on the therapist his patterned neurotic defenses against authenticity (the transference neurosis). In a sense, "the field is cleared" somewhat of other types of resistances, and it is possible to make more impactful interpretations. Let me illustrate this by describing the sequence as it worked out with Hanna.

> Hanna had worked through a great deal of her resistive inauthenticity. Concurrently she became increasingly focused emotionally upon me and was convinced of her great love for me.[2] Nevertheless, she found herself increasingly asking de-

---
[2] By phrasing it this way I do not mean to belittle her genuine emotional feeling for me. I value this feeling and am not trying to rob it of the dignity it deserves.

partures from the interview routine to secure advice from me about her children, to get suggestions for outside reading, and for a variety of other reasons. The strange thing about these requests was that Hanna was a very competent woman who, earlier in therapy when much more disturbed, had not had nearly as many questions of this type. Yet each of these questions was in its way genuine. They were not the type of spurious questions that patients ask early as a resistance designed to take over control of the interview. As Hanna asked questions I would tell her, "I will not answer the question now; tell me what you're thinking. Perhaps I can answer it later." (As an aside let me say that when dealing with patients' questions in this fashion, I generally try to stop a few minutes early and talk about the questions, although not necessarily giving answers.)

In this manner of dealing with Hanna's questions, we came more and more to associated memories and feelings having to do with conflict between her parents and with her mother's efforts to keep Hanna from forming an emotionally close attachment with her father. Particularly important seemed to be a memory from when she was six or seven years old: her mother objected to Hanna sitting on her father's lap and said this was not a "nice" thing to do. Aside from the Oedipal aspects of this (which were also important), there was also the learning for Hanna that access to her father through affection and physical contact was bad. She could, however, have his attention through getting his help, through bringing problems to him while avoiding the emotional plane.

After one particularly stormy session in which Hanna had objected to my deferring response to her questions and had found that an undue amount of anger and fright was arising, it was natural to point out to her, "Hanna, you're trying to find your way to me through asking my help, just as you did your father." Hanna was thunderstruck, but she could recognize immediately that the feeling was indeed the same as she had had with her father. From this disclosure flowed other memories and other present feelings. For several weeks thereafter, Hanna and I frequently pointed out her use of the same mechanism in a variety of ways with me and with other current figures in her life.

The important thing to recognize about this example is that the task of interpreting the transference was much simplified because so many of her other resistances had been dealt with in advance. It is also significant that what was involved here was Hanna's responsibility for making decisions in her own life. From this interpretive sequence it was possible to get rather directly into Hanna's terrible fear of not knowing enough to make important decisions affecting her children and family. She felt a tremendous weight of responsibility, even an undue weight. She was convinced that she was quite inadequate to handle that responsibility fully. She sought in me, she sought in education, in reading, and in many other areas, the authoritative answers that would relieve her of ultimate responsibility in the decisions and choices she was making. She was an excellent student, a very bright person, and had often been able to find those who would offer these answers.

Now the transference material began to come through like a flood released from a dam. First were a series of fantasies of and seekings for intimate, personal relationship with me; here Hanna found that she was in a kind of anguish of embarrassment and frustrated longing. She was sure that unless we could be much closer she would be utterly miserable. She wept, when she told me this. Again I allowed her to immerse to a point where the feelings were very clear in her awareness, and then it was possible to point out to her that this yearning was, in large part, frustrated longing for her father and for a warm emotional relationship with him which had been denied by the mother's prohibitions. It had been a less than satisfactory substitute to get father to answer questions and be a helper.

Hanna experienced but little real relief in this interpretation, although it did help to bring things more into perspective. Instead of finding relief, she found herself more than ever convinced that the pain of wanting me physically and emotionally was so great that she could not bear it. Now the way was open for the key interpretation of her existential transference. In a series of relatively brief interpretations I brought out to Hanna that what she suffered from was not the deprivation of not having me but rather the fact that this was imposed upon her, as by her mother, making her an object. She was calling on me to make all the decisions. I pointed out that if she had made a real effort to seduce me, or if she had herself decided that it was an unwise thing for us to be intimate, she would not be the object but the subject. Thus again she was really enacting the relationship with her father and her mother while seeing herself as one who could not make decisions. The next session or two Hanna was very demanding in challenging my determination not to have sexual relations, questioning my right to set limits unilaterally. Then rather abruptly she dropped the idea of a sexual relation and found, with some surprise, that she no longer felt the pain.

MULTIPLE TRANSFERENCES

Hanna's transferences were really dual. She projected on me the earlier symbiotic relation with her father in which he was the one who helped but was unavailable emotionally and physically. She also related to me as she had to her mother, who set standards of right and wrong and who denied access to the father. She sought to get to me in an emotional relationship as she had wanted to get to her father, and she fought my refusal of a physical relation as she had wanted to fight her mother's prohibitions.

Many times the therapist will find that this multiple transference situation obtains. The patient has formed his ways of relating in terms of the powerful, important figures of early years. The therapist comes to represent these several figures at various times. Indeed, there is reason to believe that transferences which are difficult to resolve are so because a second transference may be hidden under the more obvious one.

Conclusion

Each of us emerges into life in essential dependency on our parents and others. Our early learnings, the teaching of the people on whom we depend, and our experiences of fear combine in obscuring the existential reality of our situation. Among the most potent of apparent protections from contingency and tragedy are our relations to certain others. We learn and are encouraged to use symbiotic partnerships to disavow responsibility for our choices, to displace guilt for our failure to actualize our potentials for authentic living. These symbiotic relations become patterned around certain key figures in our experience and provide us with a relationship repertoire that we attempt to reemploy with other figures who enter our lives in later years. The result is that we enter into relation with our psychotherapists in a manner which inevitably includes much that is parataxic. The mature psychotherapist seeks to discriminate that which is authentic in his encounter with the patient from that which is distortedly carried over from the patient's past. In doing so, he is enabled to appreciate deeply the subjective life of his patient and to help the patient win free of the encumbering "dead hand of the past" and achieve genuine presence in his own right in the now.

9—*Tragedy and the psychotherapeutic processes*

A leading manufacturer of ladies' cosmetics uses a design on the boxes in which his products come that is eloquent in expressing much of our cultural attitude about tragedy and joy. The design is a representation of one of the classic dramatic masks, that of comedy. The traditionally paired mask of tragedy is absent! It seems fitting that in addition to the manufacturer's name, the only other word on that cover is "Hollywood." This is characteristic of much in our society, which seeks only comedy, which attempts to deny tragedy, and through which we rob ourselves of the full flavor of our being while placing ourselves in genuine and terrible jeopardy.

The existential view is that tragedy is very much a part of our being in the world, that it is one expression of the significance of our being, and that the denial of tragedy means the debasement of our being. Tragedy says that what we do matters, that our choices make a difference, that living is truly a life-and-death matter. The fully aware person can no more deny tragedy than he can deny gravitation.

EXISTENTIAL JOY

Joy, in turn, has suffered from the suppression of tragedy. We find ourselves expending more and more of our substance, our time, and our energies on "amusements" that provide little genuine joy. Passive spectators uninvolved with performances by people paid to be funny seldom experience much true joy. Meantime, with tragedy we have shelved our capacity to take joy in so much that is potentially joyous: a child's impishness, a friend's conversation, a tussle with a resistive problem, singing to one's self, awe in the presence of the stars, and so much else.

In this chapter I will give greater attention to tragedy than to joy because it is tragedy that has been more directly suppressed both popularly and professionally in our culture. However, this emphasis should not be taken—as it sometimes is—to indicate that the existential view is gloomy per se. Indeed, it is our contention that only through reincorporating tragedy into our awareness of being can we regain the more genuine experiences of joy. Arthur Miller (1951) writes, ". . . tragedy implies more optimism in its author than does comedy, and its final result ought to be the reinforcement of the on-looker's brightest opinions of the human animal" (p. 50).

In Chapter 20 we will discuss the fulfillment of one's being that comes with actualization of one's potential and that brings existential joy. As I will point out, when one celebrates his authentic being through his faith, his commitment, his creativity, and his love, he finds a sense of fulfillment, even of transcendence, which is the very essence of existential joy.

It may be noted in concluding this introduction that the concept and phenomenon of tragedy are not frequently found in the American psychological, or even the psychotherapeutic,[1] literature. One suspects a process of repression is generally at work, just as it was regarding sexuality in Freud's day.

Meaning of Tragedy

Man finds himself thrown into a world of infinite possibilities where each moment is a choice point, each act gives life (actuality) to some possibilities and condemns others to oblivion. From each such

---
[1] A quick look into the indexes of one hundred current books in psychotherapy and psychoanalysis disclosed the astonishing fact the words "tragedy" or "tragic" occurred but three times. All three such references were to literary matters; none dealt with tragedy in the lives, personalities, or treatment courses of patients.

choice branch unimaginable consequences. It is this very unimaginable quality that is at the base of man's living in contingency. Contingency here means that any act has an infinite array of possible outcomes and man can at any point recognize only some finite part of this infinite array. Man organizes his choices, his adaptations, in terms of his estimation of the possibility of various outcomes and tries in the process to increase his chances of actualizing that which he wants in his life, while diminishing the probabilities of that which he does not want. The impossibility of assuring the outcomes of one's actions, the consequences of one's choices, means that always there exists the possibility of tragedy ensuing from any choice which one makes. This is a possibility against which we can never be completely insured.

Tragedy, then, resides in man's nature. Tragedy resides in the fact that we can never know enough to protect ourselves and those whose welfare we cherish against the unfortunate consequences of our own conscious and unconscious choices and actions.

An Example. It is easiest to demonstrate tragedy in its more extreme and dramatic forms, as when a father tries to safeguard his child's welfare and perhaps chooses to have that child inoculated with a serum, only to have an unfortunate result issue. Those who early sought the Salk vaccine to protect their children from polio certainly did so with every intent of reducing the likelihood that their children would ever be afflicted with the dread disease. Certainly they had the hope that their foresightedness would mean that contingency was greatly reduced. And yet some of those children were given defective vaccine, with the result that the parents' choices actually resulted in the children being stricken by polio, and in some cases those children died. This is the essence of existential tragedy. We can never know enough, our best efforts can never be enough, our strongest intent can never suffice to assure the outcome we desire.

In its ultimate conception, tragedy is simply this, that the undesired and even feared outcome ensues despite all avail and because of some choice we have made. However, our understanding of tragedy and its role in human experience must fill out this overly skeletal statement.

THE CLASSICAL VIEW OF TRAGEDY

Aristotle observed (Cooper, 1947; Magill and McCreal, 1961) that there were three main elements to the tragic situation: the reversal of fortune, the discovery, and the suffering. Tragedy, Aristotle held, comes about as a result of *hamartia*, which is variously translated as a "tragic flaw" or "error in judgment" of the central figure. Existentially these two meanings are close, for it is the "flaw" of being finite that underlies many of our "errors in judgment."

The classic view often referred also to *hubris* or pride, holding that the tragic figure had brought about his downfall through his arrogance. Arthur Miller (1951, p. 48) comments on this point in a pungent fashion, "The flaw, or crack in the character, is really nothing . . . but his inherent unwillingness to remain passive in the face of what he conceives to be a challenge to his dignity . . ." Miller argues that it is the commitment to the attainment or maintenance of one's dignity which is crucial to the concept of tragedy. While this may be most pertinent for dramatic tragedy, a broader concept better characterizes the tragedy potential in daily living. This is presented in the following analysis.

THE TRAGIC SEQUENCE

We may conceive of the tragedy as a single event, as a reaction to an event, or—as proposed here—a sequence of human experience embracing choice, event, and emotional response to the event. For purposes of exposition, let me list these as steps:

1. I make certain, committed choices in my life.
2. As contingencies work out, those choices are pivotal in bringing about a result I would have forestalled had I but known it would occur.
3. I recognize and take responsibility for the pivotal role my choices played in bringing about the result. This is the acceptance of existential guilt.
4. I suffer the consequences, emotionally and otherwise, of what I have thus occasioned. This is the existential grief.

This conceptualization implicitly recognizes that all untoward happenings have in them something of the tragic, since almost without exception we could link the outcome back to choices at least distantly ours. However, we need to make a realistic distinction between those linkages of choice and outcome that are casual and distant and those that are immediate and crucial. Much of the therapeutic task lies in this latter area, for our patients try to persuade themselves that their choices were really only remotely connected to the outcomes when in fact they may have been pivotal.

An Example. Let us examine an oversimplified example in order to grasp better the tragic sequence:

> Arnold insists that the failure of his marriage is due to the conflict between his wife and his mother, in which he has had little part. Arnold tries to avoid the tragic recognition of how his life has been embittered by his choice not to insist his mother live by herself.

The tragedy exists, though muted by Arnold's suppression. You will observe each phase of the defining model presented above.

1. Arnold's choices, first to marry Betty and second to have his mother live with them.
2. The destruction of Arnold and Betty's marriage and all the hopes, love, and promise it once held.
3. Arnold seeks to deny the pivotal role of his choices, but obviously at some level of consciousness he is aware of his part in the situation.
4. Arnold's suffering is transmuted by his self-deception (resistance) into a general bitterness and irritability that brings him to psychotherapy.

Tragedy and the Therapeutic Work

The outline of the tragic sequence in the case of Arnold will make evident that the therapeutic task is basically that of resistance analysis. However, it is worthwhile to elaborate on the particular significance of the tragic element in conditioning the work that must be done to resolve such resistances. Similarly, it is useful to spell out the constructive consequences that may be attained by the effective carrying through of this therapeutic process.

For convenience in thinking about the matter, we may consider five facets of the therapeutic work: Disclosure of the general resistance pattern, identification of the particular points of focal emotional significance, working through to the acceptance of tragedy and guilt, facilitating the "purging" effect of the grief, and confronting the existential tragedy of the loss of being.[2]

DISCLOSING THE GENERAL RESISTANCE

In Chapters 6 and 7 I elaborated on the nature of the resistance and the work of the therapist in aiding the patient to reduce the resistance's disruption of his authenticity. Usually the therapist is first alerted to the presence of an evasion of tragedy when he is engaged in helping the patient become aware of his resistances. In the work of "peeling the onion," as we have called it, the therapist will often note that important sources and reinforcing focal events for some of the layers of the resistance reside in certain experiences of the patient. Concurrently, patient and therapist are often recognizing these—and possibly other—experiences as landmarks in the patient's life. The patient's associations may return to such events again and again, sometimes to the patient's conscious surprise.

> When Wally was first married, he tried to do everything in as nearly an ideal way as possible. He avoided any conflict with his young wife, whom he loved deeply, and he made no demands on her. When she was moody, he showed his hurt but said nothing. She evidently needed to try to break down what must have seemed a wall of reserve or even disdain. She became argumentative, rebellious, and undependable. Sometime after their first child was born, Wally and his wife had their first fight. Bursting through the months of suppression, Wally's anger was violent and extreme. He called her terrible names and ended up hitting her. She looked at him through tears of fear and hopelessness and walked out of the house, never to return. In his therapy, seven years later, Wally came back again and again to that fight and his wife's last, long look

---

[2] As I have frequently pointed out in these pages, such analyses as this do some violence to the actual transactions of the therapeutic interview. Such an analysis is a heuristic aid only if the reader recognizes that these aspects are all part of the same process and are separated out chiefly to facilitate the communication between writer and reader. By no means is any step-by-step procedure implied.

at him before she left. Also in his therapy, the resistance analysis soon came to Wally's efforts to be "nice." From his childhood he had had those words drilled into him, and they clearly meant to avoid conflict, violence, and demandingness. With the therapist, Wally was always "nice," even at the cost of being genuine.

This synopsis of Wally's experience highlights the relation of his resistance of "being nice" to the tragic fight with his wife, which ended their marriage. It should be made explicit that this connection was not as simply brought out in Wally's actual associations in the therapeutic hours. There, the pattern of Wally's constant efforts to keep all relations "nice" emerged in many different contexts with only occasional linkage to his first marriage. Concurrently, Wally found memories of the fight that ended the marriage recurring, even though consciously he considered he had "recovered" from the hurt of his divorce.

The key resistance in Wally's case is not just the pattern of trying to "be nice," as important as that is. It is, rather, the closely related urgency to deny conflict and need. Wally's use of denial was such that he could not let himself recognize that the old hurt from his divorce still lingered. It was only when this dependence on denial became the focus of the resistance analysis that the tie to his first marriage became evident.

So it is in many patients' therapeutic courses. As the resistances are peeled back, connections between feelings and strivings on the one hand and life events on the other emerge into prominence. It is not a matter of deduction that makes these linkages. When the resistance analysis proceeds well, the connections emerge into the patient's awareness with a sense of recognition that is its own validation.

IDENTIFYING FOCAL EVENTS

From what has just been said, it will be evident that the therapist will do well to become aware of the focal events in the patient's life. In some ways this is a needless counsel. Unless a therapist is intervening so much as to disrupt the patient's spontaneous account of his awarenesses and concerns, that very report of the patient will teach both therapist and patient many of the significant events around which emotions focus.

Two codicils need to be appended to this generalization. First, there are usually some apparently focal events around which the patient's associations gather but whose significance never is completely uncovered. Second, there may be repressive forces at work that prevent a key event from emerging into awareness for some time. Thus, one cannot always use the volunteered key events as guides to focal emotional concerns. Let me illustrate my second conditioning statement.

> Zelda found herself worried persistently that her friendships for other women might turn out to have homosexual implications. She had never had mature homosexual experience or even a clear impulse toward such an experience so far as she was able to recall. She had participated in the sexual games of children but with typical disregard for whether boys or girls were involved. After some months of work with her resistances, however, she abruptly recovered a memory which helped to explain her preoccupation, which otherwise had seemed to have little foundation: When she was twenty-six years old, she had visited her uncle and his family. She slept with a girl cousin of eighteen. During the night she awoke with a strong erotic feeling and found her hand was on her cousin's body. She quickly withdrew and soon was asleep again. In reporting this recovered memory, Zelda said, "It's like I always remembered it, and yet didn't know it."

Zelda's recovery of her memory is again clearly a product of the orderly analysis of the resistance. It may even be speculated that a deductive approach (which might have reasoned that Zelda's preoccupation with homosexuality indicated some event she had repressed and thus sought directly for the event) would have brought about either a deeper repression or a recovery in which the emotional element of recognition ("I always remembered it") was lacking.

ACCEPTING EXISTENTIAL GUILT

This is a point at which the existential-analytic approach may be most readily distinguished from other views of the therapeutic significance of tragedy. Let us illustrate this by returning to Wally and the tragic event in his life, his fight with his wife that ended their marriage. Having disclosed the emotions focused around this incident, some psychotherapists may teach implicitly, "You really should not blame yourself for this fight and its consequences because you were taught that you should try always to be nice. That teaching wasn't very realistic but that isn't your fault." Another group of therapists might convey a mildly different message, "You were afraid of your anger because of your earlier experiences with it when your father was so punishing and your mother rejected you for it. Of course, you had to keep it hidden until it broke through that time with your wife." The latter approach might, in time, go further to link this event with other earlier incidents to portray the reenactment of Oedipal conflicts.

Each of these explanations has its values, but the existential-analytic view has a major criticism of them. Each makes of the patient a hapless object moved by forces beyond his control, determined by his parents and his earlier life. To be sure, this may reduce blame, and blame is an impediment to therapeutic work and authentic living. But these explanations also—sometimes, indeed, by intent—seek to reduce guilt. If one is not responsible, if one is but an object, then guilt is meaningless. This is too great a price, we would hold.

To confront tragedy in one's life, the existential view insists, requires that one seek out his responsibility for bringing that tragedy about. It means accepting the guilt for the choices one made which led to the hurtful outcome.

> Wally was helped to recognize that it was his *decision* to deny conflict, strong feelings, and his needs which directly led up to the fight with his wife. When he became self-blaming, he was helped to see the roots of his choice to be nice in his earlier learnings at home. But when he sought to blame his mother and his wife, he was shown how he had deliberately suppressed his own feelings time and again and how this had brought about a strained and ungenuine relationship with his wife. It was a painful recognition to accept, but once Wally had accepted it his whole attitude about the relation with his first wife began to change. For the first time he expressed some appreciation for how isolated she must have felt, and his sorrow for the "death" of his marriage was appreciably less tinged with the bitterness that had formerly been so strong.

YIELDING TO EXISTENTIAL GRIEF

When we spoke of the change in the quality of Wally's sorrow over the death of his marriage, we were pointing to the beginnings of his acceptance of existential grief. This grief is essential to the "purging"—as Aristotle (Cooper, 1947) termed it—that is, the freeing of the emotions from the distortions of the resistance in order that greater authenticity may become available. Aristotle also spoke of the cathartic effect of tragedy (Magill and McGreal, 1961), and this is akin to familiar therapeutic catharsis.

There is nothing mystical about tragic catharsis. What is involved is the same pattern of resolution of the resistance to a feared feeling. Once that resistance has been resolved and the feeling formerly warded off is now experienced (the grief), there is a renewed openness to experience (authenticity). It must be underlined, however, that this sequence is heavily dependent upon the patient's maintaining awareness of himself as the *subject*, rather than the *object*, of the tragic experience or, saying it differently, the *author* and not simply a *character* of the play. In other words, the patient must accept responsibility for helping to bring the tragedy about (guilt) if he is to experience a genuine catharsis and increase in existential freedom.

NON-BEING: THE TRAGIC CONSEQUENCE

Still there is one further phase of the therapeutic work connected to tragedy. Let us again use Wally for our illustration.

> The real tragedy for Wally was not the fight with his wife or the ensuing divorce. The real tragedy was the death of the life Wally, his wife, and his baby daughter could have had together, and its replacement with seven embittered years for Wally (and whatever it cost his wife and child). Between his divorce and his coming to therapy, life was frustrating, hollow, and extremely lonely.

The point to recognize in Wally's case—as in so many—is that could Wally have met the tragic event, the fight with his wife, in full authenticity, the tragic sequence would have been completed then. He would have experienced the guilt of having brought about this conflict through his own choices and would have known the grief for the destruction of his relationship with his wife. Then, having dealt with this guilt and its attendant grief, Wally would have been purged and freed to meet his life with new genuineness in the now.

Unfortunately we are seldom able to meet our experience so elegantly. Certainly Wally was not able to. Very often we react to the tragic event with a kind of search for a psychological scapegoat on which to fasten the neurotic blame that screens our actual guilt. Typically we choose a scapegoat in terms of our characteristic defenses (resistances), and thus, often, we compound our alienation from authentic being in our lives.

Thus Wally assigned the blame for the break-up of his marriage to his wife, to his lack of finances, and especially to the breakdown of his determination tightly to control and hold in his feelings. He said, implicitly, to himself: "Since my marriage ended in the fight with my wife, the difficulty is in having the feelings which led to that fight. When I kept myself in control and was 'nice' we didn't fight. Therefore I shall have to exercise even tighter control." At a deeper level, Wally had to make another decision also. This one was even less conscious: "Since it hurts so very much to have conflict with someone I love, and since it's hard to exercise control over my feelings if I'm so much in love, I will never let myself get so deeply involved with another person again." Unwittingly, thereby Wally laid down the first step of the continuation of the tragic sequence in his life.

Hubris. Wally's decision to prevent himself from getting so involved emotionally and his resolve to suppress his feelings even more rigidly are violations of his genuine being, decisions to give up some of his authenticity in favor of non-being. Such decisions are the very stuff of the classic *hubris,* or arrogant pride. It is beside the point to protest that Wally was hurt and desperate when he made his resolves. One may indeed feel sympathy for him, but one needs to recognize the arrogance implicit in Wally's decision to go against his own nature.

Wally's new choices—to be more strict in his control of himself and to avoid involvement—led to the new tragic event. In this instance, the event is more accurately a spread of seven years of many incidents. Wally inevitably lived a life of superficial relationships, promiscuity, frustration, and covert anger. When he came to therapy many of the values he once had cherished were apparently abandoned. Little in his current living gave him satisfaction.

The Therapeutic Sequence

Therapy had to help Wally first to reconfront his responsibility for the failure of his marriage and then to trace how his subsequent choices had brought about the years of non-being and emptiness.

This therapeutic sequence is necessary. Its value is not only to complete the tragic sequence and free the person for better reality functioning however. It is essential also if the patient is to reclaim autonomy and choice. When Wally denies that his choice brought about the failure of his marriage and the misery of the subsequent years he denies some of his potency in his own life. Only as he reincorporates the responsibility for these choices can he free himself to make current choices on a truly aware basis. *The repression of awareness of past responsibility inevitably requires for its maintenance additional repressions of present possibilities.*

DEBILITATING EFFECT OF REASSURANCE

Too often, we as therapists have tried to overprotect our patients from the suffering that is essential to the working-through of the tragic in their lives. We have encouraged the assignment of blame and responsibility to parents, employers, spouses, and others and in the process unwittingly enfeebled our patients and reduced their authenticity in their own lives. A therapist might say of Arnold, whom I described early in this chapter, "Poor fellow, it's hurt him enough to have his marriage go on the rocks. Why add pain by insisting he see how he brought it about? Let's just make sure he gets free of his mother before he marries again. If he needs to blame his wife, it's no harm done because she's out of his life now anyway, and it won't hurt her."

While it may be true that this seemingly humane deception may not hurt Arnold's former wife, it certainly will hurt Arnold and do much to make him less aware and open to new relations and experiences (Moustakas, 1962).

RECOVERING AUTHENTICITY

Just as with the tragic event which was our entering point in understanding Wally's life, so now with the tragic consequences: the patient must confront how his choices have brought about that which has ensued. And this, too, needs to be as clear a confrontation as may be possible. When this grief work is sincerely done, then genuine vitality of experience is noticeably gained. The patient experiences that the tragedy is indeed past, and he finds the event and its sequel no longer persist in his thoughts and feelings.

> The change in Wally was very evident. Where once he had been liked in the therapy group because of his nice ways but had not been really engaged with anyone, now he became somewhat less frequent in his participation but startlingly direct. In time, he became the undesignated patient-therapist of the group. He was turned to by the others for help in expressing feelings, for aid in correcting perceptions, or for support in threatening exchanges. He did not, by any means, always provide these. Sometimes he was too involved with his own feelings, but the group could still value his extremely genuine response when he did express himself.

Tragedy and Related Experiences

It will be useful to offer some additional observations on the nature of existential tragedy and to put it in perspective with the whole of human experience so far as we are able. Tragedy is, whether recognized or not, a part of every human life. When opportunity comes (usually in psychotherapy) to investigate any life fully, the role and significance of tragedy needs to be appreciated. Unfortunately, our cultural conspiracy to suppress tragedy means that these important, pivotal experiences are often underappreciated. For tragedy is that: pivotal. Those major events of unhappy consequence each of us contributes to bringing about in his life are the crossroads from which stem marked changes in personality and experience. Thus tragedy may be a powerful growth-facilitating influence or a point of retreat from living.

SORROW AND DEPRESSION

Tragedy is not the same as sorrow. In sorrow there is regret but not guilt. We sorrow for that misery for which we are in no way responsible but which we can emphatically appreciate. Tragedy is not the same as depression, which frequently masks anger and may be part of the suppression of the tragic. Tragedy is not an emotion but a life event or series of events.

SUPERSTITION

Each of us engages in extensive maneuvers designed to forestall the possibility of a tragic outcome. Many of these partake of the nature of magic and involve unreal aspirations to secure immunity from tragedy. For many, a belief in God is an attempt in this vein, and all too often a belief in God is a kind of deal the believer attempts to enter into with the Deity to guarantee him exceptional protection. When tragedy strikes, the believer then feels betrayed in his contract and accuses God of failing his obligations. Such a use (or misuse) of religious faith is today, I think, largely rejected by many leaders in theology (Tillich, 1952). Of course there are many other ways in which we try to forestall the dire products of contingency (see Chapter 4). A wide variety of manifestly and implicitly superstitious behaviors are engaged in by various people, all ultimately seeking to insure that which is uninsurable.

GUILT AND RESPONSIBILITY

When I cited the conscientious parents who sought polio vaccine for their loved children and pointed to the tragic effects that occurred in some instances, I was also describing a situation from which existential guilt arises. The parents who secured this vaccine for their children doubtlessly in many instances had to face the terrible fact that their actions had brought about the injury or death of their children. If they faced the matter candidly, they might well have recognized that they experienced guilt. This existential guilt is always latently present when our actions are founded, as they must be, on knowledge insufficient to prevent the undesired outcome. It is regrettable, but real, that many of the crucial decisions of our lives, whether or not they are recognized as such at the time we make them, are founded on less knowledge, less awareness than is potentially available to us at such times. In such choices we bear the load of responsibility even though we have the best excuses as to why we did not know more when we made the decision. Therein lies existential guilt: it is the product of our limitedness in an unlimited world, a product of our finiteness in an infinite universe. Existential guilt is a part of man's condition. It is a matter neither for dismay nor for inert acceptance. It needs to be recognized as a given of our situation.

Conclusion

Our emphasis upon the existential significance of tragedy is regarded by some as an instance of the unhappy or frightening aspect of the existential orientation. This is a misunderstanding of or resistance to the meaning of tragedy. However, it would be inappropriate to conclude my comments without recognizing again that tragedy is but one aspect of man's situation. When we have recognized that existential guilt and existential tragedy are omnipresent, we have said but part of the story of man's circumstance. There is an existential joy, an existential fulfillment that gains from the very trials over the contingency which surrounds us. This joy takes its root in man's freedom, which accepts openly that he is limited and does not comprehend all. Whenever we know *all* that we need to know to make a decision, we make no decision but are determined by what we know. Our joy arises from facing the unknown and affirming ourselves. Fulfillment is the flower of accepting our finiteness and yet partaking of the infinite.

To recognize the fact of tragedy is but the necessary complement to experiencing the fact of growing. We are neither hapless creatures of an all-governing fate, nor yet are we the complete masters of all circumstance. Many in our culture tend to join in the suppression of the recognition of tragedy and guilt. But it is this very lopsided view of man's situation, the emphasis on comedy and the suppression of tragedy, that makes joy and comedy themselves shallow, that robs them of dimension and vitality and consonance with man's being: ". . . a seasonless world where you shall laugh, but not all of your laughter, and weep, but not all of your tears" (Gibran, 1955, p. 12).

10 — *The existential crisis*

The existential crisis is an event of major importance that may occur in the course of intensive psychotherapy as a patient comes to the climax of his work. The existential crisis does not seem to occur in all successful cases, at least not in clearly identifiable form. However, when it does occur, its handling is uniquely demanding of the therapist's best sensitivity and skill and crucially important to the patient's successful treatment outcome.

THERAPEUTIC FAILURE: THE CASE OF FRANK

Frank was forty years old the second year we worked together. An artist of more than ordinary talent, he was beginning at long last to find recognition for his gifts. The struggle for training and then for recognition had been costly in many ways. Now an end to that struggle, at least to its more debilitating aspects, was in sight. But Frank was a homosexual.

Frank had come to me once before and prematurely fled therapy after six months. He had also had two other abortive beginnings on therapy with two other therapists. When he returned to me he announced that he wanted me "to prepare (him) for confirmation as a human being," but Frank could never quite tell me what he meant by this. At times I felt he knew; at other times I was quite sure that he could not let himself know. And then in the second year of therapy, when his creative talents were beginning to earn him recognition, when he had a sense of progress in his therapy, he began to risk expressing his regret over being homosexual. He began to do the grief work (see Chapter 9) of recognizing the loss of his life which had been, at least in part, occasioned by his homosexuality. (Let me make an aside to say that I am not implying a value judgment, nor did Frank particularly. What he regretted was the loss of a sense of complete belonging with other people, the loss of being part of a family, and particularly the loss of having children of his own.)

As he worked along in that year Frank met a young man, Teddy, who—so far as I could tell—was bisexual in practice but teetering between accepting homosexuality as a way of life and trying to break loose from it. Teddy was very attractive to Frank. He was artistically gifted in Frank's own field, and he was not coarse or "fruity," qualities that Frank despised in many of his homosexual acquaintances. Frank invited Teddy to come and live with him. Teddy did not know of Frank's homosexuality, but as they lived together Frank's attraction to the young man and the hints Teddy was dropping of his own ambivalence created a constant intrusion on Frank's awareness. At length the day came when Frank faced his intentions of seducing Teddy and yet experienced terrible conflict within himself about doing so. There was little doubt that a seduction would be successful. Frank himself could read the meaning of Teddy's flight into frantic heterosexual adventures.

We were now building to the crisis in Frank's therapy, which is to say, in his life. The major options he faced can be portrayed by paraphrases from Frank's own awarenesses. On the one hand, he was saying:

Change is possible. What will change me is not some new drug or different therapeutic technique—both of which I have tried many times—it is not something external to me that I just haven't been lucky enough to find yet. What will change me is—and always has been—within me.

I can be loved by others who are not homosexuals, and I can love other than homosexually.

But even as these awarenesses became more explicitly the expression of an emerging inner conviction, other awarenesses also were screaming within Frank:

I am indeed forty years old.

My life is half over, and, if these new awarenesses are true, it has been needlessly wasted on by-paths.

I can't bear the awful pain of thinking I brought this about; yet I no longer can blame my mother or my heredity.

This was the essence of Frank's situation. I have oversimplified it somewhat by leaving out many of the attendant awarenesses on either side of the choice. At core was the choice of taking responsibility for the past in order to have opportunity in the present and future.

Frank was in an existential crisis. I know that now. I did not know it then. In that difference lies the reason that I failed as Frank's therapist. This is the report of that failure, a failure which has taught me much.

BASIS OF THE FAILURE

Frank had been helped to work out his relation to his mother, which was, as may have been anticipated, central to his homosexuality. He had exposed and partially abreacted his anguish over his age and his futility feelings. Much time had been spent drawing forth his elaborate "idealized image" of himself and what he should be, and he had begun to relinquish this while yet confronting its shadow, the "despised image" of himself (Horney, 1950). In all of this therapist and patient had worked well together, as Frank's very movement to the crisis testifies. Work on his characterological resistances had been productive, while that with the transference was only just begun. Yet despite all this, Frank's therapy failed.

It failed for three principal reasons. The first was a completely extraneous intrusion on the transference which came at a most unfortunate juncture. It was important, but had therapy otherwise been what Frank needed it to be, this intrusion alone would not have tipped the balance.

The second reason for the therapeutic failure lay in the counter-transference. What happened, it can be recognized in retrospect, was that the therapist was not as authentically present for Frank as Frank needed. Hindsight reveals intellectual competitiveness that resulted in the therapist being more reliant at times on documented argumentation than on personal confrontation—for this and possibly other reasons he tended to be more detached and more abstract than was required.

Finally, and most importantly, the therapist's grasp of the crisis Frank was facing was too limited, not nearly bold enough to help Frank truly to confront the way his life was in the balance. The therapist accurately assessed what the issue regarding Teddy meant in terms of the therapeutic situation at that time, but the therapist missed its greater, its existential significance. Here is what happened.

> Repeatedly I interpreted to Frank that Teddy was, in truth, Frank himself of twenty years earlier. Teddy's surrender to homosexuality would be a way for Frank to try to prove to himself that his own homosexuality was not a matter of choice but of fate or biology or of the unwitting effects of his relation to his mother. If Frank chose not to seduce Teddy, I urged, he was saying in effect that he had choice and that he need not have been homosexual. Frank's fear, I insisted, was of facing the wasted years, the loss of his youth and his young maturity.

THE CRUCIAL DIFFERENCE

So far, so good. This was essentially a very accurate interpretation. Frank had to see just this to be free. This is a necessary but not a sufficient recognition. It is an incomplete, overly cautious conception of Frank's plight. What needed to be seen was that *Frank was weighing in the balance his whole being.* So detached have we grown about the most vital aspects of our lives, that sentence may not have carried all it needs to transmit. It is meant most literally: Frank was weighing his whole being in the balance. By centering his interpretations around the issue of homosexuality, the therapist cooperated with Frank's resistance to recognizing the more pervasive question: "Am I indeed free to choose my life?" Frank's pattern in his homosexuality, in his profession, in his religious life, in many ways was that of the creature instead of the creator (Fromm, 1959). His artistic work itself was probably less than it could have been had he been more able to be the creator. This, of course, was his idealized image, but it was something he dared not actualize.

The result of his limited view which the therapist pressed on Frank was that both failed to recognize the genuine tragedy which existed and from which Frank (and the therapist?) unconsciously drew back. This was the tragedy that his own choices had killed the man he could have been, had forestalled his becoming the artist his potential offered, had turned him away from being the husband and father he deeply wished to be, had relinquished more than twenty years of his life to a shadow world of incompleteness in being. Under the influence of his own training and his unconscious need to defend against his own tragic losses, the therapist encouraged Frank's tendency to emasculate himself of choice potency.

    I carefully traced Frank's symbiotic relation with his mother and how it had led to his homosexuality. I denied his sense of guilt as a neurotic residue rather than recognizing it as the existential stirring it indeed was.

    And so I failed Frank and myself. I became overly concerned to protect Teddy from homosexuality and insisted that Frank look at the decision to seduce Teddy in terms of social morality. I argued logically and well for too limited a view of what was happening. Frank did seduce Teddy, was so overwhelmed with guilt that he broke the relation with him, felt my withholding as censure, and broke off treatment.

    Before leaving this account of Frank let me recognize that I have a real awareness of guilt in thinking about this man. I do not think this is neurotic guilt since I do not feel self-blaming about it. I do feel sorrow for my part in the outcome. I do take responsibility for my counter-transference and my limited perception. From this I take, also, a renewed valuing of growth and responsibility. I shall always feel some grief when I think of Frank, but I shall also feel greater courage in confronting and increased commitment to the man who is in Frank's place in my office today.

Conceptualizing the Existential Crisis

I will make a series of defining statements about the existential crisis as it occurs in psychotherapy. From these we can build a concept of the experience that will be useful in proposing therapeutic steps for aiding the patient constructively to confront his existential crisis.

The existential crisis is an experience of heightened choice anxiety.
　　Every choice is also a renunciation. From this bilateral meaning of choice flows the emotion of concern. When the relinquishment really matters in the patient's life then choice becomes, in truth, a matter of administering death to some possibilities while giving actuality to others. Recognizing this, either consciously or unconsciously, we are in anxiety. When the recognition is undistorted, this is existential anxiety and need not result in loss of authenticity. When we need to distort the choice and its alternatives—through denial, displacement, rationalization, or other resistances—we experience a neurotic anxiety that begins the malignant cycle that destroys our authenticity.

The existential crisis involves the eruption of existential anxiety.
　　It seems likely (although my own observations are still too limited to confirm this point fully) that the existential crisis comes about when the various distortions (resistances) used to forestall existential anxiety have been dissolved or otherwise breached. This breaching of the defenses may come about because of various circumstances. In psychotherapy it would occur when the analytic work has been thorough and effective in peeling back layer after layer until the patient was released to come up against the very meaning of his life in one of its basic dimensions. This naked confrontation with the very givenness of being cannot but be filled with existential anxiety. The crisis is that of responding to the givenness of being with courage (Tillich, 1952) and incorporating the anxiety or of erecting new resistances to obscure awareness of the dread confrontation.
　　Existential anxiety, truly faced, is a fact of being, and thus there is no way to escape it. Neurotic solutions seem to offer such escape, and therein lies their seductive quality. Seeming certainty (Schwartz and Wolf, 1959) and therefore relief from ontic dread is contained in the seeking for perfection, guiltlessness, complete dependency, authority, or whatever symptom formation is used to deny contingency.

The existential crisis involves one's whole way of being in the world.
　　It is difficult to find a phraseology that can convey adequately the awful meaning of this observation. Only as one experiences such a crisis himself (or perhaps as one participates in it vicariously with

another with whom he is deeply involved) can there be genuine recognition of its terrible comprehensiveness. Here is Ken's attempt while deep in the experience to convey what it meant for him.

> I walked along a perilous bridge very high in the starless night. The path was scarcely wide enough for my feet. It had been broader. It was becoming narrower. Each step increased the sense of dizzy height, and my bowels were clutched in the wrench of my fear. Behind me—the awareness gradually crept over me—the bridge was crumbling away to nothing. And the path became narrower and higher. . . .
>
> And then there was no more bridge. I stood on a tiny point in the inky night. . . .
>
> If only there had been a star, but the stars were all gone. If a cloud had moved in the vaults above, but the clouds had evaporated. If a vague firmament had promised only to smash my falling form beneath, but the firmament had disintegrated. If another figure could hold my hand as we plunged, but no other clasp met my groping fingers.
>
> There was nothing: nothing but my terror, my aloneness, my emptiness. To draw a breath was to stir the griping cauldron of my stomach's torment. And breath itself was reluctant. And so I leaped. . . .

We face many choices, and not a few involve us in anxiety of some degree. The existential crisis is, however, a crisis of our existence, our whole being. It does not seem likely that we can experience it often. When we do find ourselves at that crossroad, everything we have and everything we are is on the scales. Such a crisis is involved in the conversion experience, whether it be religious or otherwise. It is not, by any means, an event only of the therapeutic situation.

The growth alternative in the crisis is always fundamentally unknown.

The writer of the autobiographical material quoted above describes a "leap in the dark." This is the very nature of the existential crisis. It contrasts a known but unacceptable way of being with an unknown alternative. Sometimes the expression, "a leap of faith" is used. This is an accurate characterization if it be recognized that this may well be objectless faith—not faith in something, especially something external to the person making the leap.

Basically it is an act of faith to risk a total reorganization of one's way of being in the world without having an alternative clearly at hand. It is not even accurate to speak of having "faith in one's self," because the self, as a summation of one's past experiences, is exactly what one seeks to leap away from. Perhaps, if we must specify faith in what, it is most nearly accurate to say faith in being as of the moment of leaping only.

The growth alternative includes the acceptance of existential guilt and tragedy.
Since the leap of faith is in essence an act of faith in one's own being, it follows that that from which one leaps, the previous way of being in the world, was in some measure less than faithful to one's potential. Existential guilt is the feeling aspect of the experiencing of one's self as failing one's potential. Existential tragedy is the experiential product (see Chapter 9; also Boss, 1962; Fingarette, 1962a, b). As I showed in discussing Frank's plight, the grief of recognizing and accepting the responsibility for that which has been truly tragic in one's life powerfully colors the choice situation. Yet it is essential that just this pain of acceptance be taken on by the patient, for only in this way can he preserve his own integrity of experience. To deny the tragic pain is to deny one's own freedom; to accept it is to purge one's being and free one's life for current living.

Therapeutic Procedure in the Existential Crisis

Although the therapy situation is by no means the only locus of the existential crisis, it is unique in that it is the one place where this experience is deliberately fostered by encouraging the person to reduce his resistances to natural anxiety (in contrast, for example, to a crisis that may be precipitated by religious revivals, in which the external exhortation seems to be the stimulus). It is the responsibility and the opportunity of the therapist to be prepared conceptually and personally to engage with his patient in the crisis. It is proposed that the appropriate doctrine is that of, (a) clearly recognizing the impending crisis, (b) helping the patient reduce the confusions of his resistances so that he may confront the fundamental choice as directly as possible, and (c) demonstrating one's commitment to existential freedom by refraining from implicit or explicit efforts to influence the patient's choice. We will examine each of these now.

RECOGNIZING THE IMPENDING CRISIS

From all that has been said it might seem that the recognition of the existential crisis would be a relatively simple matter. Such is most definitely not the case. There are two principal influences working to make the recognition of the existential crisis difficult, though these often combine. The first is, of course, the resistance of the patient to the recognition of the terrible choice with which he is being confronted. The second is the corresponding resistance of the therapist to involvement, even if vicariously, with the guilty and tragic experience of his patient. These may combine into an unconscious conspiracy to forestall a full recognition and confrontation of the impending crisis. Such a conspiracy is illustrated in the counter-transference participation in misperceiving the existential crisis that Frank faced.

It is worth noting here that this is a point at which the existential conception makes a genuine difference in therapeutic strategy. Many times therapists having other conceptions may rest short of a recognition of the total life-weighing that is involved in the existential crisis. Certainly this is what happened in the work with Frank. The therapist saw Frank's projection of his ideal and despised selves into the struggle with the temptation to seduce Teddy. What he did not see was the genuinely total decision about his life that Frank confronted. Looking backward, one may speculate this was the unconscious meaning of Frank's statement that was quoted early in the report, "I want you to prepare me for confirmation as a human being." It is probable that only a rather thoroughly analyzed—that term is not used here in a parochial sense—psychotherapist can risk the dialogue with his patient which will bring him to the brink of the existential crisis.

AIDS IN RECOGNITION

I can make some tentative suggestions to aid the therapist in recognizing that the existential crisis impends; however, none of these suggestions will point to such explicit and clear-cut cues as to make this recognition a precise or objective matter. By its very nature this therapeutic task calls for the therapist to be a total, sensitive human being in intimate dialogue with his patient. There is no pseudo-objective substitute for this. To say it yet another way (for it is important to make this as clear as possible): the therapist's attempt to recognize his patient's movement toward an existential crisis is dependent primarily upon that therapist's authentic engagement with his patient. This presupposes the therapist has genuine access to his own subjective processes.

Mounting Tension. From this awareness of his own subjective processes and his empathic engagement with his patient, the therapist will become alerted by a sense of mounting tension that pervades all of his patient's work in the therapeutic hour, apparently without much direct regard for the particular content being developed.

Let me specify something more about that tension. (This is a difficult area since we have no glossary of well-accepted terms for discriminating these subjective sensings.) The kind of tension that precedes the coming to the crisis feels very different from the kind of tension born of fright and guilt and more typical of an anxious patient when he is new to the therapeutic undertaking. As best one can discriminate the two, the early tension is a compressing, a trying-to-hold-everything-still sort of feeling. The kind of tension the patient seems to emanate when he is frightened and guilty early in therapy conveys somehow the impression that the patient is trying to make himself small and motionless, that he is fearful of his own awareness and can allow it little freedom and can allow even less freedom to the expression of his awareness.

In contrast, the kind of tension that occurs as we mount toward an existential crisis seems to be characterized by an opening and freeing of awareness. Sometimes, it is true, the patient finds himself frightened by that opening and freeing, which seems to proceed from an inner dedication more powerful than the discomfort of the moment. This dedication is an inspiring phenomenon in its own right. The patient who has made such a commitment to life is a challenging and gratifying person to work with for the therapist. Such a patient accepts the tension of increasingly naked confrontation of his life without the constriction that tension often brings in other patients. The impression is that the patient finds himself flooded with many associations, not a few of which may appear irrational to everyday logic or shocking to the patient's traditional morality. It is as though the patient has somehow committed himself to exploration within himself in a way that brings him constantly new awareness, and, though he may be frightened, this opening and expanding experience continues, even tending at times to accelerate.

Focusing. The second of the cues to the impending crisis is most frequently evidenced in an increasing tendency for the patient's associations to draw together around particular foci. To say it differently, it is as though certain themes (not necessarily cognitive, sometimes more emotional or even fantastic) tend to get reiterated more and more frequently. Disparate associative items begin to come into relationship, and one gains an impression of an underlying and previously unrecognized unity or consistency. Often this can be characterized as the dawning awareness of the implicit style of life the patient has followed, albeit unwittingly. Clearly, the therapist's interpretations may facilitate this process, but, as with all good interpretive strategy, it is well if they neither lead it too far nor lag too far behind.

Another analogy may help to make this process more evident. The patient's associations, which have previously seemed isolated, may be thought of as musical figures scattered throughout a movement of a symphony. Now as we approach a climax, these isolated figures begin to be drawn together by the composer's genius. Certain reiterative themes, previously only implicit or incomplete, now begin to emerge with greater and greater forcefulness until, in a culmination, one or two emerge startlingly against the background of all that has gone before.

Renewed Resistance. The third cue to the development toward the crisis is frequently a re-emergence of resistance patterns that had been relinquished by the patient earlier in his therapeutic work. To continue the musical analogy of a moment ago, it is as though the major themes of the symphony begin to emerge and are first enunciated, but then there is a countertrend to the music which once again briefly breaks up the themes into their components so there must be a re-resolution and re-emergence with new force and in new configuration. Composers use this device not infrequently to increase the dramatic quality of their music. We find also in novels and plays that the author will seem to draw toward his climax and conclusion and then introduce a sudden, unexpected disruption of events just prior to the final climactic summation. So it is that the patient often will show a convergence of his associative themes and an apparent emergence of the one or two which are most significant in his life. Then a reintroduction of his characteristic resistances disrupts the smooth course of the therapeutic development. This seems to be a kind of last defense against the full emergence into awareness of the existential crisis.[1]

From these several kinds of subjective clues, the therapist may develop an appreciation for what impends with his patient. However, there is no catalogue of clues that can be adequate to this task. Here, more than in many places, the sensitively attuned instrumentality of the whole person of the therapist is required to serve the therapeutic process adequately.

Reducing Resistances

What has just been said indicates how crucial it is to recognize that the resistances are the counterforce to the emerging awareness of the patient's existential choice. The therapist frequently does well at this point to restrict the greater portion of his efforts to interpretations of resistance, allowing the patient to make the interpretations or explications of the choice components as these come into his consciousness. The theory behind this statement is that the therapist can very easily introduce contaminating material into the associative stream if he tries to anticipate just what the alternatives in the choice are. If, on the other hand, the therapist confines his interpretation to demonstrating the resistances with which the patient is struggling in his effort to gain full awareness, then the likelihood of such contamination from the therapist is reduced. Thus, in the work with Frank, the therapist would have intruded less upon the choice had he been freer from his own needs to try to forestall the seduction of Teddy and had he not voiced what *he* thought was the essential

---

[1] Some patients seem to go through a succession of these; though I think that may be brought about by my ineptness in recognition and facilitation of the emergence of the existential crisis. Other patients will show only one or no reintroduction of resistance maneuvers.

choice Frank was facing. By casting that choice in the terms that seemed to the therapist the significant ones (to be sure, these were terms Frank had also been using) the therapist constrained the breadth of his own and Frank's perceptions of the situation. Had the therapist devoted himself more fully to interpreting the acting-out as a resistance, to interpreting as denials the bursts of anger and vagueness that seemed to alternate in those last days of the work together, then Frank might have been more nearly able adequately to phrase his own dilemma.

Respecting Existential Freedom

It will be evident that this same philosophy is given point in our third strategic phase in working with the existential crisis, that of living out the therapist's commitment to freedom by providing the patient with maximum opportunity to make his own decision. Again in the case of Frank, the therapist's efforts to prevent Frank's seduction of Teddy operated to prevent Frank from having a clear field for making his own decision. The therapist was far too concerned with the substance of the decision and far too little aware of the process of Frank's facing the act of deciding.[2]

What is meant by trying to provide maximum freedom to the patient to make his own decision? First, it means that, in terms of therapist activity, a major attention to the resistance gives the patient the greatest likelihood of freedom. Second, the therapist, recognizing a patient is coming to such a choice point, needs most soberly and conscientiously to examine his own feelings about that choice so that he may be aware of any impulses to influence the patient. Third, the therapist must help to keep the full nature of the choice in focus. This means that he will need to be aware of each of the defining aspects of the existential crisis and alert to any of these the patient may be seeking to suppress. These defining aspects as we described them were as follows.

> *The existential crisis is an experience of heightened choice anxiety.*
>
> *The existential crisis involves the eruption of existential anxiety.*

---

[2] We may speculate about a possible conflict between one's sense of social ethics and his obligation to the therapeutic task, but for me, I cannot feel this is a valid reason for my course of action in working with Frank.

The existential crisis involves one's whole way of being in the world.

The growth alternative in the crisis is always fundamentally unknown.

The growth alternative includes the acceptance of existential guilt and tragedy.

AIDING THE PATIENT

AVOID REASSURANCE

The therapist who tries to give the patient reassurance when that patient is confronting the existential crisis gives evidence that he, the therapist, does not appreciate the significance of what is happening. The difficulty with giving reassurance is not the inappropriateness of trying to ease the patient's feelings but the violation of the very meaning of the existential crisis. Any reassurance from the therapist can only be a denial of the authentic choice confrontation the patient experiences. From all that has been said above, it will be apparent that this experience of the existential crisis is irrevocably one which must be faced ultimately in the loneliness of one's own being. No other can join me in weighing my whole life's pattern against an unknown but different way of being. None can lighten my acceptance of my pain of tragedy and grief for the past. Therapists who attempt to bring their own support to the patient in this awful moment are acting on a counter-transference impulse and are serving their own resistances, not the patient's needs.

AVOID EXTRINSIC REWARDS

Sometimes the therapist will be drawn to try to find rewards for the patient in taking what the therapist deems to be the healthy alternative in the existential crisis. This would be like saying to Frank, "If you don't seduce Teddy, you'll probably find that you can enjoy his company more over a longer period of time," or "If you give up being homosexual, you'll find in time that there is much more thrilling satisfaction in heterosexual love-making." The therapist cannot know that these sorts of projected rewards are indeed so for the patient. Moreover, even if he felt highly certain that they were available, they are irrelevant to the dilemma. If the patient can sense a greater vitality or satisfaction in his living from a new course of action, this is well and good, but for the most part it is not characteristic of the plight of the person confronting the existential crisis. Much more frequently the attempt to find rewards or to get the therapist to promise them is a way of resisting full confrontation of the crisis. We are so accustomed to thinking in terms of rewards, in terms of the psychological "law of effect" that our perception of the reality of life is often askew. If ever there was a point in the therapeutic process when the concept of "is-ness" was critically important, it is in the existential crisis. There the intrusion of any extraneous concerns can only serve to vitiate what needs to be as forthright an encountering as may be possible.

BE PRESENT GENUINELY

More valuable than almost anything else the therapist can provide for his patient in the existential crisis is his own being genuinely present himself. This means a kind of rigorous self-awareness, which seeks out the counter-transference promptings that might introduce contaminants, which recognizes the emphatic sharing of dread, and which preserves for the patient his right of choice. It means a kind of concern which respects the individuality and dignity of the patient and makes of that individuality an ultimate value guiding all other functioning of the therapist. Patients who successfully confront the existential crisis, make their choice, and emerge in a more creative way of living invariably report that they were sustained in some measure by just the awareness that the therapist was there and that the patient mattered to the therapist. Sometimes, disappointingly, they have forgotten what seemed to the therapist to be exquisitely timed and phrased interpretations, but most meaningfully they have known he was there.

Summary

I have attempted to examine the nature of the existential crisis,[3] setting forth some defining statements that seem to be clinically demonstrated as essential to the concept of the crisis. We have examined a case in which the inability of the therapist to recognize the truly existential crisis the patient was experiencing resulted in

---

[3] A somewhat different conception of the existential crisis is suggested by Lasko (1963).

therapeutic failure and the abortion of treatment. We have studied some of the therapeutic tasks involved in helping the patient to confront and deal with the existential crisis most authentically.

The therapist is given the unique privilege of being with his patient in one of the most significant experiences that person will ever have. The therapist who approaches his part of this work with real humility and genuine respect for the individuality of his patient will make certain that he does nothing to contaminate or disrupt his patient's experiencing and working-through of the existential crisis. The Bible says, "Except ye be born again . . ." The therapist is given the privilege of attending that awesome rebirth of a human being. It is important, though, that he recognize he is midwife, not parent.

PART THREE *The ontogogic phase of the therapeutic work*

For most of man's history the greater portion of his energies have had to be given over to getting enough food, keeping sufficiently warm and dry, fighting off enemies, and otherwise simply preserving his life. Occasional bright periods have given a privileged few the opportunity to go beyond the struggle for simple survival. The monuments of those periods are the proud heritages of all men: the wonder of ancient Egypt, the beauty of Greece, the majesty of Rome, the flowering of the Renaissance, and so on. It is a familiar recognition that for the individual, as for man at large, creative expression may flower when the minimal survival needs have been met. Abraham Maslow's (1961, 1962b) contrast between deficiency-motivation and being-motivation is pertinent once again to our purpose.

The analysis of the resistance and the transference is the essential freeing from deficiency influences. The ontogogic phase of the therapeutic work is concerned with the realization of the potential for liberated being. Not only in public monuments, majestic architecture, and artistic productions, but within the individual person there is a realm for the burgeoning of potential that we rarely fully recognize. Just as the man who has time, energy, and emotion left over after fighting off physical deficiency may well turn to creative and artistic endeavors, so the man who has emerged from preoccupation with emotional deficiency may well bring forth creative and artistic expressions within the human experience itself.

Part Three concerns itself with the ontogogic phase of the therapeutic work. The term "ontogogy" is used to designate a creative effort to help a person toward greater realization of life's potential. Ontogogy is set in contrast to the reparative perspective implicit in the term "psychotherapy." In Part Three the assumptions are made that the therapeutic work of the analysis of the resistance and the transference has progressed well and that the patient is beginning to take an enlivened part in his own being with a readiness to broaden his awareness and experience. It is unlikely—and unnecessary to our present purpose—that we assume that all resistances and transferences will be resolved. Moreover we must recognize that our society is heavily encumbered with influences that work against human authenticities as well as with those influences that may facilitate genuineness. For these reasons, it is frequently appropriate when a person has had a successful analytic course to make available to him further help in the process of actualizing his being.

In this section we will first try to free our thinking of certain false equations that limit our authenticity. This is the work of *Chapter 11*, which discusses the notion of a *self* and finds it fraught with difficulties. Most of us have multiple *selves* rather than a unitary *Self*, and this self-fragmentation is in some instances a resistance to authentic being and in all instances a source of confusion if we repose our identities in the *Selves*.

The analytic phase of our work is oriented to a conception of the person in which he is assumed to have both subject and object aspects (Bugental, 1952a). The ontogogic phase calls for a recognition that this composite conception of the person is in itself a part of the resistance to full authenticity of being. Instead, the ontogogic phase insists on the necessity of freeing the *I* from its bondage to the *Self* in order to move toward true ontologic freedom. This seemingly simple distinction is of profound philosophic and psychologic significance. *Chapter 12* examines these matters and proposes a distinction between the *I* and the *Self*.

Chapter 13 identifies awareness as the basic process of being and makes a detailed study of this process. The influences of early training, of the culture, and of our own inauthenticities do much to restrict our awareness far beyond what needs to be the case. *Chapter 14* describes how ontogogy can bring aid to those of us who are beginning to recognize the restrictions on our awareness. Such broadening of awareness is an important first step toward greater realization of our potentials.

Chapter 15 begins to use the freed conception of personhood, provided by the previous chapters, to explore the levels of ontologic freedom that are potential for us. This is an area about which we know very little. We may recognize that reduction of the handicapping bonds of equating the *I* and the *Self* is an important step toward attaining to such freedom, and I will offer some observations on how that reduction may be aided.

Chapter 16 carries the investigation of ontologic freedom into two other aspects, which we call actualization and transcendence. Maslow's studies of self-actualizing people (1954) provide our best-known explorations into this fascinating realm. Our own discussion will designate and describe eight forms actualization has been found to take in persons having a successful existential-analytic experience.

Having this general structure to guide us as to levels of conception, we are ready in *Chapter 17* to inquire more substantively into the life areas in which the basic issues of our being reside. In this chapter we will pick up from our earlier (Chapter 3) assessment of the givens of being and amplify in some detail a theoretic structure designed to facilitate our understanding of the human experience in both its inauthentic and its authentic aspects. The essence of authenticity, it will be postulated, lies in man's accord with his ontologic situation. Many of us, however, pull back in dread, and the consequence is the prevalence of feelings of powerlessness, blame, absurdity, and estrangement.

Chapter 18 employs the structure thus developed to examine what may be termed the existential neuroses. These, I believe, more typify the concerns of patients seeking intensive psychotherapy today than do the symptom neuroses. Characterized by feelings of powerlessness, blame, absurdity, and estrangement, these patterns result from falling back in dread from confrontation of the givens of being.

Chapters 19 and 20 build upon the structure thus developed. We propose that ontogogic aid may be given the person (no longer truly a "patient") in expanding his awareness and in employing that expanded awareness to confront and make choices among the ontologic options of life. Figuratively speaking, we may say that life puts questions to each of us in each of the major areas our study of being has disclosed. We answer those questions with our lives. The questions are concerned with such matters as endings and death, identity, creativity or destruction, and isolation or relatedness. When we are authentic we live in faith, commitment, creativity, and love.

In the final section of the book, *Part Four* will look at the sorts of meanings the therapeutic process may have for the therapist himself. We will then pick up from the considerations we have been covering in Part Three to speculate about the further evolution of man as he frees his being and becomes more authentic.

Problems in Discussing Ontogogy

As we now discuss the procedures and phenomena of authentic being we find our communication encumbered by difficulties of language and conceptual habits. To say that a neurotic person tends to be generally unaware in the conduct of his life would be regarded as an appropriate if unexceptional report. To say that the more-than-usually-authentic person is more aware in the conduct of his life is apt to be looked upon as undistinguishing of authenticity. There are numerous subtle reasons why this is so.

First of all there is the false assumption of normality. Our language perpetuates a myth that the average person is "normal" (whatever that means), but even more important is the myth that normal people are routinely aware and therefore the neurotic is distinguished by his unawareness. If, then, I say the authentic person is aware, "What is distinguishing?" some may ask. In point of fact, I believe it true that the average person is largely unaware in the conduct of his life and is much closer to the neurotic, while the authentic person's awareness is a genuinely discriminating characteristic.

But having made such a statement I may well have triggered a second set of difficulties for our communication. (Certainly I am aware of a kind of visceral reaction to the last sentence of the preceding paragraph.) This second type of problem has to do with a preconscious or unconscious pseudo-equalitarianism. To describe the authentic person's greater awareness runs into an implicit attitude that may be paraphrased as, "Who do they think they are? What makes them so much better? I don't think we ought to draw invidious comparisons," and so on.

Of course, if the reader (or the writer) has already decided that he is more authentic than most, then these sorts of resistances will be less effective. Then, however, we may trigger an unconscious and neurotic guilt, which must reject the propositions because they give too much pleasure!

It would be interesting to know whether Europeans, particularly from central Europe, who have not had such an extended indoctrination with the myth of indiscriminate equalitarianism would encounter the same difficulties.[1]

STATE OF THE ART

This section title probably involves some distortion of the usual use of this phrase, but I like its flavor and it is emotionally valid

---

[1] I remember reading some time ago that Leta Hollingworth found it impossible to secure funds for research on the gifted, although money was readily available for the study of the feeble-minded. This is but another instance of our false conception of democracy, which seems to operate to try to bring all extremes toward the middle.

for what I want to say. In writing about the ontogogic phase of the processes involved in helping a person toward realization of his personhood, I am writing about an area of speculation and hypothesis. Much of what I am going to say awaits both empirical validation and theoretical elaboration and documentation. At some points there are tremendous gaps in the theoretical structure I will describe. It would be more comfortable if this were not so, but it is. The stage of development of technically worked out answers to the basic human questions is still very early. Moreover, I am quite sure that this is as far as my own understanding has progressed. I would rather offer this incomplete statement now and hope to communicate what I have worked out thus far than wait until I can make a finished presentation and perhaps never communicate with others.

This is life on the human frontier at this point in time. I am sure others have penetrated further into some areas than have I. I hope that I can offer some new perspectives to some others. We have a vast continent ahead of us. Let us not wait until it is all surveyed before we begin exploring.

11—*What is a person?*

This is an intake interview. The patient called last week to say that he was referred by his minister. Meeting him now in the waiting room and walking to my office, I find him tense, quick in motion, not really meeting my eyes, agitated. I motion him to a chair. "Tell me about yourself."

"Well, I . . ." He pauses, pulls out a cigarette, lights it. "I don't know where to start. I've thought of going to see someone for a long time, but somehow . . . It's just that sometimes I get the feeling that . . . Well, it's like I get mad too easily and over little things and . . . And I was divorced just recently but I want to marry again, but I don't want to . . ."

And so the person begins telling me about himself. And though there may be hesitances and pauses, the person will fill most of an hour with material about himself, and many more hours too. And what shall I do with it? What shall I write on the fresh paper on my clipboard? Shall I set up the tape recorder? What am I to do with all of this?

But as much as the words come tumbling to inundate me, my perceptions are also unleashing another torrent: "This person is sitting on the edge of the chair. It's a big, comfortable chair, but the person doesn't seem to know that; he's not being comfortable in it. The person blinks his eyes a lot. I think he blinks them more when he talks about his ex-wife or his intended wife. The person has pulled another cigarette out but isn't lighting it. He is moving restlessly and . . ."

Now what shall I do with all of this? Sometimes I feel like I want to say, "Wait! wait! just do or say one thing at a time. Let me think about it!"

THE THERAPEUTIC ENCOUNTER

The unrelenting realities of psychotherapeutic practice confront us with a phenomenon for which our training gave us no language but whose literally vital significance is inescapable in the lives we are encountering. What is this phenomenon? It is the fact of the person whom I encounter. When I come up against the fact of that other person, *qua* person, I am suddenly without preparation. My psychology of habits, of defense mechanisms, of learning and of dreaming, of reinforcement, attitudes, superego, and archetypes is largely sterile to meet this person—not person-*ality;* person, the whole, unified, actual being.

This is no play on words or carrying a point to a ridiculous extreme. I mean what I say most literally. My training has not prepared me to deal with this person in the uniqueness of his being here with me. I can get an educational history; I can measure the memory for digits; I can determine the W-to-D-to-Dd ratio; I can do any of a hundred or more useful things to deal with parts of this person, but I cannot call upon my training to help me deal with the person, as person.

And so what I do is to meet the person as a person myself. But now, is the problem solved and have we so belabored the point only to indicate that one must be a person first and psychotherapist second? By no means!

APPREHENDING THE OTHER

The point of the foregoing is this: There is no way in which I, *purely as psychotherapist*, can grasp the totality of the person whom I am encountering; nor is there any way in which I can, *as psychotherapist*, respond with the wholeness of me. Moreover, I cannot totally grasp him or totally express myself as a man (in contrast to a woman), as an adult (in contrast to a child), as an American or a Democrat, or a professional person, or anything else. Each of these describing concepts (not defining, describing) is partial and incomplete. It is only with my awareness of the process of myself-and-the-other-person-in-the-situation-of-encountering-each-other-in-the-world that I can apprehend this event.

In simplest terms, what I want to say is this: Most of our concepts in personality theory and psychotherapy are concepts directed toward part-functions of the individual. They deal with elements. There is, usually, the implicit assumption that if all such part-functions were brought together and somehow organized, we would then have a conception of the whole person. However, no system has ever truly integrated all these concepts, and candidly we may doubt that such a true integration is possible to any present system.

The Patient's Self-presentation

Now, let us for the moment set aside the thoughts we have just been having and consider another set of phenomena. We will study several instances:

> John says to me on Tuesday, "I can see now how my wife's crying reminds me of the way my sister used to use my parents' sympathies against me. When I flare up at my wife for crying, I'm really still trying to get even with my sister. I don't think it will make me so mad any more." On Thursday, John tells me: "Well, it happened again. I tried to talk sensibly to my wife, and she began bawling, and I blew my top. I don't know what's the matter with her."
>
> Edna lies on the couch with fists clenched, muscles taut, and her tone of voice almost grating as she says, "No, I'm not aware of any particular feelings right now."

Contrasting Selves

Now what is going on in these people? John and Edna are not mentally deficient, psychotic, or otherwise incompetent. Indeed, their educational, vocational, social, and economic levels are well above the national average. Yet each seems to be trying to perpetrate a manifest inconsistency. John in two days has "forgotten" his insight about the source within himself of his anger at his wife's tears and is putting all the responsibility back on her. Edna, even more strangely, is dramatically portraying a set of intense feelings while she verbally reports no awareness of them.

We can talk of "repression," "suppression," "logic-tight compartments," and so on, but we are only naming and may actually be obscuring important phenomena by doing so. Only in a segmentalist approach to a person does such naming serve as explanation. When we look at the person as a whole, what Edna and John are doing is astounding, for they are somehow each trying to be more than one person.

But there is still more to the story. Suppose we now say to Edna, as she lies with tightened muscles, fists clenched and voice tense—suppose we say to her, "Edna, are you aware of your hands right now?"

She replies, "No, I wasn't, but what about them?" And as she does so, we may note the hands relaxing.

Now, we press a further question to Edna: "Are you aware of any feeling in your hands or that has been in your hands in the last few minutes?"

Edna says, "Yes, they feel hurt and tired like they'd been lifting a weight or holding something very tightly."

And then we say to Edna. "Can you recapture what your hands were doing just before I directed your attention to them?"

Edna answers, "Yes, they were clenched tightly into fists. Now why would I do that?"

What is going on? But a minute ago Edna didn't know what her hands were doing. Now she knows. Where did the knowledge come from? But let us watch what happens if we push on. "Edna," we say, "use that awareness of your hands clenched tightly into fists. Feel it again, and see what else comes into your awareness."

"Why, I'm tightened up all over. My legs ache, and my jaw is sore, like I'd been clenching my teeth." So, she can recover the whole pattern that we witnessed.

Now, let's consider what we have seen and what Edna has told us. We have seen two Ednas: one was the one she described with her words; the other was the one described by her physical tension. Both were "real" in the sense that they were manifested to an observer.

Perhaps I should pause and recognize that the phenomena being described are not new to experienced psychotherapists or even to normally sensitive people in many walks of life. However, the point is not the newness of the phenomena; the point is the great ignorance we have of the dynamics of such important processes. Familiarity does not mean genuine comprehension. Electricity, light, gravitation are all familiar, and each is imperfectly understood. Moreover, a breakthrough in understanding one of these can be very important because of its very familiarity.

"DYNAMIC EXPLANATIONS"

It may satisfy some to say that Edna has suppressed or repressed her awareness of her physical tension because of the threat of the breakthrough of her feared hostile impulses, and that the transference situation gave her sufficient reassurance that she would not be left alone in handling these feared impulses so that with the therapist's help she could recover the repressed tensions. Fine! More, probably true!

But back up a step and take a broader view of what has just been said: Who feared the breakthrough of the hostile impulses? Who repressed the tensions? Who decided the therapist gave enough support so that the repression could be removed? The answer each time is Edna.

It is no wonder that Freud was driven to invent homunculi and that his language creates images of the bestial id, the harried executive ego, and the blue-nosed superego. It is indeed tempting to divide Edna up into several Ednas in order to try to make sense of the phenomena with which she confronts us. But, it may be argued, it is in this very fragmentation of herself that Edna's neurosis seems to lie, and when the therapist participates in such subdivision of the patient he may reinforce rather than reduce pathology.

What Is a Person?

What is a person? What is the nature of the experiencing subject or object that the patient wants to change when he comes to psychotherapy? Who is this "patient"? These and similar questions are, obviously, basic to the whole psychotherapeutic enterprise, yet they are often overlooked because of our unrecognized assumptions about the nature of the human experience. Existential-analytic psychotherapy cannot afford to by-pass these issues for they are fundamental to the whole conceptual base of our work.

When we begin to try to answer such questions we are confronted with an apparent paradox. We generally assume that each person is a unity, a single ontological given. We regard as pathological the phenomena which suggest that the patient is not unified and single, such as when he has conflicting impulses, divergent attitudes, and multiple conceptions of himself. Yet when we get down to the facts of self-awareness and unprejudiced observation of ourselves and others, we always find some evidences of just such disunity. Indeed, all people seem to experience some degree of internal dividedness, as represented by such terms as conscience, reason-vs.-emotion, and better judgment. Similarly, most theoretical systems postulate multiplicity within the person, as shown by such concepts as id-ego-superego and self-concept vs. self-image.

The central concern of existential-analytic psychotherapy and ontogogy is, of course, the person who is the patient. The central agency—other than the patient himself—of aiding the patient make the changes or growth that he seeks is the person who is the therapist. What is a "person"? I will contend that most of us have unthought-out presuppositions about what a person is and that reexamining our ideas will do much to free them of confusions and constraint and to facilitate clearer delineation of what we are doing and how to do it.

A basic—and in my view, erroneous—assumption is that the words "I," "Me," "Self," and "person" all point to the same psychological entity. Instead, we find, much is to be gained by differentiating among these terms. I will do so very briefly here and then enlarge on these distinctions in later pages. The *I*, I will hold, is pure subject and a unity. The *Me* is pure object and really only an adjective applied to certain perceptual experiences. The *Self* may be nearly synonymous with the *Me;* although often it is used in a sense that is more accurately named the *Self-concept:* that is, as the common element in otherwise diverse perceptions involving one's own person. *Person* is a term to designate any single individual and as such indicates the composite of his *I, Me, Self,* or *Self-Concept* loosely grouped together. *Person* is a heuristic concept.

With this clarification of terminology comes also an appreciable gain in clarity of conceptualization, from which we may hope for improved sensitivity and skill in the analytic and especially the ontogogic work. Certainly, these clarifications are also essential to movement toward authentic living in ontologic freedom.

SELF-FRAGMENTATION AND THE EXISTENTIAL SITUATION

Now let us see what I have been saying thus far. First of all, I argued that our usual psychological glossary was inadequate to the conceptualization of the event of my patient and I encountering each other. The glossary was inadequate in that it could specify part-functions but seemed consistently lacking for the totality of either person involved and certainly for the processes of their mutual confrontation of each other.

Then we began to look at some patients. Edna and John demonstrated behavior which when fully examined was astonishing, in that it seemed that each acted as though he were more than one person or had within his skin more than one person. Indeed, we found ourselves tending to break Edna up into her verbal self and her physical self and John into his Tuesday self and his Thursday self.

Why should this be? Why should the patient seem to fragment himself in this conflict-producing way? To answer these questions, we must return to our view of man's situation.

CONTINGENCY AND THE PERSON

Man finds himself in a world which he always knows incompletely, which he cannot comprehend, in the fullest sense of "comprehend." Yet it is truly vital—essential to the life or death issue—that he understand his world. Thus man finds himself in anxiety.

Because of the anxiety of his existence, man seeks absolutes that will insure him against the contingencies of his world. Man attempts to read into ambiguity a variety of deities, virtues, natural laws, magical incantations, scientific rituals that will somehow prevail against contingency. But this effort to control fate is vain because the universe comprehends (encloses) man; man does not, cannot comprehend (enclose or fully understand) the universe. Thus, the best-laid plans and the most faithful adherence to what is good cannot insure the outcome.

CHOICE

So far we have recognized the fearsomeness of the infinitely unknowable that encompasses our finite knowing. This is the root of true anxiety. But there is another and equally important side of this picture of man's condition. This may be summed up in the single word, *choice*. Where there is no uncertainty, there is no choice. If I can demonstrate to your complete conviction that the room in which you sit will collapse in five minutes, it will be empty in four. From contingency arises anxiety, but equally it is integral to the possibility of choice.

So it is that when man invests in charms, rules, beliefs to forestall the anxiety of contingency, he is at the same time disenfranchising himself of choice.

RESPONSIBILITY

Let me illustrate this at a more concrete level. When John in our earlier example says that his anger is caused by his wife's tears, then John has given up choice and is—if you will—a "dependent variable" to be manipulated by his wife's crying or not crying. If, on the other hand, we can help John reclaim the experience of having choice and accepting responsibility for his own emotions, then he can no longer "blame" his wife for his anger.

But let us see some other ways in which this diminishing of one's self may occur.

> Listen to George: "When I was only five and a half my father was crippled in an accident, and we had to change our whole way of living. Then two years later . . ."

> Linda tells me: "It was all I could do to stay with him when he began to hit me, but I knew my duty . . ."

And so on. And what are they saying? George is telling me what a hard life he has had. Linda was brave. Why do they tell me, or anyone? What about it?

Magic. Sometimes they are telling me as an intermediary of the universe; sometimes they are telling the universe directly. In either case they are bargaining. They are putting gifts on an altar. They are reciting magical incantations. They are acting out superstitions.

Wait! Magic, superstitions? Linda has a graduate degree in a rigorous science. George is a successful professional man. Nevertheless, each is trying to practice magic.

George is offering his hard life, Linda her courage. Each is offering this living part of himself as a gift to some unknown god or demon whom he hopes to appease or bribe into making things better for him. Listen to the way each tells his story, and you hear the entreaty plainly. They are trying to use some aspect of themselves to ward off contingency and to guarantee some desired future. It is implicit in the way they describe their offerings.

> We can well add Thelma, who sobs out, "I was mean . . . and vicious. There's something in me that is mean and will do anything . . ." Thelma is offering her badness just as Linda offered her courage: to try to escape the responsibility of choice.

Morality. Is the sense of what is said here amorality? No, but neither is it a morality which holds that certain virtues and vices exist in and of themselves. The view here advanced is in some ways more moral, within the present perspective, than the traditional view, for it holds that each person is responsible for his choices and may neither claim a virtue nor deplore a weakness to explain away such choices.

Summary. Self-fragmentation thus may be recognized in one aspect as a resistance. It is a way the patient tries to cope with anxiety that seems overwhelming or with guilt that he seeks to avoid. This form of self-fragmentation must be dealt with psychotherapeutically as any other resistance, if the patient is to gain authenticity and reclaim his ability to choose.

CULTURALLY DERIVED RESISTANCE

When we have recognized self-fragmentation as an idiosyncratic resistance, however, we have said but part of the story. Division within the self may also be a product of cultural learning and development, and this aspect will be examined now. There is a further practical consideration, that has to do with the aid that can be given the patient who has begun to relinquish the resistive employment of self-fragmentation and to seek greater wholeness in his being. We will examine this form of aid to the patient in Chapter 19. At this point, let us only pause to recognize why such aid is needed.

One of the main areas from which influences stem that make the resistance of self-fragmentation more likely is the culture in which the individual lives. In some ways any society is a resistance, any society is a banding together to reduce certain contingencies (not in itself an inauthentic goal) that can (and often does) easily slide over into a denial of existential reality. This is clearly evident in the social institution we miscall "life insurance." A life insurance policy taken by its name would be a policy designed to insure one's life, to protect or preserve it, to defeat death. One may question whether life insurance would be as popular if it were more accurately named "death compensation" or even more precisely, "partial-payment-on-your-death."

Now let me be clear: no devaluing of the genuine values in such policies is intended. It is good to make provision so that the sudden death of a wage-earner does not leave his family impoverished. It is, indeed, a confronting of contingency and of the existential anxiety of death to do so. But what so often happens is that this valid intent is lost sight of and a very inauthentic sequence of denial and disguise of the realities is substituted. One need do no more than note the deception of the "slumber room" as a place for seeing a dead body before interment, the reluctance of many—not only morticians, but many others including, incredibly, ministers—to use the words "death," "died," and so on, and their preference for "passed on," "is asleep," and similar phrases.

The point need not be belabored. In very many ways, society practices denials of the existential anxiety that is our natural condition. Indeed, psychotherapy has been employed many times as a social device for trying to escape guilt and responsibility. Creativity and unorthodoxy are suspect in many circumstances. Psychology, for example, numbers among its "scientific" ranks no few highly trained and respected people who flee from meaninglessness by relying on statistical devices and arguing for the collection of facts for their own sakes. But probably in no area is our culture's effort to deny existential anxiety more pervasive and yet more patently futile than in relation to the anxiety of separateness and loneliness. The proliferation of various entertainment forms, the countless organizations one may join, the great emphases on "belongingness," all of these give testimony to the great threat we are naturally under. Yet one may well question whether we are not as alone and lonely as any people have ever been (Reisman, 1950).

The foregoing paragraphs have indicated how culture contributes to our resistances to existential authenticity. Yet it needs to be re-emphasized that culture is not the culprit. Culture did not pre-exist, man invented it. Men, at least as we exist today, must band together to sustain life. Banding together, we must relate to each other in terms of but parts of ourselves, for we do not yet know how to relate as whole persons. Perhaps some day we shall, but certainly that day is distant indeed. Each cultural institution collects and serves some aspects but not all; all the institutions together probably could not serve all. If they could there would be no need for any institution, for we would not be able to distinguish ourselves from the composite institution or the composite institution from the world.

So it is that the resolution of our resistances to authentic being in the world is not a job to be done once and then it is through. Nor may we assume that once the job is done as well as possible the person's need for help is at an end. Much can be done to aid the person in confronting the existential anxieties, incorporating them, and going to meet his life with a more creative perspective. This is the work of ontogogy which I will discuss later in this part of the book.

12 — The I, the me, and the self

As the previous chapter demonstrated, we will understand human experience better if we distinguish, *I*, *Me*, *Self*, and *Person*. Unthinkingly we treat all four of these terms as though they were essentially interchangeable except for the constraints of grammar. We regard them, also, as essentially pointing to the same entity (whether we construe that entity to be ultimately a psychophenomenological object, a physiological organism, or a metaphysical creation [Allport, 1955]). While I certainly accept the fact that all four terms point to phenomena which are intercontinuous, I will argue that they do not point to the same entity—at least insofar as existential-analytic psychotherapy and ontogogy are concerned. I will briefly set forth my conception of each of the four and then we will examine some of their significances in greater detail.

"*I* am aware. I feel (emotionally) as part of being aware. In my awareness I can choose among actions I will take or not take. I am a part of other men and yet apart from other men." These sentences are the closest one may come to describing the *I*. The *I* is the subject, never the object. Were it possible to describe the *I* it would have to be an object. The crude analogy may be made to the vain attempt to specify the specific location of *movement*, the exact hour of *enduring*, or the precise color of *white*. A pure process cannot be identified in terms of that which it negates or that which it includes totally.

Freud used the German word *Ich* (English = I) for what we have more usually translated as *Ego* in psychoanalytic theory (see Freud, 1933, for example). There are a number of points of overlap in the psychoanalytic conception of the Ego and what I am calling the *I* or *I-process* (see below); however, there are also significant differences. One of the most important of these differences has to do with the psychoanalytic ego being conceived as splitting on occasion:

> The ego can take itself as object, it can treat itself like any other object, observe itself, criticize itself, and do Heaven knows what besides with itself. In such a case one part of the ego stands over against the other. The ego can, then, be split; it splits when it performs many of its functions, at least for the time being. The parts can afterwards join up again (Freud, 1936).

The *I*, as I conceive it, is irreducibly a unity and invariably a subject. It is, I postulate, the essential being.

Me is a word used to designate a perceptual object. The *Me* includes the physical body, customary patterns of behavior as an observer might note them, the memory of past actions and feelings. The *Me* of itself is inert, unaware, and it cannot make any of the defining statements the *I* makes.

Self is a word used with some overlapping of meaning with *Me*. The common element abstracted out of many and diverse perceptions of one's *Me* may be named the *Self* (just as we may speak of "tableness" from our experiences of many tables). This makes its significance synonymous with the *Self-concept*, and this will generally be my usage. I will discuss the significance of the *Self* in much more detail shortly.

Person is a word we use to refer to another individual in his composite being, usually with emphasis on his inferred but unobservable *I*. In our discussions I will use the term *person* to speak about individuals when I do not want to specify whether I particularly refer to his *I*, *Me*, or *Self*.

The difficult central point of what I am trying to describe here is the concept of the pure subjectness of the *I*. Our habits of thinking are so tied up with the physical world and our related patterns of speech are so mechanically derived that we tend to think of entities as having both subject and object aspects always. Unthinkingly we then carry this over to our descriptions of the human experience. In a truly existential-humanistic framework, these habits lead to a major fallacy in conceiving our being. To set the matter at its most extreme: Only the *I* is truly the subject in world, whether that *I* be the *I* of a given *person* or the *I* which is all awareness. All other entities are objects.

This point is of crucial importance because the present confusion results in the *person* losing his sense of being, which means his awareness as the subject, the *I*, and comes to experience himself solely as object (*Self, Me*) and thus without genuine awareness, choice, relation, and so forth. From this confusion flow the sense of hollowness so endemic today, the kinds of contacts between people that are reminiscent of billiard balls bumping rather than beings in relation, the succumbing to absurdity and inertia, and much else that bespeaks our alienation from our intuition of being subject in our own lives.

T. S. Eliot, with the poet's vision, has portrayed this alienation from one's own being in *The Hollow Men* (1963, p. 221).

> We are the hollow men
> We are the stuffed men
> Leaning together
> Headpiece filled with straw. Alas!
> Our dried voices, when
> We whisper together
> Are quiet and meaningless
> As wind in dry grass
> Or rats' feet over broken glass
> In our dry cellar.

SELF-AS-DOER VS. SELF-AS-OBJECT

It will be useful to pause in the development of my conception to recognize that the distinction between the *I* and the *Me* or *Self* has been made many times; although it has not always been given the same further implications which I will be postulating.

Murphy (1947, p. 479), Allport (1943), and others have distinguished between the *Self-as-doer* and the *Self-as-object*. Murphy (p. 482) observes of the young child, "The self could not at this stage be confused with the thing doing the perceiving; this is a later quasi-philosophical way of looking at the matter." In a study (Bugental, 1948, 1952b) in which the affective tone associated with expressed perceptions of the self was examined, it became very evident that this same difference between the *Self-as-doer* and the

Self-as-object was supported empirically even though in a very limited area.

The *Self-as-doer* is, by its very nature, unobservable. As a consequence, anything said about it tends to make an object of the *Self*-as-doer, and thus there has been the tendency to equate the *Self*-as-doer seen retrospectively with the *Self*-as-object. This, it is here maintained, is a false and confusing equation. It leads to the kind of "subject–object split" in the *Self* that is termed "self-alienation." What we are discussing in this section is *not* this sort of dichotomy. Rather, we are recognizing the fact that the true *Self*-as-doer, the *I*, is a radically different process from the object of perception, the *Self*-as-object, or the *Me*.

This is the *I–Me* distinction. The *Self*, as I am using the term now, is properly related to the *Me*, never to the *I*. The *Self* is an object in the awareness of the *I-process*. Under the influence of cultural learnings, we often regard the *Self* as synonymous with the *I-process*, but it is not. The confusion of the *I-process* and the *Me* has made us think that the *Me* is a unitary given too, and it is not. It is probable that in most of us that there are two or three *Me*'s or *Selves*. Tremendous amounts of confusion in our thinking about the nature of personality and about how people experience their lives have arisen from the confusion of the *I* and the *Me*.

The I-Process

As so often, the poets have anticipated our more plodding pace. Spender uses "I" for both *I* and *Me*, but his insight is essentially the same.

> Central "I" is surrounded by "I eating."
> "I loving," "I angry," "I excreting,"
> And the "great I" planted in him
> Has nothing to do with all these,
>
> It can never claim its true place
> Resting in the forehead, and secure in his gaze.
> The "great I" is an unfortunate intruder
> Quarrelling with "I tiring" and "I sleeping"
> And all those other "I"s who long for "We dying."
>
> (Spender, 1955, p. 8)

The I-Process: A Communications Convention

It does not seem possible to me to communicate adequately about the *I* while preserving faithful recognition of its pure subject-ness and avoiding grammatical chaos. (This is particularly so because I use this same first person singular pronoun as the writer.) It may well be that this difficulty is pertinent and represents not alone a defect of language but of conceptualization. However that may be, I propose the convention of referring to the *I-process* as a way of treating the *I* as though it were at times an object for our present communicative purposes.

What, then, is this *I* or *I-process?* In describing the given characteristics of being in Chapter 3 I identified the basic process as *feelingful awareness.* Thus, most basically, the *I* is that feelingful awareness. But, as I pointed out in my earlier discussion, our awareness discloses other aspects of our being: we are finite; we have the potential to take action; we can choose from among actions and non-actions that which we will make actual; and we are separate but related with other men. These, clearly, are the attributes of the *I-process.* The being of the individual person is what we point to by the term *I* or *I-process.* It is possible, for discussion purposes, to think of the *I-process* chiefly as combined awareness and choice-making, with the other attributes subsumed under this composite function. Awareness does not mean physiologic sensation alone, which is the tool of but by no means synonymous with awareness. Choice-making does not mean motoric or even neurologic action, these being but the symptoms, the expressions, or even the by-products of the choice-making. The light generated by an electric current passing through wires in a filament is not the electricity any more than the actions taken by a person are the *I-process* that is most truly that person.

Now perhaps it will be evident from what has just been said that if the *I-process* is conceived in this fashion, then such concepts as "health," "adjustment," "good," and "bad" are not pertinent. The *I-process* just *is.* The *I-process* is the livingness, but not just biological livingness. "Soul" or "essence" may be other recognitions of what is here termed the *I-process.* It is impossible to say at this point whether the *I-process* is an immortal, a metaphysical, or simply a bio-electrochemical phenomenon. We can only describe what appears to be the nature of being and recognize that any speculation as to the deeper meaning of these observations must depend on further inquiries.

AN ANALOGY

To make more understandable the view being presented, it will be helpful to employ an analogy. The showing of a motion picture provides such a parallel. There are three main elements in the projection of a movie: the light source, the film, and the screen. The light may be equated to the *I-process*[1], to the individual being. It is undifferentiated or contentless. The *Selves* may be likened to various films that may be shown by the projector. They may be very similar or quite contrasting. The films are highly differentiated within themselves and content-laden. Raimy, who did some of the pioneer work in developing an understanding of the self-concept (1943, 1948), speaks of the self as a "learned perceptual object." This is the manner in which the "film" of our analogy comes about, through learning. Thus, contrasting learning experiences give rise to contrasting *Selves*. Finally, since we never see a *Self* directly but only its image as we experience ourselves or one another, the image on the screen may be equated to the experienced *Self* of a given individual at a given time. Thus the image a person projects of himself may be thought of as the product of his being (*I-process*) as "interpreted" by his *Self* (*Selves*) at any given time, just as the image on the screen is the light translated by being projected through the film.

Now when we noted that there seemed to be two Ednas and two Johns, it was similar to observing a picture of an elephant on a movie screen one time and picture of a steamship at another and concluding that there were two projectors involved. The confusion of what is projected at any given point with the projection process could result in grave misunderstandings of the phenomena with which we are dealing.

---

[1] I am grateful to my colleague, Dr. Alvin Lasko, for noting that this equation of the *I-process* and light has many precedents, including a frequent Zen linkage of *satori* and light (Barrett, 1956), the emphasis on light in the transcendent experiences reported by Huxley (1954a, b,) and in Christian theology.

DISRUPTIVE CONSEQUENCES

Experiments on "learning" of the Hull-Spence variety deliberately try to avoid any entanglement with the subjects' (objects') self-awareness. They do not ask what being in the experiment means to the subjects, and, one suspects, they would rather not know (cf. Orne, 1962). The reasons are obvious. As soon as the *I-process* enters the picture, awareness and choice begin to appear. These have the effect of introducing so many "uncontrolled variables" that the neatness of the experiment is quite overthrown.

I have elaborated on these further implications of the general thesis to show that the freeing of the *I* from embeddedness in the *Me* can constitute a disrupting influence in the orderliness of things. This is equally so within the individual. Since most of us are taught to be consistent or to face ridicule, to follow suprapersonal ideals or to be thought unprincipled, we find our own ontologic freedom disruptive and threatening within ourselves, even as do the experimental psychologists with their objects in their laboratories. We, like they, tend to solve the problem by suppression of the very freedom that is our most existential birthright.

CLINICAL IMPLICATIONS

Let me pause here in my development of the conceptual structure to illustrate some of the clinical significances of what I am saying. The distinctions I am proposing do much to help our understanding of just what is involved in trying to aid another person through the psychotherapeutic processes.

When a person comes to me for psychotherapy, I conceive the situation to be as follows: The person says within himself, "I find my awareness includes many feelings that I do not want. I do not seem to choose well among the actions possible to me. I am not finding fulfillment in my relations with others. I feel I have the potential for more realization in my being than I am aware of now. I want help to open my awareness so that my choices, actions, and relations better express my being and result in feelings which I will find more deeply satisfying." In the terminology I am proposing, we can say that the person's *I-process* has made a choice to change the feeling aspects of his awareness.

Although it is the exceptional instance indeed where it would be appropriate to use the terms we are here developing or explicate the concepts in the therapeutic hour itself, there are numerous occasions when we can help the patient to develop a different awareness of his own being. This is illustrated in the following sequence with a man who had progressed some way in his analytic work.

> Gary was eloquent in berating himself. He would detail in lurid, verbal colors his own stupid, self-defeating actions: "And then, when I was working for the contracting firm and I was moving up fast, everybody said I was going to be the next general manager. I knew it. Old Halloway himself practically said so one day. So what did I do? What did I do? Just smashed the whole thing! Got sore at the accounting office, challenged the Chief Comptroller, then marched into Halloway's office and put him on the spot so he had to say 'No'. But I still wasn't satisfied. I gave him an ultimatum. I gave Halloway an ultimatum! Either he goes or I go, I told him. Oh, God, what a stupid thing! It's like when I was in the army and there was a chance to go to O.C.S., and I . . ."
> In the course of time, we worked out a really productive insight into Gary's fear of success, which indeed had made him defeat himself so often. More difficult to work through but eventually yielding was his identification with his hypercritical father (reproduced in the transference with me) which made this form of self-castigation a way of trying to win a closeness that always faded away (implicitly: "You see, Dad, I'm just like you in finding Gary stupid; so now we are together, aren't we?"). Both of these points of analysis of the resistance were fruitful, but I also found this an opportunity to open to Gary a new way of experiencing his being. Interrupting such an outburst as that illustrated in the first paragraph, I said, "Gary, you're like a guy who sits in the rear-facing back seat of a station wagon and gripes about the route the driver's taking. You can sit back there and bellyache from now on, but nothing's going to change until you get in the front seat and take the wheel."
> "I know it. That's what I keep telling you. I am so damn stupid that I . . ." I interrupted him again, roughly.
> "You're still in the back seat singing your favorite song, 'How bad I am.' It seems like you'd rather bitch than pitch."

"Well, what do you want? I admitted it was my fault, didn't I?"

"Now you're going to try to get me to drive so that you can find fault with me too, huh?"

"No, I didn't mean that. Hell, I don't know how to do anything different."

"No, I don't think you do consciously, Gary. The result is you're always looking at where you've been but never deciding where you want to go. It's no wonder nothing changes."

"Yeah, I can see that. Well (pause) suppose I try to do something else besides rehash the past . . ."

And, of course, in the very reorientation of that last sentence, Gary is beginning to act in terms of his *I-process* instead of his *Me*.

THE ACTION-DERIVATION SEQUENCE

We need to understand how the *I-process* takes action, for this is fundamental to our work as therapists. Clearly, the *I-process* does not function as pure awareness and choice in most everyday situations. There are important persistent patterns (which we call "traits" or "personality characteristics" in usual thinking) that cannot be accounted for solely as the free choices of awareness. Moreover, the *I-process* cannot simply decide to behave differently and have the change occur at once. We all know how persistent unwanted behavioral patterns can be. A basis for understanding these matters better may be had if we can trace out an array of patterns by which behavior or action may be evoked or initiated.

I will postulate a sequence describing action determination as follows:

TROPISM: The influence of an environmentally derived stimulus on the organism's physical nature fully determines the action. No awareness, no alternatives, no choice are involved. The response to gravity is an example.

REFLEXES: The influence of an environmentally derived stimulus on the organism's physical nature tends to determine the action. Awareness may supersede and raise the action to a higher level however. The knee jerk is an example.

INSTINCTS: The influence of an environmentally derived stimulus initiates a tendency to perform an action sequence. Awareness may supersede and raise the action to a higher level. The sequence from sexual excitation to orgasm is an example.

CONDITIONING: The influence of a stimulus initiates an action tendency. Awareness may supersede. Rote verbal sequences ("one . . . two . . . three . . .") are an example.

HABITS: The influence of a stimulus is interactive with minimal-awareness reference systems within the individual (for example, the *Selves* or *Self-concept*) so that an action tendency emerges as "programmed" by past experience. Awareness may supersede. The way most of us select our clothes is a possible example.

CHOICE: With or without an external stimulus, awareness selects courses of action in terms of realization of being. Improvisation on a musical instrument may be an example.

LETTING-BE: A form of choice that is the willing assent to the is-ness of awareness without striving and without effortful concentration and decision-making (which are not thereby implied to be intrinsic to *Choice*). *Letting-be* represents a broadened awareness that lets go of many of the values and concerns of our daily living while yet the individual is still very much in such living (as such, it is contrasted with the cosmic or total perspective of the next level, Transcendence).[2]

TRANSCENDENCE: Awareness of one's own being as intrinsic with all Being is expressed through assent to suchness. The subject-object split is overcome as action and reaction are one with Being.[2]

The Self

Let us return to an examination of the nature of the *Self*. Raimy has called it, "a learned perceptual system which functions as an object in the perceptual field of the behaver" (1943, p. 331). This defini-

---

[2] Because of the very nature of the action determination at the two upper levels it is impossible to cite examples. At these levels any external manifestation of the determination would be possible. What the person does says nothing of how he came to do it.

tion is really a definition of the self-concept, in Raimy's language, which is "the map which each person consults in order to understand himself, especially during moments of crisis or choice" (Raimy, 1948, p. 155). These definitions make evident that the *Self* or *Self-concept* is created from experience, is "consulted" like a map, an inanimate object, and is not the acting agent.

The Functioning of the Self

Now, in this action sequence it will be evident that the role of awareness is a growing one from the lower, physical levels to the higher psychological ones. Similarly the sequence portrays an emergence from complete reactivity to activity, from response to initiation, from being solely an object to becoming the subject.

The place of the *Self* and its very real utility are portrayed in this sequence also. The *Self* is a useful, even essential, tool to free the awareness for more creative choice. Merely on a simple, practical basis the *Self* serves as a quick reference for handling countless minor decisions and action situations.

The difficulty comes about, of course, when we mistake the *Self* for the whole of our being and thus lose true choice. This is encouraged, in a way, in our culture with its many emphases on one's "image," on other-directedness (Reisman, 1954, p. 99), and on mechanomorphic (Waters, 1948) views of human nature. The net effect of these and related influences is to bring us to see ourselves as "nothing but" reactive objects. The situation is further made constraining by the great value placed on consistency. Lecky (1951) was striving for a more psychological (as opposed to physiological or mechanistic) approach to personality, but his theory of self-consistency mistook the evident short-term efficiency of consistency for a more general value. From an existential viewpoint we must recognize that consistency is not a value in itself. Certainly marked inconsistencies and conflicts within the *Self*—that is, at the subchoice level of habit-based behaviors—are apt in many (but definitely not all) instances to lessen the convenience of the *Self* for its limited function. However, consistency can become a strait jacket when allowed to become a value having effect on choice-level action. There, it is, like other extrinsic considerations, not only irrelevant but often a resistance to full responsibility.

MULTIPLE SELVES

We have been using the terms *Self* and *Selves* interchangeably through much of our discussion. We need to recognize that the sorts of encounters with our patients which were portrayed at the beginning of the last chapter document the fact that the *Self* is not a unity. Under the impacts of learnings from each of our parents, from other significant figures such as siblings, teachers, play-fellows, we learn different *Selves*. Each of these *Selves* arises from perceptual experience and is in some measure distinct from and in some degree overlapping with each of the other *Selves*. A person usually will learn two or three of these *Selves*. Often there is a mother-derived *Self* and a father-derived *Self*, and there may be a peer-derived *Self*.

Eric Berne (1961), who has creatively dealt with this same problem of the apparent multiplicity of *Selves*, demonstrates his view that three "ego states" (p. 31) may be discerned within each person, "the Child," "the Adult," and "the Parent." These "are not handy ideas, or interesting neologisms, but refer to phenomena based on actual realities" (p. 34). Certainly, these characterizations do much to illuminate the phenomena we are here studying. Berne has carried forward the development of his conceptual system in a variety of productive and intriguing ways (for example, *The Structure and Dynamics of Organizations and Groups*, 1963); however, he retains a primary concern with what we consider pathology, and thus we can only make limited direct use of his observations for our present purposes. This is, however, in no sense to slight his very original and helpful contributions.

This perspective is akin to that advanced by Shapiro in his astute clinical observations (1962a, b). Shapiro says, ". . . There is no such thing as a single psychological 'self.' There is instead, a system of 'sub-selves' more or less unified in a personal identity, depending on the strength of the synthetic function of the ego" (1962a, p. 821). Thus Shapiro recognizes "parental sub-selves," "child sub-selves," and "intermediary sub-selves." These he characterizes by such adjectives as "the rebellious child," "the good child," "the demanding parent," and "the executive." While certain of these sub-selves may recur in many patients, Shapiro does not postulate that any set of them is always present.

THE "SELVES" AND "ROLES"

It seems useful to distinguish the *Selves* from roles because phenomenologically there is a crucial difference between the two. One plays out a role at the summoning, if you will, of an environmental influence, but does not necessarily feel that the role is the *Self*. On the other hand, the *Selves* have the feel of being "one's own *Self*." When experiencing such a *Self*, it "feels like me" and I think of it as me, not as a role. These should not be taken as completely either/or statements but as central tendency statements; however, phenomenologically this distinction between a "*Self*" and a "role" is important for psychotherapy.

Our communication with our patients will be better and our understanding of what they tell us will be improved if we recognize that there is not, perforce, one *Self* which may have conflict within it but several *Selves* which may be in conflict. Indeed, it may be speculated that much of our society is organized to support and accommodate the experience of having several *Selves*.

OVERLAP AMONG THE SELVES

The several *Selves* that each of us carries with us inevitably show some overlap. The amount shared in common varies in different individuals, but seldom does a person show anything approaching unanimity among these several images. Certainly the overlap is conflict-reducing in its effect, but it may also result in a more pervading limitation on awareness of nonsubstantive being.

IDEALIZED AND DESPISED IMAGES

Although I will not take time to develop the point at length here, I find that my understanding of the functioning of the *Selves* in my patients is greatly enhanced by the insights of Karen Horney (1950), and especially by her development of the recognition that each person is constantly checking his *Self*-experience against an idealized image of what the *Self* should be and a despised image of what he fears the *Self* will turn out to be.[3]

---
[3] Fingarette's (1963) study of the nature of the *Self* and how it may be conceived more creatively is well worth careful study.

Implications of the I-Self Distinction for Actualization and the Transference

The matters we have been discussing about the nature of the person have, of course, significant implications for other things with which we will deal. In this section we will particularly examine those implications for two important areas of the analytic and ontogogic work.

SELF-ACTUALIZATION, ACTUALIZATION

"Self-actualization" (Maslow, 1954) has been an exciting addition to the psychological glossary. The attention to "growth motivation" in addition to "deficiency motivation" brought a more positive and humanistic orientation to our thinking. Yet the concept, it seems to me, has been plagued by a dilemma. On the one hand, Maslow's own conception ("Self-actualization is intrinsic growth of what is already in the organism, or more accurately of what *is* the organism itself," p. 183; emphasis Maslow's), seemed to lead to a genetic determinism that was antihumanistic. On the other hand, disavowal of the inner fate idea made the concept a flaccid captive of mechanistic learning theory. I think the dilemma came about because Maslow was still to such an extent operating within the essentially mechanical orientation of experimental psychology.[4] (Note his use of "organism.") Thus he needed to accept the unity of the *Self*-as-doer and the *Self*-as-object. This in turn led to the idea of a substantive actualization. Today, we can cast loose from this restricting need for substantive properties and postulate the pure process, pure subject *I*. In these terms, then, we will not speak of "*Self-actualization*," which could only mean a making of the past into present actuality. Instead we may conceive "actualization" as the full and authentic being in the world, which transcends any substantive limit or characterization. (This is what we have done in Chapter 16.

---

[4] These comments should not be read as in any part devaluing Maslow's courageous pioneering. His break with stultifying tradition opened the way so that we who write today can speculate with greater freedom.

There we will see how harmoniously our observations of actualizing processes in authentic being correspond with Maslow's characteristics of "self-actualizing" people.)

IMPLICATIONS FOR THE TRANSFERENCE

We have customarily thought of transference as the patient's projection upon the therapist, without fully considering what happens with the patient himself as he makes the transference. In this fashion we have often seen only some part of the true phenomenon of transference. It needs to be recognized that when in his relationship to the significant other in his earlier years the patient developed a symbiotic bond, both patient and the other were structured by that bond. This may be rephrased: a particular *Self* of the patient and a particular *Self* of the other were bonded by the relationship. When the patient today projects that prior relationship onto the therapist, not only is the transference that projection, it is also the patient's bringing that same *Self* into the relationship with the therapist. This is to say that the patient in transference does not bring all of his *Selves* into play. The transference is maintained by the patient's need to reduce contingency in this relationship to the therapist and to accomplish this he must restrict himself to that *Self* which was involved in the earlier symbiotic relationship.

INCOMPLETE TRANSFERENCE RESOLUTIONS

This point gains significance as we recognize that the process which has just been described results in the unwary therapist seeing but one or a few facets of his patient. Often these may be important facets and much important therapeutic work can be done with them. Nevertheless, they give a limited perspective. Resolution of this transference is not the same as freeing the patient from his transference potential, that is, from his parataxic tendencies in all current relationships. Many therapeutic courses have reasonably successful outcomes but the patient still shows in his extratherapeutic life certain disorders of relationship and behavior. It is postulated here that this incomplete therapeutic result may come about because the patient has not brought all his *Selves* into the relationship with the therapist but only those involved in the initial transference dyad.

CHANGE OF THERAPIST

It is a familiar observation that a patient may have a good therapeutic result with one therapist and then move on to a second therapist who experiences the patient quite differently and who also helps the patient achieve a growth in emotional health. This may well be a product of limited transference resolution with any one therapist, or—saying it more precisely—of having worked through but a part of the patient's potential *Self*-other bondings.

GROUP THERAPY

The advantage of group psychotherapy as an adjunct or part of the total therapeutic program becomes evident in that it provides for a variety of transference relationships to be established. It is familiar that the patient makes transferences to the various group members, and we often are aware that this is its advantage. What we are less apt to note is that the patient indeed presents different *Selves* to different group members and to the therapist. The therapist who works intensively with patients in individual therapy before entering them in the group often is surprised at the different manner and behavior of the patient in the group as opposed to that with which the therapist was familiar in the individual sessions. Obviously what is involved here is that the patient has brought *Selves* into play in the group situation other than those involved in the transference relationship to the therapist alone.

SUMMARY

From what has just been said it will be apparent that thoroughgoing psychotherapy deals with those several *Selves* as they are brought into play in the therapeutic relationship. Since each transference is a resistance also, the working through of any one transference-resistance is apt to be followed by the presentation of a second transference-resistance. These in turn may be peeled back in the same manner that we see with symptomatic resistances.

In sum, then, thoroughgoing transference analysis involves working through several attempted symbiotic relations or, saying it differently, as much of the *Self* fragmentation as is resistive in function. It should be evident that this may take us beyond the immediate relation between therapist and patient.

Central to any conception or practice of psychotherapy is the question, what is a person? In this chapter I have advanced what seems to be a theoretically sound and clinically supported answer to this question. The question is difficult to deal with adequately because we have unquestioningly assumed the givenness of unity in the person, have assumed that a single entity was referred to by such words as "person," "self," "I," and "me." Naturalistic observation of ourselves and others, attention to what patients in psychotherapy say and do, soon challenges this presupposition, however. It becomes impressively evident that, although there is an experienced singleness in each of us, there is also an undeniable multiplicity. Thus we are confronted with the paradox of concurrent unity and plurality in the person.

As we study these phenomena, it becomes evident that one source of the apparent diversity is the person's inauthenticity, his flight from anxiety, responsibility, and guilt. By *Self*-fragmentation the patient seeks to resist that which he has come to feel cannot be borne.

Yet the resistance does not fully account for the multiple *Selves* we encounter in all people. Accordingly, I have inquired further into the nature of the *Self*-experience and have concluded that the very processes by which we learn to live in the world give rise to multiple *Selves*. Clinical evidence is mounting that for most of us the phenomenological reality is not a single *Self* but several *Selves*.

This recognition that the *Self* is really multiple seems to refute the postulated unity of the person which we also observed. However, we find this confusion clears up when we discriminate the *Self*-as-doer from the *Self*-as-object, or, in the terms we have employed here, the *I-process* from the *Me* or *Self*. The *I-process* is conceived to be solely that of awareness and choice without content or substance as such. The expression of the *I-process* occurs through the *Selves*, which are substantive and content-laden.

From these postulations we arrive at a reconception of the nature of *Self*-actualization, which seeks to preserve the usefulness of this concept while coordinating it with the present orientation. We also expanded our understanding of the transference.

13—*Awareness: The basic process of being*

Repeatedly in this book I will insist that recognition needs to be given to the manifest reality that feelingful awareness[1] is the basic process of being (Kelman, 1956a, b). In this chapter and the next we will explore this recognition in greater detail. My intent will be to draw out some of the meanings for the human experience implicit in the fact of awareness, to become more appreciative of how unnecessarily limited awareness is for most of us, to suggest some ontogogic aids that may be helpful in supporting the patient's efforts to expand his awareness, and finally to speculate about the potentialities of truly liberated awareness.

AN EXPERIMENT

Let us begin with a simple experiment in awareness, which the reader is invited to perform.

> Read these directions through once, then carry out the suggested procedure before reading further. Seat yourself comfortably in such a way that arms, head, and back are well supported. Close your eyes. Consistently deny to awareness any sensory impression. Imagine yourself a subject in a sensory-deprivation experiment. No sight, no sound, no touch, no taste or smell, no movement. Do not move, no matter what the provocation. Imagine yourself immobile in a complete blackness of all dimensions. This is not a blackness of something black that is present but the empty blackness of utter

---

[1] My use of "awareness" telescopes that concept and "consciousness" as these are distinguished by May (1958) and others. That distinction, useful in other contexts, is not pivotal in this discussion.

nothingness. Now extend the blackness to thoughts. Do not let any thought pattern become focal. Seek emptiness of mind.

Continue this imaginal exercise for what you feel to be five minutes. Do not interrupt to check time. Rather note the time when you begin the experiment and again when you stop. It is possible with only moderate effort to sit quite still and systematically note and dismiss many of the stimuli playing on you at any given minute. If seriously attempted, you may get some feeling for what true sensory deprivation would be like.

Almost always, if one is candid with himself, he will sense the emergence of an anxiety, and many times one will find a reason to end the experiment more quickly than he had planned, or perhaps a thought sweeps in and takes over awareness so that the experiment is "forgotten" (while the awareness of external stimuli "slips back in").

The foregoing are the instructions for the experiment. Before reading further, try it out.

As an aside we may note that the way in which the reader responded to the invitation to experiment with his awareness is expressive of the reader's whole way of being in the world. When I, the writer, propose to experiment with your awareness, you, the reader, react quite rightly as though I proposed to experiment with your very being. This is exactly so. Awareness is the basic function of being. The "projective tests" recognize, although incompletely, how very true this is.

Returning to the experience of trying to sense what it would be like to have no stimuli at all impinging on us, we can best refer to it in visual terms: It is like being in the center of an immense blackness of utter emptiness.[2]

Now let us imagine that into this blackness, this emptiness, comes a pinpoint of light. It is obvious that one would focus on this at once. The need for a *something* to replace the *nothing* is so basic that we would consider as seriously deranged a person who did not so respond, or we would be sure that he was deliberately ignoring the point of light, thus proving its focal importance.

The pinpoint of light grows, and we begin to see through the hole and to detect movement on the other side. Think how compelling the need to see more clearly, to know what moves. Grad-

---
[2] This is the "night" the person in the existential crisis refers to in the autobiographical fragment quoted on page 172.

ually the hole enlarges and becomes a window out of the blackness, looking onto the world. All is empty nothingness, except as we look through this window, the window of our awareness.

The Nature of Awareness

The window of our awareness is our point of being in the world. It is not the same as our vision or any one or all of our senses, but it is mediated by our senses. Awareness, we are saying, is not sensation. It may or may not be simply the subjective aspect of sensation. No one can prove either way at this point.

But continuing the window analogy for the moment and remembering that the window is set in the midst of emptiness, it is obvious how important it would be to us to have as large a window as possible, of as good quality and as clean glass as possible, and so on. Certainly our great concern with intelligence, our attention to correcting defects of vision and hearing, our development of instruments and gauges (binoculars, microscopes, thermometers, watches), all are efforts to improve our window on the world. Yet often we seem to think these offer us a new window when actually they affect only the same basic window. Sometimes we even seem to say they take us through the window into immediate touch with the "out there" without dependence on human awareness. This is not so either.

Defects of the Window Analogy. There are two central defects to our window analogy that should warn us against carrying it much further. First, the analogy implies an awareness back of awareness (that I am back of and seeing through the window). This is definitely not intended. I am the window. The *I-process* is awareness most basically.

The second defect of the window analogy is that it leaves out of consideration the feelingfulness which we postulate as an inherent aspect of awareness. This point is so important that I will enlarge upon it in the following section.

FEELINGFULNESS AS AN INTEGRAL PART OF AWARENESS

In this chapter I will several times deal with what I believe to be a false but popularly held model of awareness as a punched-card filing system. The dehumanization of human functions which came about with the rationalistic swing of the pendulum tended to restrict our view of this central human process of awareness.[3] By and large we have thought of awareness in terms of recognition and manipulation of verbal facts. I elaborate upon this point because it is so important to recognize the fundamental fallacy involved, and to see how it leads to much misunderstanding of human functioning.

The essential affirmative assertion to be made here is that awareness is always feelingful awareness and only neurotic distortion (resistance) or the artificial models of awareness developed for research or teaching (God help us!) divide the cognitive from the conative and the affectional. Awareness, we are saying, is an integral process, which—for heuristic purposes—we may describe as having aspects of meaning, feeling, and action potential, but awareness always has these aspects and is not simply one or the other.

The significance of this point is that feelingfulness is thus recognized as implicit in the *I-process* and is properly expected in each of the aspects of the ontologic givens of finiteness, action potential, choice, and apartness.

THE EVOLUTION OF AWARENESS

Awareness is an evolving phenomenon. We are not born with transcendent awareness; we seek to attain it. There is a tendency to conceive the human situation as one in which we have fallen from the grace of full awareness through our service to the false gods of marketing values, seeking the approval of others, and so on. In this view, society is the devil and man's need for social acceptance is original sin. (I phrase these matters in this quasi-religious manner to make evident the parallel and a possible source of this way of looking at the human experience.) So viewed, we look to analytic psychotherapy to wash away the sins of the resistances so that our natural goodness may reassert itself.

---

[3] Thus it took the creative researches of the whole group nicknamed "the new look in perception" (for example, Blake and Ramsey, 1951) to rediscover what an older psychology and everyday experience had long known: affectional states are intimately part of, and importantly influence, what we are aware of. This comment is not meant to belittle the very significant contribution of the "new look" investigators, only to highlight the extreme situation they helped to correct.

Awareness grows. It is not a static, given quantum. The sequence of action forms traced out on pages 208–209 may also be regarded in terms of the growth of awareness. Further, it is an evolutionary sequence—for the race and for the individual.

AWARENESS AND TRANSCENDENCE

Awareness cannot cope with the immensity of The All until it has matured to the point of transcendence. When awareness is first flickering into life, it must deal with but minute fractions of The All. When we, as parents, teach our child to speak, for example, we are teaching him how to deal with a limited bit of awareness. Just as this learning permits him to "handle" that limited bit, it concurrently distorts pure awareness in some measure. Some learnings, of course, introduce much more distortion than others. The learning that he is particularly related to this man called "Daddy" is important and useful, even though it will in some measure distort relations to all other men and, thus, to "Daddy" also. The learning, "You should never be angry at 'Daddy,'" may serve a short-term purpose also, but it introduces even more pervasive distortions.

But what is this "learning"? In another place I will say that I do not believe learning is a valid psychological concept. Now I am using it without cavil.[4] Learning is how we come to use our awareness. Learning is not a separate process from awareness. Learning is a word we use to describe ways awareness functions. Thus it may apply to ways we feel about awareness, choices we make, and relations we form.

When a person comes to me for psychotherapeutic aid, he comes because his awareness too often has feelings in it that he feels unhappy about[5] and wants to change. This often means that the awareness is beginning to emerge in him that there are other ways of being which are potential in him, and that he is imprisoned in unawareness (resistance) which prevents his choosing those other

---
[4] Of course, on still another page I pointed out that consistency is not an existential value (page 210, also see page 398).
[5] These awkward phrases, "awareness about awareness" and "feelings about feelings" are the artifacts of our need to make an object of that which is pure subject, the *I-process* or authentic awareness. Had we language to speak in pure subject (subjective) terms, these apparent reflexive circles would be avoided.

ways. It is a familiar observation that the first major therapeutic step is the decision to seek therapy. This is the existential significance of that observation.

A REALISTIC VIEW OF AWARENESS

We need to have a realistic view of what is the usual state of awareness of most people. Despite all our investigations of subjective experience, no clear-cut delineation of the usual state of human awareness has been well documented. In the following comments I will be offering my observations based on what my patients tell me, my subjective and introspective perceptions, and what I have been able to learn from talking to friends and others.

The usual state of awareness in most people seems to be one in which there is a moderate field of perceptions that range from sharply defined to vague and amorphous, that are in constant flux, and that show within the field at any time many contradictory tendencies. There are frequently several different figures competing for dominance, the sense of other figures potential but not in the field, a pressure from subjective sources matched by the emergence into awareness of objective or external materials.

In short, what I am saying is that the visual field, with its range from sharp figures to undifferentiated background, has given us a limited analogy for the whole field of awareness. A better analogy may be the auditory field. Here the contrast between figure and ground often is even more sharp, and yet there are occasions when the difference between the two is almost indiscernible. Instances of the pre-empting of the auditory field by some line of stimulus are more familiar also.

>Louise had an appointment in the evening during the hot summer months. Customarily I opened all the windows of the offices in those days before we had air-conditioning. One evening Louise was telling me about her struggles to win autonomy from her mother. As she talked sirens approached the building where we sat. Determinedly, I tried to attend to Louise even as I heard the sirens come to a halt just below our window, heard loud voices shouting, and a crowd gathering. I found that I was beginning to sniff for smoke, and still Louise talked earnestly on. By now there were five or six pieces of

fire equipment outside, and the sounds of voices and powerful engines told of late-arriving equipment. My attention to Louise was quite overwhelmed. Yet through it all, Louise seemed not to have heard, for she went steadily on telling me of her concerns. At length I interrupted her, explaining that I felt the need to assure myself that the building was not on fire since all of this fire equipment seemed to be immediately at hand. Louise seemed rather startled. "What fire equipment?" And then, suddenly, she seemed to hear the sounds that had been so intrusive in my own awareness.

This incident with Louise redemonstrates the familiar fact that what is in our awareness is only partly a function of what external stimuli are being presented and that internal circumstances may quite override the presence of even rather compelling external stimuli. Sometimes this is only a minor inconvenience with amusing aspects; sometimes it is the basis of grave tragedy.

A FALLACIOUS VIEW OF AWARENESS

Now what I have said so far about the usual state of awareness is in marked contrast to what we tend to believe is the "usual" or "normal." There seems to be a generally held, although usually implicit, belief that awareness is properly an orderly and even systematic collecting of all data from the environment, processing these in terms of one's rational concerns, bringing to bear the fruits of one's learning and experience, and then compounding reasoned answers. To be sure, when it is spelled out in this fashion many people would say the equivalent of, "Well, I know it isn't quite as neat and orderly as that, but certainly that is the way it should be." Most people will admit that their own "minds" or awarenesses do not work quite that way, but they usually feel faintly ashamed of the fact or tend to dwell on the rare occasions when it most approached such a model. A few, with terrible needs driving them, manage to bully themselves into a kind of reduced and overcontrolled use of their awareness that then seems to match this model. This latter pattern seems especially apt to occur in bright young men who look to science to provide compensations for a sense of personal isolation and social deprivation.

Actually, awareness for the overwhelming majority of us is more like a bunch of preadolescents playing "king of the mountain" than an orderly meeting of a parliamentary body. Varying percepts jostle for central focus, coalitions form and dissolve rapidly, emotions flow back and forth, and new perspectives are constantly overthrowing the old. This is not an orderly process, to be sure, and frequently it is quite disorderly. There are times when urgency enters like a strict games leader and organization exists for a period, but usually when this occurs some of the perceptions, not a little of the feelingfulness, and probably a portion of the creativity is pushed aside.

What I am saying may seem rather paradoxical. On the one hand I think that our very primitive understanding of ourselves is represented in this somewhat chaotic manner in which our awarenesses chiefly function. As we gain in genuine appreciation of our own potential we will almost certainly learn to participate in our own being aware in a much richer and less constricted manner. On the other hand, those more productive and satisfying manners of being aware may well involve greater apparent confusion and intermingling of percepts than we now know. Far from expecting that greater efficiency is a good to be achieved by greater organization of awareness, I am inclined to think that once we release the constraints of self-bondage and learned inhibitions and fears of our own being, we may be able to find tremendous stimulation and greatly increased creativity in allowing awareness to be aswirl with a multitude of percepts mixing and interlinking in as many ways as possible, while our intentionality gradually draws from this boiling broth that which best expresses our being at any given moment.

AWARENESS AND MEMORY

Let us return to the popular model of how our awareness should work. This model is the source of much confusion and limitation on our full employment of our awareness. The model is that information comes into us on punched cards and we file it under several different headings. Then when we need the information we check through the files under the appropriate headings as dictated by our needs and see whether we have anything. If we filed under the same heading when we received the information as we now use when we look for it, then we can provide the information back out. If we can't get it, we either don't have it, or it's misfiled, or the card has deteriorated with age so we can't read it, or it's not catalogued rightly. In any of these four instances, that's that, and we can't produce it. This is a very mechanical, static concept, to be sure, but I think most of us see it somewhat that way.

I believe the model I have just described is wrong in several important ways.

—We do not get items of information as such. We are aware of the stream of experience, which includes what we will later think of as items of information at the time we try to recollect them (or because of our idea of the way the "mind" works we may even so name them at the time of the experience, but that is really irrelevant).

—As we experience, we exercise choice in our actions, which results in making some of the possibilities actual in awareness and others not so.

—Whatever has been in awareness is in awareness. This questions the validity of such concepts as learning, memory, forgetting, and recall. Because we have language forms that suggest such processes we behave as though they existed in our awareness. Actually, I believe, these postulated processes are descriptive conventions that are chiefly useful in a mechanomorphic psychology. Phenomenologically, I doubt that anyone has ever experienced "I am learning" as an immediate recognition in awareness. Similarly with remembering or forgetting. Rather, one simply is aware or unaware of certain experiences.

—Almost as certainly, the same observations may be made about the postulated processes of the unconscious and the preconscious. These are useful descriptive inventions, but they are not experienced realities of being.[6]

The apparent inability to recall something is, I think, due to any of several influences: (a) the expectation that it will be difficult to make such recall, (b) resistances such as we have dealt with in earlier chapters, or (c) conflicting awarenesses.

---

[6] Having just cavalierly dispatched much of general and abnormal psychology, I will continue to use such terms as learning, memory, unconscious, and preconscious throughout this discussion. I am the prisoner of my own experience more than my theory and I would like. If I waited to resolve all the problems that these postulations about psychological processes present I am quite sure I should die of extreme old age without finishing this chapter.

PROBLEM SOLVING

So far I have been talking about specific "memories," chiefly of facts. The inaccuracy of our model of how awareness works becomes even more clear when we turn to other aspects of awareness, which in some ways are more important but less frequently dealt with by much of psychology. A particularly significant area is how one "thinks about subjective concerns."

> John has a conflict with his wife about whether the children should go to bed at 8:30 or 9:30. Setting aside for the moment the many false assumptions John makes about children's bedtimes and his wife's way of thinking, let us simply see how John tries to solve the problem.
>
> "Oh, I wanted to talk to you about this fight my wife and I are having about the kids' bedtime. It's silly, but it gets my goat. I don't know why it bothers me so . . ."
>
> Suppose I say to John, interrupting here, "Well, take a look and see what about this gets you upset."
>
> "Gee! I have tried to think, but I don't know."

Now John is behaving as though the answer to this question is a bit of factual information he "learned" at one time. He's now checked the file under a couple of headings: "children's bedtimes" ("mostly old memories; nothing suitable"), "upset" ("too many to wade through; have to organize that better sometime"), "wife" (same), and finding nothing immediately coded to the situation, has concluded, "I don't know."

But wait a minute. If John doesn't know, who does? Well, his transference makes him think I probably do. ("Surely they teach that in graduate school?") But if he stops and thinks about that, he may conclude that I do not know but I probably can figure out from what I know about him. Thus he implies I have more file cards on him than he has on himself. Strangely, that does not seem to bother him.

> Now that I've carried him this far I may hit another kind of popular (resistance) misconception: "Well, I don't know and you say you don't; so I guess nobody knows. Shucks, maybe it just gets my goat, you know, just one of those things. Does there always have to be a reason?"

What in the world does this mean? John is an intelligent man, well educated, but he is acting more bizarrely than a primitive who might explain the situation as due to the presence of a demon. At least the primitive is not in full flight from reason.

> Let me patiently explain to John something of the irrationality. Then what happens: "Well, I guess there is a reason somewhere. Let's see, do you suppose it has something to do with my own bedtime as a child? My mother..."

Now John is handling the problem by making himself an object for speculative study, using what bits and fragments of psychology he may have. In a sense John is taking over what he thinks my job should be, since it is apparent I am not doing it. Once more I stop him, point out the subject-object split. Some place along in here John is going to go off into some of his resistance patterns: get angry, change the subject, lose interest, whatever. However, let us suppose that I deal with these and return him to the question, "Why does it bother you so that you and your wife disagree about the children's bedtime?" What can John do now? I have enjoined or disproven memory, speculation, and cosmic chance. The reader may well ask himself what choices are open to John. Many will feel almost as stumped as he does.

> "John," I say, "stop a minute. You're so busy inside you couldn't find the answer to the question if you did 'know' it as you say." And I wait a minute or two for him to settle down. Then, "Now, just tell me about the dispute with your wife without trying to solve anything or explain it or anything. Just give me as complete a picture as you can of what you each say and what you think and feel about it and, of course, of anything else that occurs to you as you're talking."

And John begins to tell me. As he does so, I keep alert to the resistances that may enter to dilute the authenticity of his being-here-telling-me. If I am able to detect these and display them for John's awareness, and if he is able to risk setting them aside, he gives me a detailed picture that increasingly opens up and carries his awareness to the meanings this dispute with his wife has for him. This occurs without his "figuring it out," without his ever having figured it out in the past, without its ever having been told him, but with a sense of recognition and a quality of certainty that needs no rational documentation and that makes evident concurrently (indeed, intrinsically) some of the choices John has for dealing with the situation. Indeed, if we press on, the linkage of this matter to other related matters will also come into his awareness, and eventually (theoretically to be sure, but I fully believe it) from this starting point we could get to all of John's experience.

Now, of course, this is the ultimate picture. In actual practice I and my patients are not skillful and sensitive and courageous enough to follow any one thread through all the tangles of resistances to final openness of the patient's full awareness. But this is the process, and it works as clearly as I've depicted for periods. It reveals the way awareness operates; so that we can discard the card-file notion.

Awareness, we are saying, is not static and fixed, is flexible and susceptible to modulation, is creative and evolving, and is ultimately a unity.

Awareness and Causality: A Speculation

So much is safe and pretty sure. Let us go out past the frontier.

John finds that the dispute with his wife over the children's bedtimes affects him so acutely because it is a reenactment of disagreements he caused between his parents. He used to play one off against the other, and he was and is guilty and frightened (because he, the child, had such power over the parents, his source of security). John and I can nod our heads in satisfaction: We've solved it. We know why.

But is this so? Well, pragmatically at this time, it may be. I don't really think so in the long run however. In a way John was right when he said "It just gets my goat . . ." And his question, "Does everything have to have a reason?" was a valid one.

The argument with his wife just gets John's goat. There does not have to be a reason. But if John wants to change what will be actual in the future, then a "reason" is a handle for doing so (not necessarily the only handle, either).

Clearly we are not going to change what did happen. The past is static, dead, and a fiction anyway. John's account of the fight is no more or less accurate than his wife's, as far as one being what "really happened." Each is faithfully saying what he saw through his window, but each has built into his window certain qualities that help to determine what he will see. These qualities are not necessarily distortions.

Thinking of our looking through an actual window, if the window is built to magnify, does that show us more of what is real, or less?—the question is not answerable. If the window screens out certain light qualities or brings in others, is that more or less real? (Again, if you see certain rocks under "black light" they glow and show colors that "normal" light does not reveal. Which is real?)

When John and I disclose a linkage between his parents' arguments and John's own arguments with his wife we have used a certain filter on our windows that enables us to see this. We are using that filter during the event of John and I talking *now* about his awareness of the event with his wife. We are *not* using the filter on the event with his wife or on the events of his parents arguing.

MULTIPLE "CAUSES"

It might be that we could also find that the argument with his wife had important connections to John's feelings of masculinity, to his competitive desire to seem more understanding to his children than does his wife, to his feelings of impotence in so many areas of his life, to his fearing tenderness in himself so that only through fighting can he be emotionally close with her. . . . This is why speculation about the meaning of the fight is useless, and we have to roll back the resistances so that John himself can lead us to the "handle" that is pertinent.

But that handle is only the pertinent one at this point in time. We may later return to this same incident five more times and each time pick up the incident by a different handle so that we "confirm" each of the explanations offered in the preceding paragraph.

Does this mean that one explanation is as good as another or that none is really so? Neither. The "right" explanation is right in terms of the event of our (John's and my) inquiry, not in terms of the incident of John's fight with his wife.

But then what caused the original fight with his wife? Nothing caused it (as John said, though defensively), or everything that

John is and his wife is caused it. The latter is probably a better way of saying it: John and his wife caused it.

The building-blocks conception of the human person "explains" the fight by saying, "This block, John's earlier experience of his parents fighting, is still in John. Therefore it somehow produced the event of the fight with his wife." The problem of how is usually dealt with by other words that ultimately boil down to the answer that a part of John is operating separately from the rest of John and does this thing to John.

Now, the reader is probably still unsatisfied with this state of affairs. We want explanations, causes, and results. Only with these can we keep the world orderly, be "scientific." But causality is not the static, atomistic, mechanical thing that the sentence, "John fought with his wife because of his reactions to his parents' fights," would require. Causality must be the constant creative act of awareness. By opening his awareness in such a way that he can experience his fear and guilt regarding his parents' fights in a forthcoming situation in which he and his wife are concerned with the children's bedtimes, John will be able to deal with that situation for itself rather than as though it were an earlier event. To the extent that one can think in terms of causes in this new situation, it is a matter of John's awareness causing a different outcome. However, it will be recognized, this is really an unusual extension of the term "cause."

IMPLICATIONS

The implications of what we are saying are these:

Awareness which is freed of resistances ("free awareness") is full awareness of all that has been or is in awareness.

Free awareness recognizes the is-ness of each element within itself; that is, an event is experienced as it is in awareness, not as some other event.

Of course, we are now approaching a characterization of transcendence. Transcendence implies, in its fullest form, the full and free awareness of being in all its aspects, in which the givenness of each aspect is the givenness of the whole. At this point, choice is the glad assent to the given. This does not mean choice is meaningless, for that very assent is the creation of the given even as it is the recognition of it. Choice, creativity, and recognition thus become synonymous in transcendence. Similarly, action is participation as contingencies are dissolved in wholeness.

Varied Experiences of Altered Awareness

We can now speculate about the further reaches of awareness that may be potential to us. We have no real survey of the probabilities, but varied kinds of experiences can suggest some possibilities.

The unusual perceptual experiences of the sensory-deprivation subjects, the altered consciousness of those who take the psychedelic preparations, the delirium of the desperately ill, the mystic experiences of religious persons, the dreams of normal sleep, the altered consciousness of those who practice meditation (Deikman, 1963), the peak experiences of those who contemplate scenes of great natural beauty, the reports of remarkable perceptions by persons practicing yoga or certain of the Gestalt therapy exercises or having "bodily awareness" training—all of these and probably many others; what, if anything, have they in common? I believe that many, if not all, are related. I think the common element is an opening of awareness beyond the bounds of our heavily conditioned, daily perceptual limits. Each person interacts with world in his own way, and thus the marked variety of reported percepts. But each person discovers more of world than he has known before, and thus the striking similarities of many of these percepts.

The attempt to list common features is hazardous at best, but it may be useful to note some of the frequently reported aspects:

—an intensified experience of color, form, and movement;
—a reduced preoccupation with usual, utilitarian meaning;
—a reduced concern with the self;
—a heightened recognition of linkages or relatednesses where they are not usually expected;
—an increase of emotional response;
—a feeling of "cosmic consciousness" or "oceanic awareness."

Constraints on Awareness

We have seen something of how limited our awareness usually is in contrast to what seems potential. Let us consider now some of the sources of this limitation.

RESISTANCES

A first important source can be identified in the resistances and transferences, with which I have already dealt. We find ourselves experiencing overwhelming anxiety, and we constrict awareness as a way of trying to reduce that anxiety. Rollo May speaks of "shrinking one's world space, which is the neurotic pattern of repressions and inhibitions described classically by Freud" (1959b, p. 6). In the extreme this is the "ostrich with his head in the sand" pattern, which far more of us practice than we like to admit. Recognition of the enslaving nature of this pattern is implicit in the teaching, "You shall know the truth, and the truth will make you free," and in the existential recognition that confrontation of the actual increases choice.

LEARNED INHIBITIONS

Related to the manner in which the resistances constrict awareness, and frequently overlapping with that influence, are those learned inhibitions which produce similar constraints. It needs to be recognized that the combined effects of resistances and learned inhibitions can be very powerful in its influence on perception itself.

Ken, at nineteen, was timid and mother-dominated. He was intensely curious about girls and sex, but he was very ashamed of his curiosity. His dating was circumspect and frustrating. Looking back on it later when he was in therapy, Ken observed, "I always hoped something would happen so that we'd have to get undressed or something, but I never could make even a little pass at a girl." One night something did happen. Since it was a warm summer's night, Ken and his date drove to the beach. The girl decided to take a moonlight swim and invited Ken to join her. He was beside himself with a whirling maelstrom of feelings. He was tremendously excited sexually as he realized she meant to undress right there with him, and he would soon see a nude girl for the first time. He was terribly ashamed, for he was convinced that his sexual response would reveal him to the girl as base and unworthy of her trust. He was eager to join her and yet completely convinced that he could not do so. He was terrified that someone would discover them, and finally he was nearly sick with the fear that he might have the chance or be expected to act on the erotic fantasies and hopes which he'd so long known in secret.

Making some vague excuse, Ken held the girl's clothes while she did indeed strip, run into the water for a bit, come out and dance about to shake the water from her body, and then dress again. Telling me about it, Ken said, "I wanted to see her more than anything in the world, but I thought she'd be angry if she knew that. Anyway, when I did try to look—you won't believe this—I couldn't see her. I mean, I really couldn't make my eyes focus. I haven't any idea what she looked like!"

In the therapy group Julie constantly protested that the others were attributing hostility to her remarks when she only had the desire to help. Again and again she felt wronged when others protested that she had hurt their feelings. To the therapist it was clear that Julie could not let herself hear the constant belittling and condescension with which she reported her perceptions of the other patients. She was quite sincere in reporting her conscious awareness of an attempt to help, but her limited awareness was very evident to the group and the therapist.

The line between the resistances in their effect in constraining awareness and the learned inhibitions is a vague one. It is important, however, to recognize that there are these several kinds of constraints upon our awareness.

LACK OF TRAINING

A third source of constraint lies in the fact that we are given little, if any, training in using our awareness. Generally it is assumed that awareness is a spontaneous capacity. While this might be so in ideal circumstances, it is certainly not so under our usual living conditions. People show tremendous ability to learn to use their awareness more broadly, more deeply, and more effectively. This is evident, for instance, in one's learning to appreciate various art forms, particularly those that are somewhat esoteric. People who come to enjoy certain forms of classical music (such as chamber music), of graphic arts (such as impressionistic painting), or of dance frequently report that their whole experience of awareness is that of enlarged appreciation and receptivity.

It is reasonable that each person can find his life enriched as he increases his range and scope of awareness. Particularly in our culture, much can be done to increase sensitivity in interpersonal relations, to free one's capacity for empathic understanding of others, and to learn more trust of one's "intuition" or unreasoned perceptions. The work of Bruner and others (McCleary and Lazarus, 1949; Postman, Bruner, and McGinnies, 1948) in demonstrating the process of "subception" suggests what is otherwise supported, that nearly instantaneous perception is possible and available when we let ourselves use it. So-called "mathematical wizards" can briefly examine a long column of three- and four-place numbers and write an accurate additive total. Many who have become expert in certain kinds of visual tasks can perform them with extreme accuracy and unusual speed. One can be trained to read in excess of one thousand words a minute with excellent retention. Certain visual discriminations can be made by motivated people with a speed that seems incredible. All these and many other instances may be cited to show that much more speed, efficiency, and clarity of perception is possible than we have traditionally recognized.

Recognition of the high probability that our awarenesses are capable of very great expansion is a clear-cut instance of the "new world" that awaits us. The discovery of an easily reachable and hospitable planet could afford us less enrichment of our being than could the attainment of greater range and depth of our awareness in our daily living. This is, of course, a major purpose of the analytic work, but it is also a central concern of ontology, as we shall see in the next chapter.

14 — Ontologic aids to expanding awareness

Ontogogy is the process of leading a person out into greater realization of his being. This conception is nowhere more pertinent than when we undertake to facilitate the patient's own efforts to enlarge the compass of his feelingful awareness. The implication of that statement needs to be made explicit: ontogogy may aid the person who seeks to broaden his awareness, but the intent of that person is fundamental to any hope of success. This necessity of the person's own intent being directed toward broadened awareness has two significant consequences. The preliminary work of the analysis of the resistance is usually essential not only because it in itself does much to free awareness but because it is often only through such an analysis that the person can get free enough to grasp genuinely and to pursue actively the life meaningfulness of broadened awareness.

From one perspective all the work of the analytic phase of the therapeutic course is directed toward the resolution of constrictions of awareness. The therapist's interventions are designed to bring to awareness percepts that have been potential but not actual to the patient's consciousness. As these interventions are well presented and as the patient effectively incorporates the reclaimed perceptual material thus presented to him, the "healing" effects are to be observed in greater range and depth of awareness, in more aware experiencing by the patient of his own life and feelings, and in his more perceptive relations with others and the nonhuman environment. In short, the analytic phase concerns itself with the release of awareness and its success is evidenced in broadened awareness. This is not really surprising, of course, but it is a reminder of the fact that awareness is the central process of our being.

PURPOSES OF ONTOGOGIC EFFORTS

When we come to the ontogogic phase we must build on the foundation of effective analytic work and with the expectation that such work will continue throughout the therapeutic course. The ontogogic work seeks to supplement the analytic, not replace it. In offering such supplementation, several functional purposes may be identified.

> Faulty concepts of the nature of awareness may be disclosed and more useful ones taught in their place. In this fashion much can be done to ensure that the growth is supported by the cognitive resources of the patient. Further, the patient is aided in taking responsibility for the further development of his awareness once the therapeutic relationship is terminated.
>
> Experiences can be capitalized upon or even evoked to arouse an emotional and attitudinal recognition of the restrictions now confining one's awareness and of the greater range that is potential.
>
> The patient's direct intuition of his own being—the *I-process*—is a matter of his sensing his centeredness in his awareness and his aware choosing. Awareness training may help in dissolving the false equation of the *I* to the *Me* (or *Self*) and facilitate non-self-conscious being in the moment.

Although the analytic and ontogogic phases overlap greatly in all areas, the concurrence is greatest in this aspect of fostering greater awareness. The resistance constrains awareness, and the analytic work seeks to lift that constraint. At the same time, we gradually begin to supplement the analytic interventions with ontogogic aids designed to expand the patient's appreciation of free awareness. Because this overlap is so great, the suggestions that follow will be seen to be chiefly limited aids rather than major strategies.

TEACHING A NEW CONCEPT OF AWARENESS

In earlier pages of this chapter we have described an implicit and frequently held conception of the nature of awareness. As we saw there, what the patient feels as the way his "mind should be" is roughly akin to a well-maintained library card catalog. Often there will be an overlay of reflexive shame, anger, or guilt that the patient may be conscious of without ever having fully examined its basis. Inquiry will often disclose that the patient, knowing his awareness is not as orderly as he thinks it should be, feels this is an evidence of his inferiority, inadequate self-discipline, or his "neurosis." There is a relief of internal conflict and discomfort as well as a gain in effective therapeutic motivation possible once the patient begins to adopt a more realistic conception of awareness.

> Henry is trying to understand why it is that he is so short-tempered with his family when he is known in his work situation for his evenness of disposition. He is well motivated now to try to solve this problem, yet he is experiencing great difficulty in focusing his attention. He complains of many distracting thoughts, of ideas that seem momentarily available and then disappear. At length he bursts out in exasperation,
>
> P: Oh hell, I can't think worth a damn. I don't know what's the matter with me.
> T: You're pretty sure something's the matter with you.
> P: Of course, I can't get my fool mind to settle down and think about why I'm so nasty to the family.
> T: Perhaps this is the way you can best find the answer to your questions.
> P: How do you mean?
> T: Well, you seem to feel you should get the answer like drawing a certain paper out of a well-organized, alphabetical file, and you're angry because it's more like trying to assemble it from a jumbled jigsaw puzzle.
> P: (Henry is surprised.) Gee, I never thought of it that way. Maybe it is more like a jigsaw puzzle...

This is a simplified instance of the kind of teaching that can facilitate the patient's ability to use his awareness constructively.

THE SEVERAL STREAMS OF AWARENESS

A second teaching device I have found helpful involves giving the patient greater appreciation of the omnipresent diversity of his awareness.

The therapist will gain much understanding of his patient that may later enable him to know how best to make his interventions in "the patient's own language" if the therapist does not try to alter the patient's own manner of reporting his concerns and awarenesses at first. However, later on, and usually well before we enter the ontogogic phase, it is well to note the ways in which the range and variety of the patient's awareness—as revealed in his associations—are unduly limited and to begin to teach the patient about other aspects potential to his consciousness. A device that has sometimes proven helpful this way is illustrated below.

>I ask the patient if he has visited the "Nickelodeon" at Disneyland. If so, I use his memory of the unusual little motion picture house. If not, I describe it to him.
>
>There are no seats in the Nickelodeon. Instead one stands on a central platform raised less than a foot above the floor. Arrayed around the circular room are six small motion picture screens, set several feet above head level so that all viewers can see each screen. On each screen a different picture is playing, and all are playing at the same time. One may be showing *The Perils of Pauline*, another an old Betty Compson feature, a third an early animated cartoon, and so on. The viewer may watch any one he chooses, may switch from one to another as suits his fancy, or as the action on the screens attracts him.
>
>This, I tell my patient, is something like the way it is within one's awareness. There are a variety of forms of awareness all going on at the same time. The person may choose to which to give his focal attention, and he may choose to switch from one to another.
>
>Usually there is one aspect that is the explicit content of the moment as my patient and I talk. A second would be his continuing perception of his *Self*. In some manner his *Self* is always present, even though explicitly he may deny this. A third aspect usually is an affective-evaluative appreciation of what is under consideration. Sometimes this may be a mild interest in what is being discussed, sometimes it may be an intense emotional response. There is always some measure of feeling tone, and frequently this is linked to judgmental attitudes toward the experience. A fourth aspect of awareness, one that seems often to be largely outside of consciousness, is the anticipatory or conative. Each moment we are making minute adjustments and preparations for each succeeding moment. Very often the patient can learn that he is phrasing what he is saying now in anticipation of what future things

he will want to say or want to avoid saying, or perhaps in terms of intended impact on me. The fifth area has to do with memory. Very often, when the patient's attention is called to it, he can find memories either quite distant or quite recent that relate to the stream of his awareness at this given moment. A sixth area has to do with fantasy. For many patients it is hard to find the day-dream extensions of that about which they are talking. It seems that this aspect or dimension of awareness is much devalued for adults in our culture, and they have difficulty identifying it. Those patients who are freer or more artistic or those who have achieved some therapeutic progress may show more ability to identify the fantasy aspects in what they are discussing. Finally, it is possible to recognize the ongoing stream of physical awarenesses. This, I usually find, is one which most handily may be used to illustrate the whole process of discovery of one's awarenesses. For, as I point out to the patient, the pressure of his back against the couch was not in the forefront of his consciousness until I called it to his attention, but once brought to attention as an example the patient often can find many other physical awarenesses that are ongoing. This can serve then as a model for trying to locate the other dimensions I have listed.

EXPANDING AWARENESS

Our description of the stream of physical awareness leads us to the recognition of how often the physical can inform both the patient and the therapist. The presence of many pressures in our daily living which operate to focus our attention on externals usually means that the greater portion of the therapist's efforts will need to be given to bringing to the patient's attention his more internal experience. Thus the therapist will frequently do well to reflect back to the patient evidences of emotions, physical tensions, or implied meanings in what the patient is saying.

Many patients are quite cut off from genuine awareness of processes within themselves, so that I often find it helpful to call on them from time to time to give attention to bodily sensations: "You seem all tensed up as you tell me about this," "How do you feel physically right now?" "Notice the way you gesture with a closed fist as you speak about that," and so on. Similarly, attention to the patient's facial expressions as he talks may prove enlightening to both the patient and the therapist.

Grace tells me of her feeling of estrangement from her parents and her life-long belief that she was less valued than her brother. As she talks, however, there is a pleasant smile frequently on her face, and her whole manner conveys a good-natured indifference. However, when I repeatedly call this to Grace's attention, a change occurs: "You seem to need to be so very tolerant as you tell me about your parents' preference for your brother." Grace protests, "It's all so long ago now, it doesn't really matter." But I persist and continue to note the good-humored smile which somehow has a flavor of forcedness about it. "It's very important to you to regard that hurt as something in the past." At length Grace herself begins to wonder and she finally reports, "Today I tried to talk to you without smiling, and, do you know, I can't." Grace's awareness is expanding, and her resistance to true awareness of her experience is being resolved in this interchange. Moreover she is learning to use additional clues to deepen her awareness.

**DEVELOPING AN EXPERIENTIAL BASIS
FOR BROADENING AWARENESS**

Not infrequently patients will protest my efforts to bring them to greater awareness. They say, in effect, "What's the use of being more aware when I know I'll only be more frightened if I am? What I don't know won't hurt me." Over the years I have used a homely device for dealing with this attitude and have found it a genuine aid.

First of all, it is important to emphasize that I only use this device when the patient has achieved a clear recognition of his fear of greater awareness and his clinging to his own resistance. I regard that recognition as a major therapeutic gain in itself. To use the device when the patient is more inauthentically protesting would, I imagine, be futile and only lead to specious argument.

"I want you to imagine that you are going to cross the street in front of this building at one of two times. You may choose which after I describe the two. In either case you must cross in the middle of the block. Your first choice is to cross it at 5:10 this evening just after the university offices and classes close, the stores begin emptying, and just when traffic is most frantic along the street. The other time will be at 2:00 in the morning when only a very occasional car comes along.

However, if you choose 2:00 a.m., you will be thoroughly blind-folded and your ears stopped up completely. Now really imagine yourself crossing at each of those times, and tell me which you choose."

In many, many presentations of the problem, no one has ever seriously chosen the unaware crossing. Moreover, without my elaborating the moral, person after person has recognized the human truth that we are less anxious when we know the hazard than when it is unknown. In this same vein, I have sometimes enjoined a patient, "See your enemy's face. Look at him full on. Don't terrorize yourself with the unknown." In such instances the patient has known clearly that I meant the enemy within, the feared aspect of his own being.

TALKING AS A WAY OF EXTENDING AWARENESS

Earlier, in Chapter 13, I talked about the fallacious views of awareness that are generally held. The file-card view of the mind often is implicit in the patient's understanding of his own experience and the unwary therapist may find he is unwittingly agreeing to it. This is particularly apt to be the case when the patient seems aware—and even so reports—but without affect (feelings). Authentic awareness is feelingful awareness.

> Pete had heard another member of the therapy group describe his greatly improved relation with his wife. The account was a warming one and was meaningfully received by all. Pete said nothing, but his manner showed he had been listening intently.
>
> T: Pete, you seem involved in Harold's description of what is happening with his wife.
> P: Yes, I am, but only intellectually. I can see what he means and recognize the connection with my own marriage, but it's all pretty abstract.
> T: Why don't you say it anyway?
> P: Well, it's just that I have the feeling that once I could have had that same sort of closeness with Mary, but now too much has happened and I've pulled away too much, and it can never be like that for us.
>
> Pete stopped talking, his tone was level, his manner composed. Then abruptly he sort of collapsed in his chair, and a great sob burst out of him.

P: Oh, my God, I'm so sorry for what I've missed. I guess I don't really know whether it's too late or not. But I'm afraid to hope or to try to change things. But I want so much more . . . And I know Mary does too. . . .

The point is this: Pete thought he knew the facts and his feelings about this matter. In a way, his convincing himself that he did know was a resistance to facing the still-alive hurt and guilt. Avoiding that, he also avoided the possibility of recognizing that there might yet be an opportunity to do something to make a better relation with his wife. The therapist's encouragement to say it out once again demonstrated the nonfixed nature of awareness. In the very saying of what he felt he knew, Pete found himself saying and discovering what he had feared to know.

It is often useful to have the patient say out in full that which he says he knows so well there is no need to talk about it. The patient who learns that he can broaden and deepen his awareness by expressing what he is aware of as completely as possible is the possessor of a powerful aid to his own growth and enrichment.

TEACHING PRECONSCIOUS EXPLORATION

Some patients find it very difficult to explore their nonfocal awarenesses with the therapist. Very often these patients come with an agenda in mind, either consciously or unconsciously. This is a way of controlling what will come into awareness, what will be reported. Some of these patients seem to be blind to the realm of awareness that is the background for the figure of what it is they are expressing. Several devices are available for illustrating to the patient what it means to explore their nonfocal awarenesses.

T: I want you to count aloud from 1 to 25, with a deliberate pause between each number.
P: 1 . . . 2 . . . 3 . . . 4 . . . 5 . . . 6 . . . 7 . . . 8 . . . 9 . . . 10 11 . . . 12 . . . 13 . . .
T: Now interrupt your counting. The numbers are in the front of your mind. What thoughts are in back of them?
P: Well, I was wondering what you were having me do this for and whether I was going fast enough and . . .
T: Now these words you are telling me have moved to the front, what's in back now?

This procedure, when repeated several times, will help some patients to gain more awareness of preconscious thinking and of the figure and ground relationship in their thoughts.

With other patients it is helpful to teach them to recognize the background awareness by using a different analogy.

T: You paused just now as you completed that thought. What were you thinking of? What was in your awareness back of the thought?
P: How do you mean?
T: Well, do you recall the experience of being stopped to let a train go past and then you sit in your car watching the train? You may be looking to see what the road is like ahead of you so that as each car goes past you try to get a quick glimpse of what lies on the other side of the train. You look between the cars very quickly. In somewhat the same way your thoughts that you're most conscious of and that you're telling me about are coming along one after another, but there are brief gaps between them. In those gaps, if you are aware, often you can sense some background thoughts, some background awarenesses. See if you can catch any of these and tell me what they are.

Group Methods and Expanding Awareness

Although anything like an adequate discussion of group methods would take us greatly beyond the purview of this book, I cannot leave the topic of aids to the expansion of awareness without at least mention of this important field in which so much that is creative and exciting is happening.

Two forms of work with groups need to be recognized. They are not distinct and much overlap exists between them. On the one hand is the whole field of group therapy, which has grown up as an offshoot of psychotherapy (Bugental, 1962b; Hora, 1961a). On the other hand is the burgeoning work that originally was called "group dynamics" and that now has its center in the National Training Laboratories programs (National Training Laboratory, 1953). Some of the earliest clear-cut instances of what I am, in this book, calling ontogogy have occurred in this context as programs were developed for the effectively functioning, growth-seeking leaders in the community. Quite recently this orientation has been explicitly extended to try to find ways of extending awareness and fostering positive growth (Bugental & Tannenbaum, 1963).

The Therapeutic Relation and the Therapist's Example

The foregoing suggestions are in the nature of devices or aids. Each assumes an effective working alliance between therapist and patient. When this exists the use of an illustrative anecdote or a demonstration is received by the patient as a facilitation of his own purpose rather than an imposition on him. Where such a relationship does not exist, these same procedures will be experienced as "gimmicks" and manipulations and their net effects will be anti-therapeutic. What I am saying, of course, is that authenticity in the therapist and genuineness in the patient–therapist encounter is the *sine qua non* of the growth process.

Indeed, I can carry this point a bit further and illustrate a further truth of the whole process with which we are concerned. When the therapist is authentic in his own being in the situation and when a genuine dialogue is developing between patient and therapist, the therapist will find his own awareness providing him with the materials for illustrations and demonstrations congruent with his own nature and harmonious with the patient's dominant emotional theme and current needs. This is more than a matter of convenience also; it is the kind of living example of open, creative awareness from which the patient is most apt to gain and which may need no elaboration in words to have its maximal effect.

Implicit in the foregoing is the belief that the technology which is most effective is that which is most authentic. This means that the therapist will certainly recognize his responsibility and opportunity to improve his sensitivity and skill in disciplined and growing ways. It also means, however, that the therapist will seek his own emergence into spontaneous being with the patient in which the procedures are expressions of that "being with" and not self-conscious introductions into the ongoing process. Let me be quite clear: I believe this stage of spontaneity comes about only after self-discipline and not instead of it. Learning, practice, and much attention to one's own self-awareness are fundamental to spontaneity that is genuine and not license.

15 — *Ontologic freedom: Emancipation from the* Self

Before me four regularly spaced and gracefully tapering columns rise to a roof high above. The columns seem to be of beautifully grained and prepared wood. The roof is of another substance, however, apparently a cloth spread on a wood framework. Above the roof is the most fantastic and clearly alien feature. We are accustomed to the roof being the topmost feature of our buildings; not so here. At the far side of the roof a perpendicular wall rises monumentally as high again above the roof as the roof, in turn, is above the base of the supporting columns. What a marvel of engineering to raise that immense wall in such perfectly balanced fashion that these, after all slender, pedestals will sustain the whole in sturdy equilibrium. From each side of that upper wall extend long bridges or runways, which come forward paralleling the roof but well above it to a point nearly to the front of the structure, at which place the forward ends of these bridges are supported by uprights of impressive size. Both the bridges and their supports are of that same fine timber that forms the columns beneath. The back wall, on the other hand, seems to be of the cloth or hide-like material (stretched on timbering) that is used in the roof.

This is the account of a space traveler describing a native structure discovered on an unfamiliar planet. Is the space traveler from earth landing on the third planet of Alpha Centauri and examining there a native temple? Or is the traveler (three inches tall by earth scale) from the third planet of Alpha Centauri landing on earth and describing a chair in my office?

The existential perspective on man's situation brings about new and sometimes startling awarenesses concerning some of life's most familiar aspects. When faithfully retained, these new awarenesses disclose to us a realm of much wider possibilities than we usually recognize. Familiar issues are revealed as having broader implication, and accepted statements of the "way things are" become obvious fictions. This transcending orientation can prove at once frightening and exhilarating. Just as it bestows greater choice and freedom, so it exacts the price of our sense of familiar, comfortable knownness. Endless possibilities unfold before us, but the certainty of calling any one real is denied us. Even our example of the space traveler is misleading in that it suggests a definitive reality (Earth or Alpha Centauri III).

In discussing the resistance and the transference, I necessarily concentrated chiefly on the influences that disrupt the patient's authentic being in his life. I tried to keep in mind that the therapeutic task in dealing with those distortions is not alone that of helping the patient rid himself of malignant influences but is also that of encouraging his greater choice and authenticity in being. Now, however, we are exploring aspects of the therapeutic process in which the balance changes, and increased emphasis is given to that which opens greater possibility and expanded being to the patient. Ontologic freedom opens areas of choice and actualization in which and through which the fully functioning (Rogers 1961a) or self-actualizing (Maslow 1954) person celebrates his being.

I am convinced that we are on the brink of a breakthrough in our understanding of the human condition which may be as pervasive and significant as any which have emerged in the physical sciences. I feel drawn toward the ideas I will set forth below by such an array of varied influences that I am like a surfer riding the strong wave of man's emergence. The general trend in much thinking and writing today is clearly toward fundamental re-evaluation of what it means to *be*. My own notions about this are presented with the full expectation that they may be faulty in many aspects but with the sincere hope that they will add their iota to this tremendous evolution.

I will first review briefly some of the diverse elements in this general trend. Thereby, I hope, the reader will be aided in recognizing both the extreme variety of such questionings about human potential and certain common features that seem to emerge. Then we will speculate about three phases of more ontologically liberated being, sending our awarenesses venturing over the mountains that wall in our colonies of the familiar, seeking report of the vaster realms awaiting man's exploration.

The Nature of Ontologic Freedom

PATIENTS' DESCRIPTIONS OF THEIR INNER LIVES

As John, Edna, Greta, Harold, Wally, and so many more talk to me hour after hour about their thinking and feeling and experiencing, I accumulate a composite image of the world of our inner lives. That image is lacking in precision, organization, or the refinement of systematic structure. It has many points of incompleteness, ambiguity, and self-contradiction. Withal, it is not mute in conveying a "feel for" the subjective life which leads me to believe that many of our models for "psychological processes" are either in error or so extremely oversimplified that generalization from them is impossible. At first I told myself that this was because the accounts I heard were distorted by something called "psychopathology." I had been taught that the "mental processes become confused because of emotional disruptions." But as the hours of listening to self-descriptions mount into the tens of thousands, I become convinced that those who so taught me were in error, for never have I heard someone talking about himself just as the theories imply one would if he were truly self-understanding. Moreover, as patients progress and show in some cases truly remarkable increases in self-confidence, self-acceptance, social effectiveness, vocational success, marital fulfillment, and so on, they still do not begin to describe their inner living as it seemed to me the theories said they should.

The impression I had gained from my studies was that the "normal" person would think rationally, keep emotion in its place, act in terms of his best judgment at all times, not be troubled with competing impulses or feelings, have deep and instantaneous self-knowledge, be free of guilts and anxiety, and establish wholesome relations with others in which he would never be constrained by them or in conflict with them. Obviously I looked for normal people and successful patients to achieve that which I had not achieved myself.

Sometimes this seeming failure on my part was a source of guilt for me. I would redouble my efforts to study the experts' writings or to rework my data on the patients or to inquire into my own confusions and countertransferences. Often these strivings produced some gains but never did they appreciably increase the matching of my patients' progresses with what I expected should be the case. In a kind of desperation, at times, I would decide the "depth methods" were too cumbersome or beyond my skill and try to teach or directively counsel my patients toward the approved ways of being. Usually such efforts were futile. In a few instances they were successful in a way which more than ever demonstrated the fallacy of the goals themselves. The patients in these latter instances began to describe themselves as I wanted them to, but the descriptions were so patently forced and designed to please me that I knew they were but actings-out of transference feelings.

In time, and especially with the help of my personal therapeutic experience, I came to realize that many patients were living richer lives and were well pleased with their therapeutic experiences without their ever attaining the seeming ideal. I came to appreciate the deeper richness of the kinds of growth that were occurring and to sense their intrinsic validity within the human situation as opposed to their correspondence or lack of it with some abstracted ideal. Now I could see that the same situation existed within my own inner life: I did not find my *I* and *Me* and *Selves* merging into a smooth unity. I still wrestled with conflicts within myself. Even though I find increasing genuineness, effectiveness, comfort, and relatedness, there are confusions and frustrations within me as always. I find fear and anxiety are still with me. I have gained much but much remains to be won.

Farber (1956, p. 109) quotes Kierkegaard in a metaphor that says it all very well.

> In relation to their systems, most systematizers are like a man who builds an enormous castle and lives in a shack beside it; they do not live in their own enormous buildings. But spiritually that is a decisive objection. Spiritually speaking, a man's thought must be the building in which he lives—otherwise everything is topsy-turvy.

EXPERIMENTAL PSYCHOLOGY'S INCOMPLETENESS

The same things that I have been saying about theory in the realms of psychopathology and psychotherapy can be said of most of the work in experimental psychology. The multitude of researches into topics such as learning, memory, motivation, perception, and so on have yielded vast quantities of information that are admittedly incomplete. We can speculate that eventually this material may be summated into larger theoretic structures which could describe significant aspects of human experience; yet I think that many would agree that this is not likely in the foreseeable future, and some would maintain that it is probably neither likely or possible. Experimental psychology is part-function psychology (Bugental, 1963b, c) and as such is a legitimate scientific interest, but it should not be confused with human psychology, which is concerned with the whole person.

A second major limitation on the sorts of information about the human experience which experimental psychology can provide is that it is almost completely information about response behavior—in other words, about the person as an object (*Me*). It is my contention that the most distinctly human activity is that which is initiative and active (*I-process* action). Experimental psychology is mute about this realm.

RESEARCH ON SELF-PERCEPTION

A great many investigations have been conducted of the manner in which people see themselves (for example, Jourard, 1963, 1964; Moustakas, 1956; Wylie, 1961). In these studies the *Self* is varyingly conceived as subject and object, although for the most part the latter aspect has received greater attention. As a result, all too often the person has been viewed in terms of attributes and responses rather than in terms of awareness and choices. In a series of investigations (1948, 1950, 1952b, 1955, 1962f, 1964a) of the way in which people identify or describe themselves, I have been increasingly drawn toward the point of view enunciated in these pages. However, I am of the opinion that neither my own nor many of the other inquiries have ever adequately mined the rich ore of knowledge about the potentials of human experience which might be obtained from carefully obtained accounts of self-perception. The nearest we have to this is, of course, the information derived from psychotherapeutic work. A very small start on the sort of investigations I have in mind has been possible with the experimental procedure of asking people to give multiple responses to the question, "Who are you?" Among other easily anticipated findings which were demonstrated was the difficulty respondents had in answering "Who" not "What." Clearly the nonsubstantive nature of the I-process is involved here too. Only the answer "I am I" is truly a "Who?" answer.

LITERATURE SUGGESTIVE OF ONTOLOGIC FREEDOM

Literature of every form may be found which hints at or explicitly enlarges on conceptions of the human experience which are much more expansive than that which guides most of our daily living. In addition to scientific and professional writing, fiction and poetry, religion and metaphysics, accounts of Oriental and Hindu philosophy and the extraordinary feats associated with them, science-fiction and fantasy, and still other writings express man's concern to find his potentiality, to push beyond the barriers of tradition and convention.

Thomas Hora has written some of the most provocative and evocative studies in the realms of human potential opened by the existential perspective.[1] In "Beyond Self" he demonstrates the constraints on being that the *Self* imposes through his definition of the meaning of the *Self*.

> *The self is a conceptual center of being, built up from accumulated assumptions about the nature of reality as mediated by the sensory apparatus and discursive thought.* . . . The self is then built up from what appears to be and what should

---

[1] A cross-sectional sampling of Hora's writing will be found in the references at the back of the book.

be. Moreover, what "should be" insists on ignoring what really is.

Concepts are statements *about* reality. They have no reality of their own and their location is in that unknown place which is called memory and mind. Thus the self, or the "I am" can neither be localized nor does it have actual reality of its own. Yet ordinary man spends most of his life in an unceasing effort to confirm this abstraction as a concrete reality. The need to confirm the reality of the self is in itself evidence of a lurking doubt existing in the awareness of man (Hora, 1962a, p. 85; emphasis Hora's).

It will be evident that Hora equates the *Self* and what he calls the "I am" in contrast to our distinction between the *Self* and the *I-process*.

Mention needs to be made also of Aldous Huxley's concept of the "reducing valve" (1954a, b). His belief was that the mind serves chiefly to screen out much of the immensity of potential awareness but that under the influence of the psychedelic drugs this effect may be offset. Thus, he felt, the transformed awareness of those affected by such agents was a truer awareness of ultimate reality.

PEAK EXPERIENCES

A. H. Maslow (1954, 1962b) has given us the concept of the "peak experience" to characterize those times of exalted being in which there are feelings of enriched awareness of one's own life in the whole of the world. From time to time a patient will report such an experience. This seems to occur more often as we progress past the major characterological resistances, but it is by no means restricted to that zone of experience. I have, myself, on occasion sensed this same sort of illumination, but I feel equally at a loss to communicate with any precision my own or my patients' full experience.

I think, however, that many, if not most, of us have these peak experiences in which we sense that we are more than our narrow, familiar selves. We may feel a kind of embarrassment about these when we think of them retrospectively. Not infrequently we hesitate to talk with others about them, and we may even regard them as temporary aberrations of reality sensing. However I believe these experiences may be moments in which the *I-process* breaks free of the *Self*, and in which one senses what true ontologic freedom may mean. Almost always it is impossible in such moments of illumination to report the full meaning of one's experience. What one can say has certain qualitative, though not necessarily substantive, parallels to what subjects of the psychopharmacological experiments report. One senses deeper meaning and richness in all things and all experiences, and yet concurrently there is a reduction of entanglement, obligation, or imprisonment by experience. It seems to approach a cosmic perspective in which everything matters greatly and yet no one thing matters crucially.

Reconceiving the Inner Life

In the preceding pages we have reviewed a number of different sources of speculation about the human condition and the range of potential that may be open to an expanded conception of our being. Let us now briefly list some of the main implications for a reconception of the human situation that are suggested from these sources. The following will be my own first attempt to summarize this motley collection of straws blown by varied winds. The reader is invited to prepare his own list as well.

1. Our perceptions of what we think of as the "usual, everyday world" are misleading when they seem to say this is all there is to world or to existence.
2. Our perceptions of ourselves as over against world, as different from world, are misleading and obscure the essential unity of observer and observed.
3. The "*Self*" we know in terms of memory chiefly is not the same as the *I* who experiences this moment.
4. All experience is somehow related or a unity and that unity has qualities of beauty, of just rightness, of wordless meaningfulness.
5. The seemingly critical concerns on which I pour out my life and which so feverishly engross all around me somehow seem two-dimensional, transitory, and so much less crucial.
6. Livingness (not organic life) and awareness seem so very precious and far too little recognized for their quality of making us all truly related.

THE CONCEPT OF ONTOLOGIC FREEDOM

It should be apparent to anyone who considers the matter that most of us in our culture live out our lives within bounds which are much more restrictive than is inherent in our nature. Whether one's vantage point is that of the anthropologist or sociologist looking at man's constitution and culture or that of the individual psychotherapist listening in on the individual's contending for his own destiny, the impression seems to me inescapable that it is the rare individual indeed who even approaches the limits of his potential. Moreover, this seems true whatever the realm of human experience to which we turn our attention: the intellectual, imaginative, inventive, artistic, relational, mystical, or spiritual. It is usual to estimate that the average person uses less than a quarter of the potential of his intelligence. Thinking about the way we tackle most problems that we encounter, we would surely grant that we are ill-focused, restricted in attack. Every lover knows how clumsily and incompletely he gives himself to his beloved, how easily he lets himself hurt and be hurt where he would give warm understanding.

Ontologic freedom is the name I suggest for that realm of greater realization of our potential which is latent to every one of us. In this chapter and the next I will set forth observations and speculations about what this realm may be like. Before doing so, however, I would like to remind the reader of what is the stage of the development of our knowledge about this matter. I have suggested that we are at about the point which can be equated with the planting of the first permanent colonies in the exploration and development of the Western Hemisphere. The notions set forth in this chapter will be the equivalent of the reports of exploratory trips into the interior. We may have seen something of the Ohio Valley, certainly not much more. The human frontier is immense, and we have but begun to meet the challenge it presents.

THREE CONCEPTIONS

When we come to conceive what is meant by genuine ontologic freedom, we find that conceptions are possible at a number of different levels, ranging from the simple opening up of our familiar perception of being to quite metaphysical and speculative reaches. In this chapter and the next I will present three conceptualizations of the nature of ontologic freedom. In sequence these will be termed: emancipation, actualization, and transcendence. These titles are used solely for our ease in reference. They describe ways of grouping our observations (not discoveries) of systems of ontologic freedom. The conceptualization of ontologic freedom is capable of an infinite variety of approaches. The three here employed seem useful in aiding communication, but they are by no means advanced as the only ways of grappling with this difficult problem.

It will be helpful briefly to characterize each of these three forms of conceptualization before going further. *Emancipation* will be used to refer to the process of freeing one's awareness of being from the false equation of the *I* and the *Me*. *Actualization* carries the understanding of freedom into a different area as it suggests the greater scope of choice available to the person in expressing his being in the familiar world of experience. "Actualization" here is used in the same general sense as it is used by Maslow or as "fully functioning" is used by Rogers. *Transcendence* brings us to the realm of metaphysical speculation; probably the nearest equivalent of transcendence as here conceived would be the Buddhist concept of *Satori*.

Emancipation

When a person is able to free himself of the false equation of the *I* and the *Me*, he is open to experience his life in a new fashion. In Chapters 11 and 12 I described in detail the reasoning on which this distinction between the *I* and the *Me* is based. There are a number of concrete ways in which this emancipation is experienced and from which greater choice can flow. In essence what emancipation means is that the patient can recognize himself now as the subject of his experience instead of the object.

> Lucy had many times described how her plans for running her home were interfered with by her mother, who seemed unable to relinquish her attempts to control Lucy, although the latter is now in her thirties. Lucy's mother overrode Lucy's instructions to her own children, dictated the choice of decoration for Lucy's home, and constantly reduced Lucy to a fuming, inarticulate child.

After Lucy had worked through her guilt for her anger toward her mother, had reduced her resistance pattern of avoiding responsibility by letting her mother take over, and had achieved some recognition that her *I* and *Me* were not the same, she began to see her relationship to her mother entirely differently. Once she protested helplessness to change her mother, since her mother was determined to do things in a certain way. Now Lucy found that she could say to her mother what it was she, Lucy, desired in such a way that she would be heard.

Earlier Lucy would say, "What can I do? Mother told me that the children should be in bed at seven, and I didn't see any point in making a big fuss by telling her to keep her nose out of it." In this plaintive inquiry Lucy revealed the confusion of the *Self* and the person. Since her mother told her something, she could only react to what her mother said. She could react either compliantly, as she chose to do, or rebelliously, as seemed to her to be the only alternative.

Today Lucy says, "When mother told me that the children could not go visiting with us, I suggested that she take her car and I would take mine since I intended to take the children along. Then mother changed her mind and decided it would be nice to have the children with us." With her *I* freed to be the subject, Lucy can make a decision that is not simply reactive to her mother but is active in Lucy's own right.

ACTIVE VERSUS REACTIVE BEING

This simple example needs to be elaborated a bit. In Lucy's change from being only reactive to her mother to being active in her own right resides an expression of the very meaning of emancipation. Lucy-as-object can only listen to her mother and feel whatever is evoked in her by her mother's words or actions. At the earlier point in her therapy this is clear when we try to lead Lucy toward discovering a nonreactive way of handling the situation.

"What can I do?" Lucy asks. "Either I do what mother tells me or I get in a big fight with her. I can't win either way."

"Are there only these two choices, Lucy?" I ask.

"Well, I suppose not, but it certainly feels that way. I suppose I could try to explain to mother why . . ."

Now the therapist should not be fooled. Lucy is still being reactive, still being an object. She is being reactive to the therapist and trying to produce a "third way," and since she is bright, she may succeed. With encouragement she may even try it out. Usually the results are disappointing. Sometimes there is a success with the plan worked out in advance, but the next exchange with the mother shows the patient still responding in the old way. Counseling methods or re-educative therapy may, with much persistence and effort, gradually teach ways of handling these situations, but usually the therapist, if he is candid, will recognize that the basic passive-reactive stance remains, and the personality still seems without style or liveliness.

An adequate analysis of the resistances to authentic responsibility (which usually, but not always, are found underlying this reactive pattern), coupled with interpretations which bring out the false equation of the *I* and the *Me*, produces an entirely different therapeutic change. This is deceptively simple on the surface but phenomenologically and existentially is tremendously significant. Practically, too, the contrast is important: re-educative counseling tends to generalize to other relationships or situations in a limited way and may not persist once the support of the therapist (to which the reactive patient is now reacting) is ended. Free awareness of being the subject (the *I*) of one's own life tends to grow and become a basis for yet other gains in autonomy and authenticity (including the resolution of the transference to the therapist).

Perhaps I can illustrate the significant difference in Lucy's experiences with her mother by a heuristic overelaboration: in the first instance, when the mother says the children should go to bed earlier, Lucy hears this directed toward her *Me*. It is as though it then adheres to the *Me* until Lucy can "clear" it in some manner. Since the *Me* is equated to the *I*, then the *I* also is obligated by this statement of the mother. Thus Lucy can only think of ways of acting that are *re*-actions, that deal with what her mother has said. In the second instance, when Lucy's mother says the children can not go visiting, Lucy can recognize that this was again directed toward her *Me*, but since the *I* is not tied to the *Me*, Lucy can think what she wants to do—consulting the *Me*, the record of past events, including her mother's opinion—but not being bound by it.

EITHER-OR THINKING

Either-or thinking is typical of the patient who cannot discriminate his *I* and *Me* functions. Since he can seldom find sources for initiating action within himself, the patient is chiefly reactive in his relation to his world. Often we see such patients as highly dependent, and indeed they are; however, it is suggested here that it is more functional to recognize the basis of the difficulty in a perceptual pattern which confuses the *I* and the *Me* than in an alleged trait of dependence.

LEARNED DESCRIPTIONS OF THE SELF

When the patient sees the *I* and *Me* as the same, then the self-as-object is seen as embodying the nature of the *Self* totally. This has important consequences. As the patient has learned to see himself (as an object), he has learned that he has certain attributes or characteristics. Thus, Ben's mother called him "lazy" constantly; Sally's father told her repeatedly she was "stupid"; and Henry's whole family insisted he was "brilliant." These are but simple examples of the kinds of characterizations that in our present thinking are applicable to the *Self* or *Me*, rather than to the *I*. Ben found himself repeatedly acting-out his mother's instruction that he was lazy. Sally had great difficulty making decisions because she had learned that she was stupid; while Henry exerted himself sporadically to enact his brilliance. It should be clear that these patients did not consciously carry these names for themselves around, but they were clearly present at the preconscious level.

These kinds of *self*-descriptions, as cited in the foregoing examples, are simple to recognize, and their contaminating effect on the spontaneity and authenticity of experience is readily evident. In most cases, however, the kinds of *self*-descriptions the patients are attempting to actualize are much more subtle, complex, and even contradictory.

> Actually, Henry's learnings about himself from his childhood were quite complex. He had been told repeatedly by his mother that he was brilliant and that he was expected to perform brilliantly. Being members of a very small Jewish minority in a small town, the mother felt that all eyes in the com-

munity were focused on the family and that they had to justify their presence in a variety of ways, one of which was Henry's brilliance. But the mother also had the idea that Henry was not very strong and that he needed to husband his energy and to look after his health. She transmitted this to Henry too. The result was that he learned a kind of implicit injunction to perform brilliantly with as little effort as possible. These learnings from his mother collided with his father's expectation. The father was working exceedingly hard to establish his family and to raise their socio-economic level. He frequently became incensed at Henry's apparent "laziness," which was in good part an acting-out of his mother's implicit injunction to conserve his limited energy. Henry learned then that though he was brilliant he was somewhat inclined to be lazy and that he must watch himself carefully, both to protect his health and to be sure that he worked diligently, for he learned a suspicion of himself also.

Henry's progress through school was marked by occasional outstanding performances, as when he was a class officer or editor of the school annual. But there were also many periods of mediocre or inferior work in areas, especially mathematics and science, where he could not perform brilliantly with little effort. Teachers often implored Henry to study harder, assuring him that he had great possibilities. But these injunctions only served to enforce the learning that he was brilliant and, implicitly thereby, that he must husband his energy carefully. When, in his late thirties, Henry entered therapy, he was the despair of his professional associates. At times he performed exceedingly well, and at other times he failed utterly in his obligations to them. Henry had by this time added to his self-description the ideas that he was sporadic, undependable, and should not be too close to anyone.

When Henry was able to free his experience of the false equation of the *I* and the *Me*, he could accept the fact that indeed these various adjectives had characterized what he had done, but that they were not necessarily characterizations of his basic nature. With this recognition, he became able to respond to situations in a fresh fashion, without carrying the weight of past self-descriptions constantly with him. The result was that he became more able to do the work he wanted to do in a consistent fashion, that his frantic need to prove his excellence and brilliance diminished, and that he got much more satisfaction from his relationships in his work and in his social life.

DETERMINISM

It will be apparent that what we are saying here is that a person ultimately is not the sum of his own or others' perceptions of him. These are, so to speak, a collection of his memories and experiences, a sort of scrapbook of photographs and other mementoes, but they are not the essential nature of the person. Under the influence of radical determinism we have tended to see the person as but this collection of past perceptions, and we have taught each other well so that we come to see ourselves in this same fashion. Then we try to act consistently with our history and so continue this self-deception. Once we are able to recognize that what *has been* so has no mandate over what *will be* so, we regain choice.

> I recall a personal experience some years ago that illustrates this essential truth in an homely way. Driving to my office one morning along a relatively narrow road I found my progress slowed by a driver who seemed to be poking along. Watching for an opportunity, I sped up and got around him, only to come up close behind a second car. Again I found a chance to speed around him, and by now was moving at more than an ordinary clip and overtaking further traffic. As I passed the third car I realized that what I was doing was responding to an image I thought I had created in the eyes of the other drivers and certainly had created in my own inner eye. I was "a fast driver." It was as though I said to myself, "Wouldn't I look silly, having passed several cars so speedily, if I now settle down to the pace of the rest of the traffic? I have to keep going fast." This kind of yielding up of one's choice to the image one feels he has created in himself and others can easily rob us of real autonomy and represents the kind of destruction that confusion of the *I* and *Me* can occasion.

THE CENTRAL CONCEPT

The *I-process*, when most truly understood, is essentially independent of the *Self* and of the world of familiar experience. In turn, the *Self* is an instrumentality, used by the *I-process*, but having no *be-ing* of its own. A tremendous oversimplification is to say that the *Self* is a vehicle employed by the *I-process* in order to express its being in the world, but the *Self* is no more identical with the *I-process* than the automobile is identical with its driver.

It is clearly important to our being in the world that we have access to memories of our own past experiences. The *Self* as a composite of such memories is certainly a useful aid, but when it becomes a mandate for the future, then it is no longer useful but enslaving.

A FALSE DILEMMA

There is an apparent contradiction or dilemma into which one falls when dealing with this matter of the separation of the *I* and the *Me*. We need to render this explicit and to demonstrate why it is fallacious before proceeding further. On the one hand, we are well persuaded that the false equation of the *I* and the *Me* leads to the loss of choice and a reactive stance in the world. It is essential to an understanding of the nature of ontologic freedom that one recognize that his present awareness is not necessarily subordinate to his past experiences in their cumulative, descriptive significance.

On the other hand, patients very frequently are caught in the "subject–object split" at the intrapsychic level. This split is an alienation from one's being that results in a pathologic lack of self-awareness (not knowing what one feels, wants, intends) and an inability to make choices (because of not knowing one's own needs). People who show this form of alienation tend to treat themselves as objects to be manipulated, observed, and "traded in the social market place" (Fromm, 1947).

Superficially, it may seem that the subject–object split typical of self-alienation is the equivalent of the emancipation of the *I* from the *Me*. Actually it is the opposite. This contrast is of sufficient importance for me to enlarge upon it in the next section.

ALIENATION: THE INTRAPSYCHIC SUBJECT–OBJECT SPLIT

Some time ago the *New Yorker* ran a cartoon of a puppet that manipulated its own strings. This was not, to my mind, a funny cartoon. It graphically portrayed a disease endemic in our American middle-class culture: alienation from one's own being. The alienated person breaks himself up into a tragically ludicrous self-manipulating puppet. He has lost the immediacy of being that is the birthright of human life.

Let us examine the sequence which brings about such alienation in order that we can understand its meaning and contrast it with the emancipation of ontological freedom.

Experiencing anxiety, existential or neurotic, one may find the discomfort such that he attempts to "shut it off." I have said that the awareness which is our basic process of being is *feelingful* awareness. Anxiety is experienced through the feelings, and so the "shutting off" is a matter of shutting off the feelingfulness of our awareness. Now, obviously, the feelings cannot be truly shut off, but awareness of them in the present moment can be withdrawn, and this is what happens. The alienated person escapes anxiety by suppressing current awareness of his feelings and only experiencing them retrospectively.

By suppressing current awareness of feelings some relief from anxiety may be obtained for a time, but the cost of this relief is enormous. The sense of centeredness (May, 1961a), the consciousness of presence in one's own life, is a part of this very feelingfulness of one's awareness. It is this that underlies the concern which is essential to our feeling of identity (see Chapter 3). Suppression of the feelingfulness of awareness leads to suppression of the feeling of identity and presence in one's own experience. The result is the alienation in which one *knows* but does not *feel* that he is the one who is doing thus and so in his life.

The alienated person, in the terms I developed in Chapters 11 and 12, becomes chiefly aware of his *Me* (or Self) and only abstractly aware of the *I-process*. But the crippling process does not end even here. Cut off from direct experience of his feelings, such a person comes to treat himself as an object. He must speculate about why he does things, set traps or tests for himself to figure out what he is up to, reason what it is he must want. The "shutting off" of the feelings cannot be done for just the anxiety, just the unpleasant, unwanted feelings. Feelingfulness is really all of a piece; the savor as well as the threat of living is suppressed. The alienated person typically complains that he does not have much joy, can not be sure that he loves those he is close to, wonders if he really likes what he does.

The sorry sequence has one further extension. The sense of relatedness with others depends in appreciable part upon the feelingfulness of awareness. Experiencing another with empathy gives the person an appreciation of the deep bond which bridges our aloneness. But the alienated person, treating himself as an object, soon is treating those about him so also. This is Buber's (1958) "It–it" relationship. Like billiard balls clicking against each other, not like human beings interpenetrating with each other, such relationships are frustrating and incomplete.

Summary

This then is alienation. It is the loss of true, feelingful awareness of the *I-process*, of one's own presence in his life. It is, it will be evident, the very opposite of emancipation, in which there is heightened feelingful awareness of being the *I*, the subject of one's living.

16 — Ontologic freedom: Actualization and transcendence

In the last chapter we began the consideration of what greater freedom in the realization of our human potential might mean. Diverse sorts of evidence and speculation converge to encourage the recognition that we live within an exceedingly constricted psychological range. One of the major constraints bringing this about is the *Self*, and I have described some of the influences that seem to arise from this bondage to the *Self*. Now, in this chapter, I will describe two other aspects of ontologic freedom, to which we have given the names "actualization" and "transcendence."

Actualization is the name I am suggesting for a way of being in one's life in which there is greater realization upon the potentials of human existence than is usual, at least in our culture. Actualization, to phrase the negative side, is a way of being in the world in which the needless constraints of the personal resistances and cultural inauthenticities are eliminated or markedly reduced in their limiting effects.

The effort to understand the characteristics of actualization is handicapped by language and conceptual habits that are more adapted to dealing with pathology than with health. Indeed, this very phrasing of the matter in terms of the dichotomy of "pathology–health" is a case in point. Similarly, much confusion of the *I* and the *Me* or *Self* is built into the words and syntax with which we will discuss these matters. No better instance of this can be cited than Maslow's use of the term "self-actualizing" when he clearly intends to go beyond a static self. His characterizations of self-actualizing people have long demonstrated a much more dynamic conception (1954). Since I have already dealt with this matter of the false equation of the *I* and *Self*, I will assume that work on dissolving this handicapping bond is going ahead as we now turn our attention to other aspects of actualization.

Maslow's Findings

The most thorough inquiries into this area are, of course, those of Maslow. As in so much that has the effect of restoring dignity to the human condition, Maslow has here demonstrated his enormous creativity and far-sightedness. The following quotation gives Maslow's own view of actualization (1962b, p. 109).

> ... a development of personality which frees the person from the deficiency problems of youth, and from the neurotic (or infantile, or fantasy, or unnecessary, or "unreal") problems of life, so that he is able to face, endure and grapple with the "real" problems of life (the intrinsically and ultimately human problems, the unavoidable, the "existential" problems to which there is no perfect solution).

Maslow's main approach to actualization has been his study of those unusual people who showed in their lives this quality. Our own studies are coming at the matter from a somewhat different angle. I have been trying to observe in more usual people those evidences of unusual realization of their potentials that would suggest what is latent to the human condition. A rough analogy might be that Maslow has talked to explorers who have gone beyond the frontier of the known and brought back reports of what lies out there. I have questioned those who live on the frontier and make occasional trips into the unknown areas. Each kind of report has its values, and the overlap between the two is sufficient to be heartening indeed. Let us look first at the characteristics Maslow reports (1954, Chapter 12).

> 1. *More efficient perception of reality and more comfortable relations with it:* . . . They live more in the real world of nature than in the man-made mass of concepts, abstractions, expectations, beliefs, and stereotypes that most people confuse with the world (pp. 203–205).

2. *Acceptance (self, others, nature):* . . . They can take the frailties and sins, weaknesses, and evils of human nature in the same unquestioning spirit with which one accepts the characteristics of nature (pp. 206–207).
3. *Spontaneity:* . . . Their behavior is marked by simplicity and naturalness, and by lack of artificiality or straining for effect (p. 208).
4. *Problem centering:* . . . These individuals customarily have some mission in life, some task to fulfill, some problem outside themselves which enlists much of their energies (p. 211).
5. *The quality of detachment; the need for privacy:* . . . They positively *like* solitude and privacy. . . . It is often possible for them to remain above the battle, to remain unruffled, undisturbed . . . (p. 212).
6. *Autonomy; independence of culture and environment:* . . . They are dependent for their own development and continued growth on their own potentialities and latent resources (pp. 213–214).
7. *Continued freshness of appreciation:* . . . The wonderful capacity to appreciate again and again, freshly and naively, the basic goods of life, with awe, wonder, and even ecstasy . . . (p. 214).
8. *The mystic experience; the oceanic feeling:* . . . Feelings of limitless horizons opening up to the vision, the feeling of being simultaneously more powerful and more helpless than one ever was before, the feeling of great ecstasy and wonder and awe, the loss of placing in time and space with, finally, the conviction that something extremely important and valuable had happened . . . (p. 216).
9. *Gemeinschaftsgefuhl:* . . . They have for human beings in general a deep feeling of identification, sympathy, and affection in spite of the occasional anger, impatience, or disgust . . . (p. 217).
10. *Interpersonal relations:* . . . They are capable of more fusion, greater love, more perfect identification, more obliteration of the ego boundaries . . . (p. 218).
11. *The democratic character structure:* . . . They can be and are friendly with anyone of suitable character regardless of class, education, political belief, race, or color (pp. 219–220).
12. *Discrimination between means and ends:* . . . Strongly ethical, they have definite moral standards . . . their

notions of right and wrong are often not the conventional ones . . . they are fixed on ends rather than means . . . (pp. 220–221).
13. *Philosophical, unhostile sense of humor:* . . . that elicits a smile more usually than a laugh, that is intrinsic to the situation rather than added to it, that is spontaneous rather than planned, and that very often can never be repeated (p. 222).
14. *Creativeness:* . . . A special kind of creativeness or originality or inventiveness that . . . seems rather kin to the naive and universal creativeness of unspoiled children (p. 223).
15. *Resistance to enculturation:* . . . 1 . . . apparent conventionality . . . yet they are not really conventional . . . 2 . . . an accepting, calm, good-humored everyday effort to improve the culture, usually from within, rather than to reject it and fight it from without. 3 . . . they select from American culture what is good in it by their lights and reject what they think bad in it . . . 4 . . . ruled by the laws of their own character rather than by the rules of society (pp. 224–227).

CLINICAL OBSERVATIONS

Every patient who progresses well in his therapy is a pioneer on the frontiers of our knowledge about the human experience. Each such person with whom I have had the satisfaction of working has contributed out of his very life to my accumulating appreciation for what fuller realization of our potential may mean. Different patients, because of various influences, portray different aspects; although there seems to be a certain underlying commonality that encourages the hope of making useful generalizations. In the following pages I will describe some of the observations that are supported by being present in several different patients and that seem to me to represent expressions of the nature of actuality.

CHANGED NATURE OF CONCERN

Almost without exception, the person who moves toward greater realization of his own potential shows a succession of changes in his feelings of concern. Both the substance of what elicits concern and the form in which that concern is expressed show this evolution.

Early in therapy the patient is often much involved with the question of his basic "goodness" or "badness" or with his guilt for violations of social codes or with his strivings against his feelings of impotency. These all—and the many other forms such concern may take—have to do with fear of what may be revealed to be the essential (inborn) value or quality of the self.

> Howard feared that he was basically a coward; Sally that she was "born stupid"; Greta that she was innately promiscuous; Bill that he was "just constitutionally no good." Each expended much of his life in attempts to prove that what he feared to be true was not so, in efforts to disguise or hide anything that might confirm what he feared (Horney, 1950). Each hesitated to move out into his life because only in the familiar and trite was there any hope of continuing the seeming escape from the feared disclosure. So each lived like a fugitive in an unfriendly country, never daring to be himself, to be intimate with another person, to relax and let down his guard.

When the distortions of the resistances are resolved and the person enters into more authentic being, concern is less preoccupied with *Self* and becomes an involvement with living in a broader sense. In a somewhat oversimplified fashion, we may say that the person attaining to actualization is concerned significantly with much in his life but that no concern seems crucial.

Authentic concern seems to be a matter of being willing to make commitments, to let things matter, and yet to retain sufficient perspective so that one is not catastrophically imperiled or even overcome by reverses in any one or any group of concerns. This characterization picks out another aspect of neurotic concern which may be contrasted with the authentic: the neurotic often is so threatened by his restricted, covert concern that he is unable to allow himself investment in that which is truly important to him.

> Lucy's fear of how people would regard her if her house were not spic-and-span so pre-empted her emotions that she had but little left to share with her children who were hungering for her more than for a clean house.

> Although Tom deeply wanted to write his novel, his constant nagging fear that it would reveal he was effeminate or

neurotic kept him from bringing to bear on his writing the creative potential he had.

. . . . .

As Lucy freed herself of her neurotic concern, she began to discover a world of experience that seemed to her incredibly new. "Tim (her son) called me to come see the circus on television. He was just delighted with it. Suddenly I knew he just wanted me to be delighted too. Usually I would have explained to him why we couldn't afford to go or done something else, but this time I just could see how he imagined himself at the circus and what fun that was. He didn't really expect any more than that, and I really liked imagining it with him. I mean I really did! When I went back in the kitchen I found myself starting to cry because I never knew before that sometimes that's all he wants, just for me to be delighted with him."

Tom started to college during the second year he was in therapy. This was the fourth time he'd entered college. Each time before he'd given up because his need to do exceptionally well had foundered on his fear of really trying (for if he really tried and then failed he'd be shown up so terribly; while if he wasn't really trying then of course there was no real test). Now he could say, "It's a funny experience just to listen to a professor to hear what he's saying. It may sound crazy, but I've never really done that before. I always was listening to prove to myself I already knew what he was going to say or to find out the trick he was going to pull on the exam or with the expectation that any minute I'd discover I really didn't know what it was all about and that I had no business being there at all. Now I just listen, and, you know, it's really interesting, and I get most of it, but not all, and that's alright too."

"Now I just listen," Tom says. This is the essence of authentic being. The changed concern of authentic being is that concern is directed toward that which one is intending, not dispersed on what one may be disclosing or other irrelevent matters.

SELECTIVE COMMITMENT

What we have just pointed out about authentic concern being directed toward what one is intending instead of being dispersed on extraneous matters is an example also of a second frequent characteristic of the person coming to greater actualization of his being:

the ability to commit himself selectively and effectively. The authentic person seems to have at his conscious direction the energies and emotional involvement that may be scattered and uncontrolled in the neurotic.

> Edna longs, she says, to become a better pianist. She wants to practice regularly, but somehow she has trouble doing so. As she talks about it, it becomes clear that Edna is distracted from her practice by daydreams of how her friends will admire her when she plays exceptionally well, by speculations as to whether she can "go professional," by a dozen minor tasks (writing a letter, shopping for socks for her son, and so on), which somehow she must perform before she can really settle down to the piano.

Now it is certainly true that we can see the resistance pattern in Edna's dispersion of her energies when we look at this segment of her life, but this is a focus only on the pathological. We may help Edna more if we recognize and deal with the resistance but also go beyond looking at what is wrong to catch a wider perspective.

> Edna is the treasurer of the P.T.A. at her daughter's school. She is active on a committee of a liberal social-political group, and she teaches Sunday School. She and her husband are part of the neighborhood social group, and they also are "in on" the activities of her husband's business association. She seems to enjoy most of these, but she does recognize that she tends to have too little time for all of them. "But what can I do?" she protests, "They're all important. I don't do any of them just because I want to. Not that I mind doing them, but they're also good for our family."

Each of Edna's activities is a constructive one, but none is just because she wants it, as she says. This is the point, of course; Edna's investments of her life are for many, good, external reasons but not for Edna's own reasons.

Authenticity frequently involves a more selective commitment of one's energies. The person who is aware of his being is apt to be seriously concerned how his livingness is given actuality. He frequently will display what seems to be a jealousy of his autonomy or an insistence on "*I*-determination" (what is miscalled "self-determination"). More valuing of authentic, committed experience, less concern with how the *Self* is seen by others, and more selective commitment of one's time and energies seem to go together.

Over a year later, Edna is talking about her commitments again: "So I told Pastor Swenson that he'd just have to find someone else to teach the class in the fall. It's a shame because I've liked doing it at times, and I think I was pretty good at it, but it's just not for me right now. It's like the P.T.A. thing and the partying in the neighborhood. They're all real nice but I can only do so much, and I know now I really want to play the piano, and I really want to work on this next election. That and the family will take all the time I have."

Implicit in what we are saying about selective commitment is the acceptance of one's limitedness in the midst of possibilities. Clearly, many of our patients are unwilling to accept that limitedness because it is importantly linked to the fear of fate and death. To say no to any possibility is to admit one is finite. This is severely anxiety-evoking for some people.

Another implication of selective commitment is the tendency of the more authentic person to exercise his greater freedom to choose by rejecting many of the social "games" and formalities that are recognized as shallow and fostering of malignant symbiotic relations. To the person capable of genuine commitment in relationships, many of our formalized associations (clubs, business and professional organizations, service groups) may be seen as inauthentic and defeating of genuine encounter. The person achieving actualization is often the despair of busy membership chairmen or association officers, for such a person may pay his dues or otherwise lend a support impersonally but refuse to participate in a more personal (time- and energy-expending) way. Such selective participation may seem to some to be callous, idiosyncratic, or "selfish." (Of course, when arising as we have here described, such behavior is most certainly not *Self*-ish since it comes about because the person is no longer trying to build a public *Self* to win approval.)

INTENSIFICATION OF PARTICIPATION

What I have been saying about the changed nature of concern and the selective commitment which characterize the person achieving greater actualization of his being will make apparent why we will usually find that such a person participates with much more wholehearted involvement in those matters to which he does choose to devote himself.

In oversimplified form we may say, when a person is able to act in accord with his ontologic freedom he is highly selective with regard to the concerns to which he will commit himself but he tends to be deeply involved in those matters he does select. The authentic person is not a casual person.

>Tom made his best grades of his academic career in his first semester back in college after being out of school more than five years. He continued through undergraduate school to do better than average work. He never sought or achieved a "straight A" record, for as he said, "I could make better grades if I'd focus on the kinds of things the profs are apt to ask in the tests, but this takes too much time. I want to read about the things that interest me more and work on this research I've got started. If I can make good enough grades to keep them satisfied and keep my fellowship, I'm content. But, boy, this research thing is really coming. Let me tell you what I did yesterday . . ." And Tom went on to describe a research which he had developed himself and which had won the enthusiastic support of two senior faculty members, one of whom wanted to collaborate with Tom on a series of articles. This occurred before Tom had finished his bachelor's degree.

Two other characteristics of this intensified participation deserve mention also. Very often the focus of the person's involvement tends to be on broader, more challenging fronts. Thus, Edna chose to develop her artistic potential at the piano and to work on an election campaign, while Tom brought his involvement to bear on his research interests. Secondly, and somewhat paradoxically, along with the greater intensity of involvement there seems to be more resilience of involvement. The actualizing person retains his own being and is not made the object of that in which he chooses to participate. Edna's view was soundly defeated in the election. She was disappointed, furious at some of the tactics of the opposition, and eager to plan for the future. She was not "destroyed" as she had once described herself when she made a social blunder with the neighborhood group. And, of course, this is almost literally the state of affairs. With the neighborhood group, Edna had been busy constructing an image (a *Self*), which the blunder literally destroyed. In the election, Edna participated but she did not lose her own identity in the public issue.

DECLINE OF THE GOAL OF HAPPINESS

In Chapter 9 we described a general cultural trend to deny tragedy and pursue happiness. This near deification of happiness as a life goal has resulted in a gross distortion of existential validity and in no noticeable increase in happiness. Coupled with this exaltation of happiness has been the false assumption that material advantages provide the route to such happiness. Only the most casual comparisons of our own and earlier times, of American life and that of "primitive" people, or of the wealthy and the poor within our own society are necessary to demonstrate beyond any question how ineffectual for attaining happiness are material advantages. (The continued pursuit of such advantages by so many in our society derives from quite different dynamics, of course.)

Authentic living is characterized by the dropping away of happiness as a goal in itself. The actualizing person is busy with the concerns to which he has chosen to commit his living and seldom stops to assess his happiness. Very often, of course, it will be apparent that he is a happy person—although by no means is this always so—but it seems to be only the neurotic and the unhappy that expend their concern explicitly and directly on their happiness. The impression is inescapable that happiness is a state that is pushed away by the hand that would grasp it but that tends to accompany the person who is alive to his own being.

APPRECIATION OF SUCHNESS AND AESTHETIC LIVING

The authentic person seems to have a perspective on life which enables him to take satisfaction in the very fabric of being. This is a difficult matter to describe, but it is evidenced again and again in my patients as they begin to arrive at greater actualization of their potential. What is involved may be likened to the "closure" of a good gestalt, the appropriate fitting together of experience. It is often found most clearly in art forms: in the evocative words of the poet or novelist, in the skillful use of form and color of the painter or sculptor, in the composer's effective architecture of rhythm and tone. It is the experience of "Aha!" when the puzzle is satisfyingly solved, the mathematical proposition elegantly demonstrated, the philosophical issue cleanly developed. For many it is present in the contemplation of natural scenes of beauty and grandeur, or in meditation on God and religion, or in studying scientific developments.

What seems to be involved in the experience of suchness includes: (a) a personal awareness of an area of experience in a state of tension or incompleteness; (b) an emotional investment in the tension system, a willingness to let it matter; (c) a personal participation (perhaps vicarious or imaginal only) in the resolution of the tension, in the achievement of closure; and (d) a sense of the appropriateness of the closure, an appreciation that the resolution is faithful to the original tension.

It seems to me that the popularity of the detective story may in some part be an illustrative instance. The good "who-done-it" sets a tension system in motion, evokes the reader's identification, leads him through the steps to provide the materials for resolution, and then using these materials (and no others) provides the tension resolution. In citing the mystery story as an example, I do not mean to imply that it is necessarily the prototype of authentic fiction, only that it certainly is a familiar example of the attraction and satisfaction of suchness.

The person who is actualizing his own being seems to have a style to his living, a certain artistic quality. Often this quality is not externally obvious, but to intimates it is apparent. Such esthetic living uses the participation in suchness as one of its ingredients. For example, such a person willingly accepts certain tension states, participates in them, and sees them through to satisfying closure. Living so, the person would not want to seek the intervention of someone else to bring about the closure any more than he would want to read the last chapter of the mystery novel out of sequence in order to have the solution early.

> Dave was a research scientist who had been hesitant and uncomfortable in many interpersonal situations, especially where there was any competitive element. As we worked through his resistances and he came into more actualized living, the time came for Dave to make a presentation to a panel charged with allocating funds for research projects. These had often been difficult and even terrifying occasions for

Dave. Sometimes a colleague had made the presentations for him on one pretext or another, and sometimes Dave had taken a collaborator (when he really didn't want one) so as to have someone to "front" for him. This time when a friend offered to make the presentation for Dave, he was surprised to hear himself reject the offer. As he explained to me, "Hell, that would spoil it, really. You can see, can't you, that all we've been doing here is preparing the way. If George does it now, then I'll miss out on something . . . something . . . I don't know, something important to me. I'll be scared stiff, I know. I wish I wouldn't be, but that's not the point. I want to do it myself, and I'm going to." And he did. Later he reported that he'd been rather tense until he was through the formal presentation but that when the questioning began afterward, "I suddenly realized I knew a hell of a lot more about this whole thing than anyone else there, so I relaxed and had a whale of a time. Besides, they asked good questions which were fun to deal with."

RECOGNITION OF THE WHOLENESS OF EXPERIENCE

The appreciation of suchness is probably closely related to the recognition that so many people who come to actualization make and that Betty put so very simply:

> It's all one really. I just opened my eyes and looked, and I can see it so clearly now. Mom and Dad were trying so hard, but they were so scared. And I was scared too. We've always been such frightened people. And what were we frightened of? Just of being ourselves! Isn't that awful? All that pain and all that unhappiness, just because we were afraid to be ourselves! (She is weeping hot, quiet tears as she talks.) And that's what I've been running from: by being so bright or pretty or popular or sexy or successful or all the other things I've tried to be. I've been trying to be those things instead of just being me. It's all one, isn't it?

Betty has discovered her own wholeness and her relatedness to her parents from whom she has been long estranged. She will no longer be the hapless creature of her fear of being herself. She can lay claim to her own being in a newer, fresher way. For others, the wholeness of experience is discovered on a broader scale: a recognition of the essential humanness of those who formerly seemed so different or so hostile, an empathy with the human experience of people in general, a feeling for one's own participation in the general and of the universal human outlook being present in oneself.

FREEING FROM THE SUBJECT–OBJECT SPLIT

Except for its immense importance, this overcoming of the subject-object split might be subsumed under the recognition of the wholeness of experience. It is certainly a part of that recognition. Discovery of one's essential rootedness in all mankind gives a sense of being uniquely oneself while yet related to all others. World no longer seems out there and in opposition; rather the boundary between *I* and world is experienced as fluid and changing with one's awareness and experience. Similarly, one no longer feels the split within himself. The *Me* or *Self* is recognized for what it is, a scrapbook of the past, interesting, personal, but static and not binding upon the liberated *I* that lives in this minute.

CENTEREDNESS

This is Rollo May's term (1959b, 1961a) to express an awareness of being in one's own life. It is expressive of the direct intuition of being which replaces self-consciousness when that handicapping sort of awareness is surmounted. The centered person (not "*Self*-centered") is the person who is actualizing his being with aware choice. He recognizes the possibilities open to him, the contingencies that are within his ken, the responsibility of commitment, and he chooses knowingly.

Centeredness is the positive aspect of the same process I have characterized as the freeing of the *I* from the false equation with the *Me*. As this handicapping linkage is dissolved, the person becomes centered in his being in the moment of actuality and leaves behind the diffuse concern with the past or fruitless apprehensions of the future that characterize the inauthentic. Actualization occurs only in the moment, Now. Centeredness is the active core of actualization.

SUMMARY

Actualization is a way of being in one's life in which there is greater than usual realization of the potential inherent in our ontologic freedom. Clearly, what this implies is that the person who is actualizing his life is confronting and incorporating existential anxiety in a more authentic fashion. In this section I have discussed eight characteristics of actualization. In the next two chapters I will be talking about the manner in which we respond to the various forms of existential anxiety. As might be expected, these are interrelated aspects of the same matter. We may illustrate this by identifying the aspects of actualization that are most closely associated with each of the forms of existential anxiety. Each of the characteristics of actualization expresses the manner in which the individual confronts each of the forms of existential anxiety, and I am only picking out some of the particular linkages to aid our thinking and therapeutic work.

Centeredness and winning free from the subject–object confusion within one's own being are importantly tied to a courageous response to the anxiety of fate and death. As we shall see, it is only through such actualization that one can experience that faith which is part of overcoming the dread of powerlessness.

When one confronts the anxiety of guilt and responsibility authentically he is able to change the nature of his experience of concern and give up the futile pursuit of happiness for its own sake. In this way he makes his commitments in life without the constant oppression of fearing blame.

Of course, the selective commitment of the actualizing person is a part of his handling of responsibility, but I am here emphasizing the element of selection that is so important to confronting meaninglessness and emptiness. The appreciation of suchness and an esthetic quality to living similarly are part of confronting this form of existential anxiety. These courageous responses overthrow the dread of absurdity that otherwise threatens.

Finally, we may link the intensification of participation and the recognition of the wholeness of experience to the manner in which one confronts the anxiety of loneliness and isolation. These two characteristics are aspects of the response of authentic love that replaces the dread of estrangement. Love for another person or a loving approach to all relationships is most meaningful when the person shows in his love a readiness to participate deeply and a clear recognition of his fundamental oneness with all others.

Transcendence

Transcendence is an hypothesized point of full authenticity of being in which the person would emerge into oneness with The All. There is no nonmystical language really available for describing this concept. By its very nature it partakes of mystery or mysticism —it is unknown to our usual understanding. Transcendence implies the complete confronting and incorporating of existential anxiety in all its forms (Lasko, 1963). It includes, by definition, the overcoming of the subject–object split both within the individual and between the person and his world. Transcendence is complete awareness and full feelingful assent.

We choose to include the concept of transcendence in our thinking because it is essential to put into perspective the other forms of ontologic freedom, emancipation and actualization. When these are set against the background of transcendence they may be seen as the significant but incomplete forms of being that they are. This is by no means to devalue the meaningfulness of emancipation and actualization. Each represents a truer affirmation of life than most of us now know. But transcendence provides the further value of opening our awareness to the true immensity of our potential. Perhaps this will be even more evident if I try to spell out further what this conceptualization means.

Hora's Conceptualization

Probably the most free speculations within professional writings are those offered by Thomas Hora. His inquiry into the range of transcendent being potential to human experience is at once an illustration of his courageous thinking and a stimulation to the conceptions I will be advancing.

> From a psychotherapeutic standpoint, then, the following definition offers itself:
>
> *Transcendence is a broadened state of consciousness enabling man to cognize reality in dimensions which are above and beyond dualities and multiplicities.*

In relevance to healing, the following phenomena of transcendence have been found to be of significance in the psychotherapeutic process:
1. Transcendence of the subject–object dichotomy between therapist and patient.
2. Transcendence of the body–mind dichotomy.
3. Transcendence of dualistic thought.
4. Transcendence of the ego.
5. Transcendence of disease as expression of the pleasure–pain duality.
6. Transcendence of causal and teleological thinking.
7. Transcendence of the motivational split of means and ends.
8. Transcendence of the temporo-spatial coordinates of experience.
9. Transcendence of the epistemic barrier between mind and world.
10. Transcendence of the duality of being and nonbeing.
11. Transcendence of the separation between man and Ultimate Reality (God).

(1961b, pp. 501–502, emphasis Hora's)

The important point to bear in mind in examining such a truly challenging conception as this of Hora is not whether he is right or wrong. In a very real way that question is meaningless. Rather it is essential to open one's awareness to the conceptual impact of such thinking. Such a way of approaching human experience, if truly received, sets that experience in so much more significant a scale than do many of our more usual approaches (such as those of the customary theory of psychotherapy or, even more so, the usual approaches of experimental psychology).

ENLIGHTENMENT

It may well be protested that I am going to extremes when I attempt to deal with this concept of transcendence. Of course, that is exactly what I intend doing. Transcendence is the extreme of human potential so far as we can conceive it. In other areas of our thinking, conceiving the extreme is a useful heuristic device (for example, speculation on the behavior of matter at the speed of light), there is every reason to feel the same will be true in this area. Certainly if we can overcome some of the cramped, reductionistic, and mechanomorphic thinking that usually inhibits our thinking about human experience, we will have gained something.

I have never had a patient who approached true transcendence. I'm not sure I would recognize the fact were it to occur before me. I think it may be the same as the transfiguration of such figures as the Buddha and the Christ. Doubtlessly there have been others who have attained to something similar to transcendence. Certainly the person making such an attainment would have no need to trumpet it about unless to offer something to others (as with the religious leaders), so there is no reason to be surprised that we do not hear about such instances.

In Asian terms *Satori* or enlightenment has long been recognized as a part of the human potential. Suzuki (Barrett, 1956, p. 21) speaks of Satori as "the power to see into the nature of one's own being." This is an easily equated statement to our own concept of transcendence as the fullest realization of one's being.

In Chapter 12 I used the analogy of the motion picture projector to illustrate the relation of the *I-process* to the *Self*. There we likened the former to the light and the latter to the film. Now we may return to that analogy and suggest that transcendence would be pure light without the form-giving but constricting effects of the film.

Conclusion

STATUS OF THE CONCEPT OF ONTOLOGIC FREEDOM

It hardly needs stressing that the speculations offered in this and the previous chapters are most preliminary and subject to extensive revision. Nevertheless, it is hoped I have been able to suggest the directions in which inquiry must go, to point out some of the obstacles to our perceptions, and to excite interest in more thoroughgoing inquiry into this tremendously important matter.

Numerous questions need to be answered before these speculations will warrant the dignity of the title "theory." While I am convinced that the *I* does not have substantive attributes, I am unable to say yet how it is that the *I* can become a prisoner of the *Me*. In the foregoing pages I have spoken of the learned misidentification of the *I* and the *Me*. But this presupposes a learning function of the *I*. I think this is somehow inaccurate. I believe that *I*-awareness is atemporal and universal, that the kinds of learning which are involved in memory are *Self*-learnings, not *I*-learnings.

RELATIONSHIP

Another whole area needing tremendous exploration is that having to do with relationships. I am loath to conclude that love is solely a *Me*- or *Self*-level experience. It seems that love can be an expression of choice, and yet I find that there is much to suggest that love at the *I*-level is universal love and nonselective. One view that must be considered here is that at the *I*-level, separate identity does not truly exist. Individuality, some would assert, is simply a "hole through which The All shines." Whether this makes of individuality truly nothing or whether individuality represents "nodules" within The All is something I cannot guess at this point.

RELIGION

It will be apparent that these speculations bring us to the borders and the realm of metaphysics and religion. I regard this as a tremendously exciting and encouraging development. Too long has psychology tried to deny centuries of man's devoted, intelligent effort to know the meaning of his being through the avenues of religion. There needs to be an end to the artificial separation of the scientific and the religious that reduces our perspective on such important questions. Such provincialism as is represented by separate camps of religionists, scientists, psychotherapists, and philosophers is a luxury that man can ill afford at this point in his history.

I do not pretend to have any competence to speak on such matters as the reality or the nature of God, but I do not feel this issue can be settled by fiat as some attempt. I do not have competence to speak on such matters as whether the *I* is the same as the "soul," but I think that it is tremendously important that we not be handicapped by superstitions masquerading as scientific attitudes, which would prevent our using whatever insights and recognition on these points man has been able to bring forth.

Summary

It is essential to the development of existential-analytic psychotherapy that the psychotherapist maintain an openness of perspective on the nature of the human condition. The psychotherapist who is burdened with a closed mind on religious or ontologic questions cannot be adequate in serving his patient. Ontologic freedom is an estate to be aspired to but seldom achieved. It is probable that it is not a single level or condition. Rather, one increases in ontologic freedom as he frees himself, first of the "deficit" influences of his resistances and transferences, and second of the confusions about the nature of being that arise from the false equation of the *I* and the *Me*. The psychotherapeutic task needs to become that of ever-deepening inquiry into man's nature, more than trying to impose a theoretically derived condition upon him.

17—Courage or dread: The existential issue

So long as one only asks questions, one can remain existential and phenomenological. When one begins to give answers to the questions, he leaves the purely existential realm and "gives notice" on his phenomenological foothold. When one systematizes his answers, he has left both the existential and phenomenological positions. This is all true, and yet in another sense it is false. Existentialism, most broadly and most meaningfully conceived, makes a place for all modes by which man enters into the encounter with Being (The All-ness of existence). The abstract, conceptual, or constructual approach is certainly a part of the dialogue of man and existence. If one can use conceptualization as a tool to expanding awareness and not confuse the tool with that which it serves, then he is facilitated in his encounter with Being.[1]

The basic fact of existence is existence. The basic significance of existence is the potentiality of being. The basic experience of existence is awareness. This much is the framework within which I write; all that I say hereafter is derived from the intercourse of awareness with existence, is the creation of our being from the isness of existence. Existence is, period. One can say no more of

---

[1] This is akin to the semanticist's dictum that "the map is not the territory." The existentialist goes one step further, however, and says, "the map is not *the* map!" This is a way of saying two things concurrently: (a) there is an infinite number of possible maps; and (b) any map—any construction about existence—is already a fiction. The mapmaker would need to be outside of the territory mapped to have any genuine perspective on it, and it is a manifest absurdity to speak of being outside The All. Only The All itself is an adequate map of The All.

existence, as existence. The meanings and descriptions we write are neither purely discoveries about the givenness of existence nor yet are they purely our inventions imposed on existence. They are the outcomes of our being and of our being aware as a part of existence.

Awareness is the medium through which we invent-discover our being. Awareness is our being, in the process of be-ing. Being without awareness is never be-ing, though it may exist. When we come to write of man's existential situation and to postulate needs, anxieties, therapeutic procedures, and hoped-for outcomes, we are, perforce, emphasizing the "invent" aspect of the "invent-discover" process that is awareness. This phenomenological outlook is the point of departure for our attempt to understand man's distress in being, the therapeutic procedures which seek to reduce that distress, the nature of the authentic being which is sought, and the aid we can bring to that seeking for greater actuality. When we undertake this task, we build on the foundation of our recognition of the basic actuality and oneness of existence, of the potentiality of being, and of awareness.

So oriented, we must recognize that there are no necessarily "right" or "real" answers to such questions as "What is the nature of existence?" or "What are the given dimensions of being?" Various sets of dimensions, contrasting descriptions of the attributes of man's situation, have equal claims to validity; though this means none has any ultimate claim. The more useful question becomes, "What way of understanding our existence, what manner of interpreting our awareness most facilitates our realizing our being?" My way of answering this question is given in this and the next three chapters.

The Confrontation of Existential Anxiety

"There are many ways to cut a pie," the old saying has it. Indeed, at least theoretically, there are an infinite number of ways. The pie we must cut is the fact of existence. Just as the decision the housewife makes in cutting the pie takes into account the number to be served, the amount of the pie to be saved for another meal, and so on, so our decision is based on the needs of the therapeutic enterprise. We must consider what any particular way of ordering our awareness of being offers in terms of insights into important sequences of therapeutic work and into significant appreciations for the person who is our patient. In this perspective, as we saw in Chapter 3, four attributes of man's existence seem pertinent: the sense of our finiteness, the recognition of our potential to take actions, the realization of our autonomy, and the discovery of our separate-but-relatedness. It should be evident that these are not truly discrete categories, for they are importantly interrelated at all points.

ESTABLISHING OUR BASE LINE

I want to present a relatively simple schema for thinking about the human situation, one that will permit a coordination of the given characteristics of being with some of the main forms of inauthentic and authentic being. Our communication will be more adequate and our work with our patients more effective if we have a modest vocabulary of terms whose interrelations we know and which point to meaningful psychological experiences.

To give us a framework of this kind, I will draw on the germinal observations of Erich Fromm and Paul Tillich.[2] Then we can derive certain further extensions of those observations that will let us consider common human experiences and the ways we react to them.

EXISTENTIAL NEEDS

Erich Fromm (1959) has examined man's situation in terms of the basic needs that must be met for man to be fully human. In a penetrating analysis of human experience, he arrives at the conclusion that four such basic needs may be recognized: rootedness, identity, transcendence, and relation. We will examine each of these in somewhat greater detail below; however, we may be able to gain a greater appreciation of their significance if we speculate on parallels between these existential needs and yet another astute observation about man's existential situation.

---

[2] In this, as in so much that I am presenting, I am building on the prior contributions of a number of writers in works too numerous to list here but included in the reference list at the end of the book. Among the many gifted observers particularly contributing to the views we are presenting but not specifically cited must be listed Buhler, Farber, Hora, Jourard, G. A. Kelly, May, and Rogers.

FORMS OF EXISTENTIAL ANXIETY

Paul Tillich (1952) has proposed that there are three main sources of existential anxiety: the threat of death and fate, the experience of guilt and condemnation, and the confronting of emptiness and meaninglessness. Although Tillich does not explicitly recognize a fourth, it may be argued that it is implicit in much that he says. We will propose that the human experience includes an additional source of existential anxiety, that of the threat of loneliness and isolation.

ATTRIBUTES OF AUTHENTICITY

Finally, on the basis of clinical observation as well as logical inference, we may postulate that full authenticity in being seems to be characterized in the individual by the attributes of faith, commitment, creativity, and love. I will enlarge on these in later pages.

It will be evident that I am speculating on certain parallels among these several sets of observations. These parallels are set forth in Table I.

It is my experience that this ordering of the several different observations is useful in conceptualizing the patient's experience as

TABLE I

Existential Needs, Anxiety, and Authentic Being

EXISTENTIAL GIVENS	EXISTENTIAL ANXIETY	EXISTENTIAL NEED	AUTHENTIC BEING
Finiteness	Fate and death	Rootedness	Faith
Potential to act	Guilt and condemnation	Identity	Commitment
Choice	Emptiness and meaninglessness	Meaningfulness[a]	Creativity
Separateness	Loneliness and isolation	Relatedness	Love

[a] I have substituted "meaningfulness" for Fromm's "transcendence" since I am employing the latter term in a more inclusive manner.

he confronts existential freedom. To say it differently, when a patient has made good progress in freeing himself from that which distorts and prevents his authentic being in the world, he still—at least in our culture at this time—must clothe that being in some manner of expressing his actuality. Perhaps under other circumstances freeing one's being from inauthenticity might be synonymous with a fulfillment that needed no specification of life applications (mystical transcendence? Nirvana?). It is clinically and practically rather clear, though, that this is not the case for most of us. What is here maintained is that the resolution of the resistance and transference is facilitated and the maintenance of those gains in authenticity once achieved is promoted if there is attention also to growth and unfolding in these key areas of experience. It will be apparent that I am here dealing with matters such as A. H. Maslow has so effectively stated in terms of contrasting "Deficit-motivation" and "Being-motivation."

Summary

I have made a first general synopsis of a schema for examining ontological authenticity and have characterized it as being that has the qualities of faith, commitment, creativity, and love. I have postulated that these attributes of authenticity are linked to the manner of response to existential anxiety and existential need. We are ready now to make a more detailed examination of the derivation of these attributes of authenticity.

The Core Dynamic Sequence

When man encounters the givens of his existence he experiences existential anxiety. How man responds to that anxiety—whether with dread or with courage—tells the story of his non-being or his being. The crossroads of life, existentially speaking, lie at the point of the confrontation of existential anxiety. In this and the next chapters we will study that response to this confrontation which leads to neurotic anxiety. Chapters 19 and 20 will look into that response which leads to authentic being.

Table II summarizes the core dynamic sequence through which the person comes to experience actualization or blockage of his existential needs. It may be read schematically as follows: The

TABLE II

The Core Dynamic Sequence

I discover world through awareness. I am in world. I am ...
FINITE ... ABLE TO ACT ... ABLE TO CHOOSE ... SEPARATE
 These are the *Existential givens*.

Because I am so, I find I am subject to ...
FATE ... GUILT ... EMPTINESS ... LONELINESS
 These are the forms of *Existential anxiety*.

I cannot escape existential anxiety. I can confront it. To confront it means to incorporate into my being-in-the-world ...
CONTINGENCY ... RESPONSIBILITY ... AUTONOMY ... APARTNESS
 These are the *Existential confrontations*.

If I find these too devastating to accept, I may seek to avoid existential anxiety. Thus I will fall prey to feelings of ...
POWERLESSNESS ... BLAME ... ABSURDITY ... ESTRANGEMENT
 These are the forms of *Neurotic anxiety* or *Dread*.

On the other hand, if I do confront and incorporate existential anxiety, I am able to realize my being in the world through ...
FAITH ... COMMITMENT ... CREATIVITY ... LOVE
 These are the forms of *Authentic being* or *Courage*.

If I am authentic in my being in the world, then I am able to realize ...
ROOTEDNESS ... IDENTITY ... MEANINGFULNESS ... RELATEDNESS
 These are the *Existential needs*.

---

existential givens of our being, once recognized, occasion deep feelings of existential anxiety. That anxiety is natural to our being, but it may seem too overwhelming at times. Genuine confrontation of existential anxiety means taking into our very awareness of ourselves certain attributes of being in the world that may seem more than we can sustain. In such instances we may try to avoid being overwhelmed by distorting the nature of the givens of existence. When we do so, we experience dread and the feelings of neurotic anxiety. If, on the other hand, we confront existential anxiety authentically and take into our experience of ourselves the aspects of being that seem so threatening, we are making the courageous response and are freed for authentic being. Only when we are authentic in our being can we truly satisfy our basic existential needs. Figure 1 illustrates this process.

FIGURE I *The Courage or Dread Confrontation*

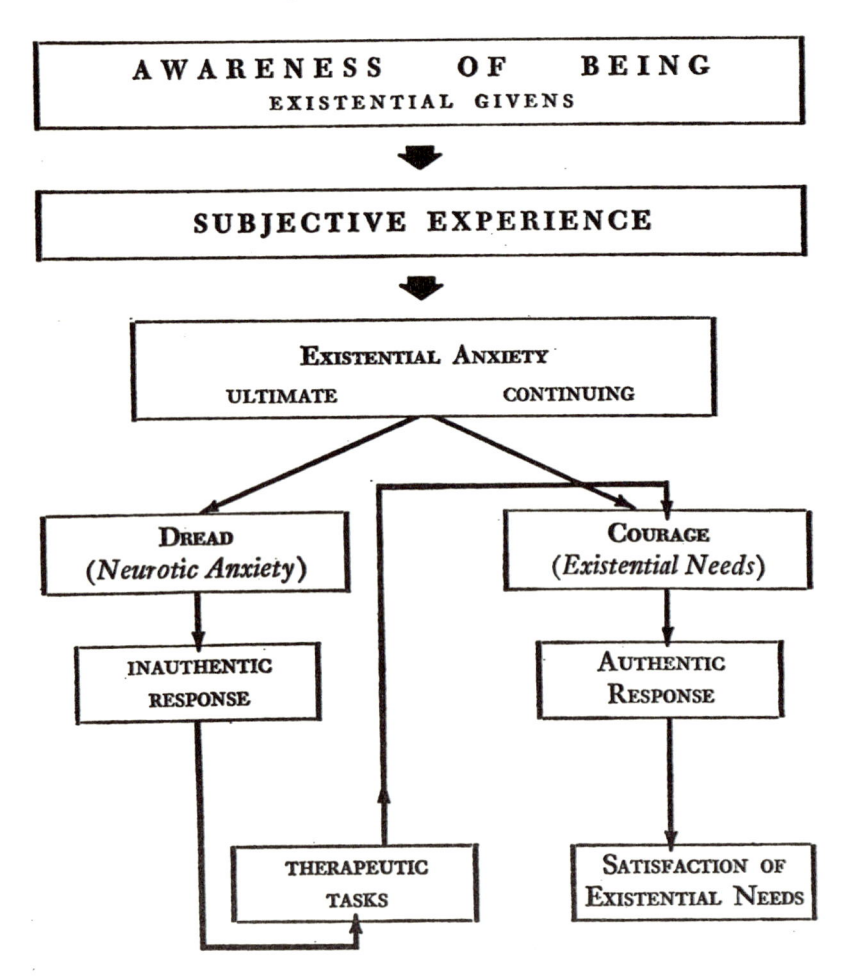

```
┌─────────────────────────────────────────┐
│         AWARENESS   OF   BEING          │
│           EXISTENTIAL GIVENS            │
└─────────────────────────────────────────┘
                    ▼
┌─────────────────────────────────────────┐
│         SUBJECTIVE EXPERIENCE           │
└─────────────────────────────────────────┘
                    ▼
        ┌───────────────────────┐
        │  EXISTENTIAL ANXIETY  │
        │  ULTIMATE   CONTINUING│
        └───────────────────────┘
           ↙         ↑         ↘
┌──────────────────┐   ┌──────────────────┐
│     DREAD        │   │     COURAGE      │
│(Neurotic Anxiety)│   │(Existential Needs)│
└──────────────────┘   └──────────────────┘
         ↓                      ↓
┌──────────────────┐   ┌──────────────────┐
│   INAUTHENTIC    │   │    AUTHENTIC     │
│    RESPONSE      │   │    RESPONSE      │
└──────────────────┘   └──────────────────┘
         ↓                      ↓
┌──────────────────┐   ┌──────────────────┐
│   THERAPEUTIC    │   │  SATISFACTION OF │
│      TASKS       │   │ EXISTENTIAL NEEDS│
└──────────────────┘   └──────────────────┘
```

THE EXISTENTIAL CONFRONTATION

It will be evident in Table II how I have employed the four existential areas developed in Table I in order to give flesh to the skeleton of the core dynamic sequence. (For ease in reference, I have shortened some of my terms also.) Table II will be our basic outline in the following pages for studying these processes of confrontation and their outcome. Before we begin that discussion, however, let us recognize what a serious matter is this very confrontation which we have made our pivot.

The confrontation of the basic givens of our being means an unflinching acceptance into full and feelingful awareness of one's limitedness and vulnerability, of one's unrelenting responsibility, of the eternal silence of world in the face of our most desperate pleas, and of the ultimately unbridgeable chasm that separates us each from the other. It is the rare person, if any exists, who can truly accept all this into his own being.

> To human eyes too much of light
> Is blinding as the blackest night
> And this is so, too, of the mind:
> In total ignorance it's blind,
> But more truth than it can absorb
> Will overwhelm the mental orb.
>
> So, lest our vision burn to ashes,
> God shows us truth in bits and flashes,
> White revelations that the brain
> Can comprehend and yet stay sane.
> And we, poor fools, demand truth's noon
> Who scarce can bear its crescent moon.
>
> (Georgie Starbuck Galbraith, 1954)

EXISTENTIAL ANXIETY AND THE RESPONSE OF DREAD

The four forms of existential anxiety that have just been detailed are the cornerstones of the conception here being set forth. Each person must deal with each of these forms of anxiety in some fashion. Obviously, the manner in which one handles his experience of such anxiety will vary tremendously from person to person.

However, as we have seen, there are two general ways of responding to the experience of existential anxiety. These are the response of dread and the response of courage.

The response of *dread* is that which gives rise to neurotic anxiety. When the recognition of existential anxiety seems overwhelming and the person cannot support incorporation of that anxiety, then he must engage in maneuvers designed to distort the reality of his awareness of being. His experience of existential anxiety is transmuted, as it were, into dread, which in turn produces various forms of neurotic anxiety.

When a person confronts existential anxiety and accepts it and incorporates it within his being, we speak of his response being that of *courage*. In such instances the forms his response takes are fulfilling of his existential needs. Saying it differently, we are postulating that *to recognize that one lives in anxiety is a part of the response to that anxiety which makes it possible for one then to recognize his basic needs as a human being and set about fulfilling them.*

Obviously this dichotomization of response to existential anxiety oversimplifies the matter. It is probably so that each person shows some measure of dread and some measure of courage in his response to each of the forms of existential anxiety. Nevertheless, there is genuine value to our simplification because it makes it possible for us to examine in greater detail the nature of neurotic anxiety and of the therapeutic tasks essential to a reincorporation of existential anxiety and a courageous response to being.[3]

INAUTHENTIC RESPONSE

Let me pause a moment to describe what I mean by this term "inauthentic response." It is my postulation that as the individual responds in terms of dread rather than courage he relinquishes authentic being in the world, and he is non-being in some measure. This non-being in turn is expressed through symptoms or resistances that attempt to deal with the dread and the underlying anxiety and that perpetuate the loss of authentic being in the world.

---

[3] I will enlarge on courage in my discussion of ontogogy in Chapters 19 and 20; the present and the next chapters examine the response of dread.

18 — *The existential neuroses*

I want to offer the hypothesis that most of the so-called "character disorders" or "character neuroses" we see increasingly today among the intelligent, educated patients in intensive therapy are more accurately denominated existential neuroses. By proposing this I do not intend to argue past nosologies or to propose a new one. I do hope to support a line of thinking and observation that seems to be promising of more effective understanding of and communication with our patients. Further, this same schema may be carried forward to the constructive phase to which we have given the name ontogogy.

In brief, my speculation is that the existential neuroses represent the person's unconscious preoccupation with one or another (sometimes several) of the givens of existence. When the therapist is attuned to conduct his analytic work in a fashion that encourages the emergence of the nuclear, existential (anxiety) conflict, he may appreciably advance the therapeutic work, sometimes in promptness of movement, sometimes in thoroughness of analysis, and many times in both regards. Further, when the therapist (consultant?) in the ontogogic phase gives attention to all four aspects of the givenness of being, he has similar advantages and clearer perspectives for his efforts.

Let me make all this more concrete: it has seemed to me that many of the patients with whom I have worked intensively have ultimately disclosed to me their preoccupation with feelings of powerlessness, blame, absurdity, or estrangement. Oftentimes more than one of these were important; usually in such cases one area was predominate in the early stages and another later on. As I come to appreciate the existential significances of these four forms of neurotic anxiety (that is, as I sense their linkages back to the givens of being, as has been traced out in the preceding chapter), I am aided in finding sooner the dominant emotional themes and in helping the patient to reduce the seeming diversity and contradictions of specific symptoms and resistances. The analytic work thus becomes more orderly and efficient. Let us examine in more detail how this works out. In doing so I will translate my theoretical or conceptual observations into more clinical terms and indicate some of the significances for actual therapeutic work.

Each of the four forms of neurotic dread represents a breakthrough of neurotic anxiety occasioned by the failure of defenses (resistances) to the confronting of existential anxiety. In this way of seeing the matter, the therapist is given the opportunity to understand what it is the patient is trying to express and to facilitate the patient's efforts to come to grips with the core conflicts of his life.[4]

DREAD AND INAUTHENTIC RESPONSE

Table III provides an overview of my conceptualization of what happens when the person succumbs to the experience of existential anxiety and undertakes the distortions of being that seem to promise relief. In this table are set forth the forms that the existential neuroses take in hypothetical "pure" cases. As we have already noted, most people show concerns that touch nearly all of these areas, although there is often a clustering in one or two. The following pages will enlarge on these points and illustrate them with case examples as we study the response of dread in each of its four major manifestations.

Response to the Anxiety of Fate and Death

"The anxiety of fate and death is the most basic, most universal, and inescapable . . . Fate and death are the way in which our ontic

---

[4] This is not to say that the therapist will want to employ the language in which I am here presenting these concepts in his actual talking with the patient. Much more effective is developing with the patient the terms that experientially convey his own personal confronting of these issues.

TABLE III
Existential and Neurotic Anxiety and the Sources of Inauthenticity

EXISTENTIAL ANXIETY	Fate and death	Guilt and condemnation	Emptiness and meaninglessness	Loneliness and isolation
CONFRONTATIONS	Contingency	Responsibility	Autonomy	Apartness
NEUROTIC ANXIETY (DREAD)	Powerlessness	Blame	Absurdity	Estrangement
INAUTHENTIC RESPONSE (NON-BEING)	Resignation	Surrender of freedom	Alienation from self	Withdrawal from others
DISTORTIONS OF BEING active forms	Activism Manipulation	Blind rebellion	Destructiveness	Dominance
passive forms	Fatalism Embeddedness	Conformity	Apathy	Submission

self-affirmation is threatened by non-being" (Tillich, 1952, p. 42). It seems reasonably safe to assume that anxiety over the anticipation of his own death is felt by nearly every person at least at some times in his life. Sometimes this fear is less for the actual fact of death itself than for the fact that one cannot tell when or in what way that death will come. This is, of course, the meaning of the sense of being subject to fate. When many neurotic symptoms are analyzed it can often be found that they have, among other meanings, something to say of the fear of death and the sense of fate.

Man is apparently a limited being in the midst of the apparent unlimitedness of existence. By the very nature of the matter we have no affirmative evidence of either the presumed end of awareness nor the assumed infiniteness of possibility. The former we hypothesize on the basis of negative evidence only (and even that questioned by some); the latter we accept as a logical inference. Whatever the defensibility of these assumptions, our lives are set in a phenomenological world in which we assume that living will have an end, in which we always experience that the possibilities in any situation far exceed our awareness, and in which we can never predict with surety. This is our experience of finiteness as a part of our very existence.

THE EXISTENTIAL ANXIETY ARISING FROM FINITENESS

Confronted with his finiteness, man experiences existential anxiety arising from his anticipation of his own death and from his sense of being subject to fate. Tillich distinguishes between death and fate, calling the former the "absolute" and the latter the "relative." This distinction is a useful one, though we choose to rename it for our present purpose to designate the anticipation of death as an ultimate existential anxiety and the sense of being subject to fate as a continuing source of existential anxiety. The difference implied is that the ultimate condition represents the end-point of a continuum characterized by the continuing aspect. Clearly one experiences the existential anxiety of finiteness not in terms of his death itself, but in terms of the anticipation of it. The fact that we live in contingency makes us recognize that seemingly chance factors may importantly affect our lives and thus makes us aware that we are always in some measure subject to the workings of fate.

Confronting Contingency

It is one thing to recognize abstractly that we are limited within an unlimited world, to say that this is logically a basis for anxiety. It is another matter to confront genuinely just what this means. It is quite another matter to look unwinkingly at the tremendous personal meaning of contingency. This is what we mean when we speak of the "existential confrontations:" not an abstract recognition but an immediate, personal incorporation of such recognition as a part of our very experience of ourselves in our world. One cannot appreciate the full meaning of the pivotal confrontation, which means the difference between being and non-being (in a sense that is scarcely metaphorical, between life and death), if he regards it only at a distance. The reader may act out his own inauthenticity if he insists on so considering what is here said. In miniature, this presentation is a confrontation.

To confront contingency means to open one's awareness to the full meaning of infinite possibility, to recognize that what will happen is always, at least in some measure, unknown. Contingency means that the number and potentialities of all the influences that go to determine what will happen in this instant, in the next hour, today, in my life are beyond my knowing. For most of us, were it possible to tear away the curtain of partial awareness and resistive unawareness, we could not endure to look suddenly and unprotectedly at the reality of infinite possibility and ultimate unknowability. The reasons this is so include the loss of our familiar world, the infiniteness of the potential, and the limited ability we have to control outcomes.

THE LOSS OF THE USUAL WORLD

Immediately in front of you the busy city intersection is tense with an all too familiar drama. A minute ago a speeding car hit that handsome young man who now twists in agony on the dirty pavement. His pain is the price of his heroism, for at the last minute he managed to shove the woman who was with him out of the car's path. Then, suddenly, you are pulling back from this scene. Abruptly, you realize this is a motion picture, as the camera lifts above the city street and the store fronts are revealed as two-dimensional. Still the camera rises, and now you can see that next to the familiar street there is another set on which savages struggle with soldiers, while further on the first moon landing is being portrayed, and in yet another area an elaborate court ball is occurring. Glancing back at the street corner, you may be aware of relief that the tragedy was only the portrayal of a skillful actor; but perhaps you will sense a hint of regret too, as though for something irretrievably lost.

Just as you adjust to the new perspective, there is again the sensation of moving back still another time. Now you can see that the studio "lot" is but one such lot and there is another on either side. On these adjoining lots the sets are busy also, the figures—perhaps it is the distance, but you don't really think so—look somehow different. As you move higher and your view embraces more, the whole of a vast panorama seems to be filled with various scenes in progress. You can't be sure there are cameras in all instances. Some of the action is so patently melodramatic and artificial, some may not be drama at all, but you realize you can't really tell which.

Yet another enlargement of the perspective makes evident that there are numerous other watchers such as yourself. It is as though the sky is full of them. Or is it that they are but actors on other sets . . . ?

Or are you but an actor on another set?

When we come to confront contingency we must yield up the comfortable sense of being in a known, familiar world. We dwell instead in an insubstantial space of the probabilities of possibilities. We no longer can be complete participants in the usual social conspiracy, which pretends that most of life occurs within the realm of the known and only some aspects are still to be worked out by science or philosophy. Instead we come to realize that only a very small portion of our experience occurs in the area of what is truly, reasonably probable, most is in the area of tradition and convention unsupported by any surety, and none is in complete certainty.

Let us pause to make explicit that the statements of the previous paragraph are in no sense hyperbole. We do not really understand the nature of heat, gravitation, light, electricity, the transformation of matter, human or other life, the relations among people whether as individuals or in any grouping up to and including nations, weather, birth, assimilation of foods, and so on and on. In some of these areas we have reasonably good pragmatic generalizations which we call laws or theories; in many we do not even have that. We cannot detect the potential murderer of the President of the United States or of ourselves. Although we examine candidates for driving automobiles, we license many killers. We do not know whether the man who could touch off atomic annihilation is now arriving in a position of crucial power or has just been committed to a mental hospital. Before this page is finished now by the writer or now by the reader the course of one or all of our lives may be completely altered for good or evil.

THE INFINITE POTENTIAL OF CONTINGENCY

Contingency flows away from us on every side as though our every act were a stone dropped in a pond. Our smallest acts, our most casual choices, have the potential of reaching to any point in their consequences. We can never imagine all the possible permutations and ramifications of our doing and not doing. Literature finds in this fact an immense storehouse of material for fiction. The unexpected consequences of seemingly trivial acts make for fascinating reading when we are comfortably reassured that it is all a story. Indeed, this may be one of the sources of the enjoyment of such accounts: a vicarious contending with dread contingencies. But there is nothing shallowly entertaining in direct recognition of the immensity and unpredictability of contingency. It may lead to the dread of powerlessness or to the exhilaration of participation and rootedness. It certainly can powerfully affect our whole way of being in the world.

OUR LIMITED ABILITY TO CONTROL OUTCOMES

A peculiar accident reported by the National Safety Council involved two housewives in separate cases. Both were using an ordinary toilet bowl cleaner. Not satisfied with the way it was removing stain, each one added some household bleach and stirred with a brush. One died quickly—the other spent a long spell in the hospital. . . .

What happened in the above cases was that a poisonous gas was liberated when the users decided to use a mixture of two or more common cleaning agents . . . [producing] a quantity of chlorine gas.

(Tenth District Bulletin, Los Angeles P.T.A.)

The other face of the infinite potential of contingency is the limited ability we have to control what will occur. Just as the most unimaginable consequences may flow from our most trivial act, so our most heroic efforts may prove fruitless, our most dedicated intentions unavailing. These sad outcomes are always possible. They are not, as some fear, inevitable. Our efforts may be wonderfully effective. Contingency does not deny our power to have some effect; it simply denies certainty.

Summary

These are three of the important threats which make the raw confrontation of contingency the threatening source of anxiety that it is and which must be incorporated by the person seeking greater authenticity of being. The person who seeks to actualize his potential is, among other things, the person who constantly seeks to open his awareness more to the reality of contingency. It should be apparent that the fuller appreciation of contingency would result in a sort of person very different from those most of us are or know.

The Dread of Powerlessness

The dread of powerlessness traces back to the existential anxiety of fate and death. When a patient emphasizes how impotent he is, it will usually be found that he is preoccupied at some level of awareness with the effects of contingency on his life and with how to handle the fact that he cannot control all the variables affecting his experience. In whatever language the patient casts the matter, what he is saying over and over again is that he feels at the mercy of forces beyond his control and even beyond his knowledge. There is, of course, a realistic basis for the patient's concern; for each of us is subject to contingency. But what the patient does who is preoccupied with powerlessness is to say in effect "Since I can't control everything that will determine what happens to me, I have no control at all." Experiencing the unpredictability of his life, the patient gives up and enacts this feeling of having no possibility of affecting what happens to himself. He makes himself totally an object.

Freda was raised by very authoritarian immigrant parents. She was taught not to question or argue but to be guided by the one, right way that was set out for her. Then when Freda was seven her father began disappearing for periods that gradually became longer until he was no longer a regular part of the family. With adult understanding, Freda can recognize the break-up of her parents' relation with each other and the vain efforts at reconciliation. As a child, Freda did not have this understanding. Her parents "protected" her from their quarrels and from the separations, until finally her mother told Freda the divorce was complete.

In her therapy Freda shows much anxiety and dread centered in the area of fate and death. Repeatedly she expresses her feelings of powerlessness. "I can't do anything about it" is practically a refrain to each concern with which she deals. Her early learnings served to make her feel quite ineffectual. Only by being very good could she hope to gain any advantage, and the standard for how good she had to be kept rising until today Freda can recognize she is quite unrealistic in what she demands of herself. Yet, even with herself, she feels, "I can't do anything about it." The suicidal thoughts which so frequently accompany this dread of powerlessness are treasured by Freda as her "ace in the hole." She literally begs me with pathetic tears not to take this possibility away from her! For even in this she feels the powerlessness.

In response to the dread of powerlessness we see various forms of resignation. These may take the passive forms of embeddedness (Schachtel, 1959) or fatalism or the active forms of activism and manipulation. In the former the individual is handling his dread by resigning from any contending with contingency for his life. He lapses into an inertness which seems to accentuate his helplessness. In the more active forms there is a substitution of a valuing of action for its own sake. This amounts to an effort to hide from the dread of powerlessness by making so much "noise" about doing that one can not hear the hollow echo from contingency, and the point of the doing is utterly lost. Another active way of handling the dread of powerlessness is to victimize other people, capitalizing on their powerlessness and apparently gaining gratification by exercising gratuitous control over them. Parents who are oppressed by the dread of powerlessness often need to make their children excessively dependent upon them and to defeat the child's efforts to gain independence.

Response to the Anxiety of Guilt and Condemnation

In taking and not taking action, man finds that he affects the stream of his awareness. Changes in that stream, moreover, have more than a casual importance. They are not solely changes in the "out there" but also evoke concurrent changes in the "in here." Man's awareness is feelingful, and these feelings are importantly affected by how he uses his action potential. Man discovers responsibility.

It is in this experience of making a difference in world and in our own subjective feelings that we discover our "being there." In making such a difference we become aware of that which we have directly intuited, that we are the subjects, rather than solely the objects, of our experience. Thus we bear responsibility. As the subject we give actuality (life) to some possibilities while denying it to others. Therein resides our guilt also. Guilt is always an aspect of our being; condemnation is the ultimate threat we must face. The guilt and condemnation here specified are natural and not neurotic. They are inherent in our human situation, not judgments against our worth. Existential guilt is frequently misunderstood as a kind of malignant or masochistic self-flagellation. Quite to the contrary, existential guilt seeks to give recognition to the fact that what one does matters. Man does have responsibility for acting or not acting and thereby determining what will be actual. Life is serious, and the power to affect what will be actual in life is a serious responsibility. It is ennobling to view man in this light, rather than to make of his acting and nonacting a triviality.

My discovery of my potential to take action is the basis for my awareness of my own being. If I were unable to influence the stream of my own awareness, but could only passively regard it, I would have no recognition of my own existence. It is in the doing and not doing that my being is expressed and evidenced in awareness. (It should be very clear that in using this term, "potential to take action," we do not imply physical or motoric action only. The action to which we refer here is implicit or explicit, perceptible or imperceptible, and includes nonaction as its obverse aspect.)

It will be apparent how the anxiety of guilt and condemnation shades off into the other forms of existential anxiety (Haigh, 1961). On the one hand our very concern becomes expressed through our choices, and this brings us to the whole matter of the need for meaningfulness. On the other hand, because we are finite and subject to contingency, we find the weight of our responsibility underscoring our concern. Moreover, concern is amplified when our relations to others are recognized as being involved at all points.

CONFRONTING RESPONSIBILITY

> For want of a nail the shoe was lost
> For want of a shoe the horse was lost
> For want of a horse the rider was lost
> For want of the rider the battle was lost
> For want of the battle the kingdom was lost
> And all for the want of a horseshoe nail.
>
> (Traditional, Stevenson, 1945)

In discussing contingency we pointed out how the consequences of our actions flow out from us on all sides, predictable only in part, stretching we cannot know to what further possibilities. The old Mother Goose jingle makes a simple chain from the overthrow of the kingdom back to the momentary carelessness of a blacksmith or groom. But that momentary carelessness is a responsibility defaulted upon, is a guilt of smith and groom.

Were each of us to look into his own life with the same pursuing eye and trace our responsibilities to their furtherest reaches we might be aghast at the wake thus revealed. Yet, far short of such an extreme, we may often recognize dimly or clearly how much our acting and nonacting has had effects we did not anticipate. Sometimes these are fortuitous, sometimes without importance one way or another, and sometimes they are malign. This is the awful fact of our concern.

Where we stop the causal chain, where we accept responsibility and where deny it, where we protest innocence or accept guilt, these are issues which are part of our confronting our concern. Clearly some seek to flee from all link to any but the most obvious of connections. They render themselves hapless things thereby. The compulsive person may insist on extremes of guilt that verge over into blame. He is too greedy. Responsibility is one side of a coin, the other face of which is opportunity. Where one has no responsibility, he is impotent. Where one takes too much responsibility, seeks too much potency, he is cursed with the Midas touch.

THE DREAD OF BLAME

The dread of blame stems basically from the existential anxiety of guilt and condemnation. Oppressed by the sense of concern the person comes to regard each action as fraught with the possibility of new blame and as a threat to his identity. Blame seems to imply defect or fault in the person himself rather than in his action. Children who are raised with heavy emphasis on blame and shame (the two often go together) become preoccupied with assessing the rightness or wrongness of each thought, each word, and each deed. The intrinsic utility, appropriateness, or effectiveness of any action is obscured as attention is focused on its rectitude, whether real or fancied.

The inauthentic response to blame is a surrender of freedom. Non-being is evidenced in the blame-laden person's inability to carry his birthright of freedom and his relinquishing of it to his accusers, whether actual or projected. Surrender of freedom may take either active or passive forms. An example of the active form is the sort of blind rebellion against all standards or principles in which some engage. The more passive form of surrender of freedom is that of blind conformity. Here the person yields up his identity and wipes out his individuality for the seeming protection against guilt and responsibility afforded by undistinguished uniformity with the social code.

> Ed had been the pride of his whole family when he was accepted at a well-known divinity school. Since early childhood he'd been singled out ("Ed's going to be a minister") so consistently that in later years he never could be sure just whose idea it was or how surely he'd thought he really wanted to go into the church. Then in his second year, Ed had a

severe cold that hung on for some time, after which he abruptly left his studies and returned to his parents' home. He was treated with worried kindness by all concerned, but he had an extended period of depression and withdrawal. The following autumn he took a business course in sales work and became an insurance salesman. When he came to me fifteen years later he was still in that work, in which he was making an indifferent living and finding no satisfaction.

Ed's life was suffused with a sense of shame. Trying to work with him, I soon discovered, was like trying to help someone who had been severely burned over his whole body. The least contact about his life experience evoked in Ed a suffering none the less real for being the expression of his neurotic dread of facing his flooding awareness of guilt and responsibility. Each topic, each relationship, each choice made or not made was a new evocation of his shame. We worked together scarcely six months before he interrupted. A year later he began again. This time he managed to hold with therapy for over a year, but then he had to interrupt for a longer period. Again he returned, and we set up a very loose plan in which he could pace his appointments as much as five to seven weeks apart. In time, we were able to increase the pace to a more usual working schedule again.

The therapeutic course in itself is not the central point of Ed's case. Rather it is his intense shame and its roots. At base what Ed had to face and yet fled from facing was that he really did want to go into the ministry, that he felt he did have a "call," that he had acted to leave the seminary for transitory reasons and then had somehow let shame and false pride intervene so that he did not go back. To face all this and to know it was really so, and to know in addition that it was now really too late (he still fantasied returning to ministerial training) to have the life he had wanted and intended and so nearly had—all this weighed so heavily on Ed that he was a continual fugitive from his own life.

If we seek to avoid guilt, we deny our identity. If we fear the weight of responsibility, the possible condemnation, we deny our choice and distort awareness. Thus is born neurotic guilt and anxiety. In the confusion of blame and guilt, lies much that destroys our authenticity of identity. Blame that attributes fault to the *I-process* is existentially invalid; more, it is not-sense. Guilt, which relates to the choices we have made, is inherent in our being, but it need be neither crippling nor depressing. Guilt is a part of the dignity of being a man. Were there no responsibility attaching to our choices, no guilt inhering in our identity, we would be inconsiderable, as unmeaningful as the chance scrawlings of a mad infant.

Response to the Anxiety of Emptiness and Meaninglessness

You are driving an unfamiliar freeway late at night. It is raining and somewhat foggy. Your headlights bore rather ineffectual holes in the cloudiness. Your eyes, although drowsy, are constantly checking the white lines on the pavement. The windshield wiper is becoming hypnotic and lulling you toward sleep with its steady, rhythmic "clack-clack." Dimly you are aware that there seem to be more than the usual number of lanes on either side of you. You no longer can really make out the edge of the road. Then the white lines disappear!

You shrug out of your drowsiness like a person who has fallen into deep water frantically thrusting himself to the surface. You watch for gaps in the fog to see if the lines will reappear. They do not. You wonder whether you should slack off the gas, but you're not sure what the traffic is like behind you. You want to edge to the side, but you're not sure you can see where the edge of the road is.

Now headlights are coming toward you and they seem closer on your left than they should be. Cars begin overtaking you on either side, but a minute later there are headlights approaching from both sides too. In the fog and rain, the highway is without guides, other cars seem to be following no discernible pattern, and you are suddenly, terribly alone in a world of chaos and terror.

We look in vain for preordained significances in ourselves and in our world. Again and again man raises the cry, "Why am I here?" "What does it all mean?" and again and again he is thrown back from the awful silence of the universe. Confronted with the terrible anxiety of emptiness and meaninglessness he may feel the very roots of his being shaken. He may feel the need to insist that he has discovered special meanings in the "out there."

Man seeks meaning in the "out there." But man discovers that the source of meaning is "in here." Thus man experiences that he has choice. Since world does not provide man with "built-in" meanings, man is confronted with the existential anxiety of ultimate meaninglessness which gives rise to the continuing experience of emptiness. The experience of meaninglessness is the recognition that world does not impose its meanings on man and thus involves the resulting anxiety from the responsibility involved in choice. Consequently, day-to-day experience can give rise to feelings of anxious emptiness when that choice is not meaningfully employed.

CONFRONTING AUTONOMY

At first thought our birthright of open choice seems an unalloyed gift that can only be a source of gratification. Certainly this has been the foreboding of many moralists who feared that men free of constraints would produce chaos. Oscar Wilde said, "When the gods wish to punish us they answer our prayers," bespeaking his gloomy prediction about autonomy. But such excesses, I believe, are the product of factors other than our autonomy. A full confrontation of autonomy is far from an intoxicating draught; it is brutally sobering. The imagery of the freeway without lines gives but a hint of the terror that can reside in the emptiness of our autonomy.

Yet there is another side also. Because man is not exclusively governed by tropisms or instincts, because man can select among alternatives, because man is not solely the creature but is in some measure the creator of his being and his experience, he can transcend being but a thing and partake of the godhead's very nature. This is not a postulation about the free-will–determinism issue, which is, after all, an invalid question phenomenologically.[1] It is, rather, a recognition that our being involves a "taking part in" all

---

[1] Periodically this free-will issue crops up again in the psychological literature (Adcock, 1961; Angel, 1956; Budd, 1960; Hartmann, 1961; Kelly, 1955; Schaller, 1959; Wolfensberger, 1961). It seems to me that the logical issue is relatively easily disposed of in terms of a recognition of the phenomenology of choice. But the underlying psychological-existential questioning is not so readily dismissed, for it is really the basic subject-object dilemma of the human experience that is involved.

existence. Choice and autonomy express our being and contribute to our being.

THE DREAD OF ABSURDITY

When man finds himself unable to confront the immensity of the meaninglessness of the world, when he finds his searching for preordained meanings to be vain, his life may seem "a cosmic triviality." Thus his fear has become distortive, and man finds himself in absurdity. Absurdity, in turn, leads to alienation from self. Absurdity means, as we are using it here, either the denial of meaning (which is quite different from the recognition of meaninglessness) or the imposition of man-made meanings onto "The All" as though they were discoveries about the nature of The All.

In the grip of absurdity, further defenses against the existential anxiety of emptiness and meaninglessness break down and the person is flooded with additional reminders of absurdity about himself and his life. The experience of choice becomes a mockery to a person so entrapped, for he feels that his choices are without point, and he finds the emptiness of the world insofar as preordained meaning a continual frustration of his own seeking for purpose. In such people the inauthentic response, the loss of being, takes the form of alienation from the self. It is as though the person said, "Since the world refuses to give my life meaningfulness, it has none, and I am uninvolved with my living." Some of the typical patterns of distorted being associated with this condition are, on the active side, destructiveness and, on the passive side, apathy. Through destructiveness the person who feels caught in an absurd world parodies his constructive and creative impulses. Destruction can be a kind of construction; destruction can serve as a kind of creativity. The hypercritical person who needs to tear down the ideas of others and devalue all institutions very often is engaged in a desperate fight with his dread of meaninglessness. The apathetic person, on the other hand, seems to have given up that battle and withdrawn all emotional investment.

In Beckett's play, *Endgame*, what may be two of the last men in the world after atomic devastation talk in a shelter where they have been awaiting death. Clov, the servant, shows through most of the play the response of apathy, as he waits on blind Hamm, the master. Clov occasionally wonders why he continues to do so, but he does continue. Hamm, feeling any constructiveness thrown back by the manifested absurdity of a devastated world, has become capricious and destructive toward Clov. In the following segment, Clov announces without any apparent reason:

CLOV: I'll leave you. (He goes towards door.)
HAMM: Before you go . . . (Clov halts near door.) . . . say something.
CLOV: There is nothing to say.
HAMM: A few words . . . to ponder . . . in my heart.
CLOV: Your heart!
HAMM: Yes. (Pause. Forcibly.) Yes! (Pause.) With the rest, in the end, the shadows, the murmurs, all the trouble, to end up with. (Pause.) Clov . . . . He never spoke to me. Then, in the end, before he went, without my having asked him, he spoke to me. He said . . .
CLOV: (despairingly): Ah . . . !
HAMM: Something . . . from your heart.
CLOV: My heart!
HAMM: A few words . . . from your heart. (Pause.)
CLOV: (fixed gaze, tonelessly, towards auditorium): They said to me, That's love, yes, yes, not a doubt, now you see how—
HAMM: Articulate!
CLOV: (as before): How easy it is. They said to me, That's friendship, yes, yes, no question, you've found it. They said to me, Here's the place, stop, raise your head and look at all that beauty. That order! They said to me, Come now, you're not a brute beast, think upon these things and you'll see how all becomes clear. And simple! They said to me, What skilled attention they get, all these dying of their wounds.
HAMM: Enough!
CLOV: (as before): I say to myself—sometimes, Clov, you must learn to suffer better than that if you want them to weary of punishing you—one day. I say to myself—sometimes, Clov, you must be there better than that if you want them to let you go— one day. But I feel too old, and too far, to form

new habits. Good, it'll never end, I'll never go.
(Pause.) Then one day, suddenly, it ends, it
changes, I don't understand, it dies, or it's me, I
don't understand, that either. I ask the words that
remain—sleeping, waking, morning, evening. They
have nothing to say. (Pause.) I open the door of
the cell and go. I am so bowed I only see my feet,
if I open my eyes, and between my legs a little
trail of black dust. I say to myself that the earth is
extinguished, though I never saw it lit. (Pause.)
It's easy going. (Pause.) When I fall I'll weep for
happiness. (Pause. He goes towards door.)
(Beckett, 1958, pp. 79–81)

A CASE EXAMPLE

Paul's parents were the least successful financially of all the family units within a group of seven brothers and sisters. The total family attempted to maintain a semblance of closeness and periodic dinners or picnics with 25 to 40 people were part of the pattern. There was much covert comparison of "success," and Paul always had the feeling of being on the losing end. Perhaps it wouldn't have been a source of difficulty for Paul if his parents could have met the issue directly. Instead they constantly invented rather feeble excuses and fed each other and their children the tranquilizer of "We're not concerned with material things," and the sedative of "You'll see, it will be different next year." By the time Paul entered college he had seen through these defenses quite completely. He handled his reactions in a different way.

Paul was an earnest, if incompletely successful, nihilist. He pronounced his disbelief in God, morality, and all values to any who would listen and with angry insistence. He made it a point to sympathize with unpopular causes and to belittle generally accepted ones. In personal relations he was a boor and a nuisance. He had engaged in a number of minor legal infractions, was proud of having been jailed in five different cities, and was flirting with the possibility of more serious criminal acts.

Without trying to detail the therapeutic course here, I am sure it is already evident how Paul was acting out his fury and hurt that the world gave him no answers, no compensation for having poor parents, no appreciation for his hidden genius (of which he was as convinced as his parents had been of their impending change of fortune). Since world was obviously absurd, Paul was determined to deface it.

Response to the Anxiety of Loneliness and Isolation

When my baby says "Blue" does she see what I see? Does my beloved feel the same deep, yearning fullness that I feel? How much can I be sure that you really understand these ideas which are so very important to me? When, in the night, I hear our silent house breathing with our family in its embrace, how can I say to you the longing, the tender fullness in me as I visit in thought and feeling each one of these I call "mine," as I feel myself one with the house which is "ours"? As Don lies on the couch talking to me, I sense his finding a courage he's never known before, a courage to meet and deal with old, old fears, a courage I had some part in helping him discover, but do I really know Don's terror, his courage, and his triumph?

These are the questions of man's apartness. In them is expressed the questioning, the anxiety of aloneness, the seeking to bridge the unbridgable gap. Yet the very questions themselves are the other aspect of apartness too. I can write such questions only because I know you will in some degree resonate with them, will likely find similar questionings you have known. Not all of you, but many. And so I am not utterly *apart* but am also *a part* of others. This is a pun, but I mean it to be more than a pun; I mean it to express the very paradox of man's being. We are always in relation and yet always separate. Authentic being confronts and incorporates this paradox.

Confronting Apartness

An ever-present aspect of awareness is that there is *I* and there are others who are at once like I am and sharing my experience and yet different from me and not fully knowing my awareness. The experience of being discrete, separable, in some measure unique, is clearly an element of the human condition. Each of the other givens is in some measure colored experientially by this fact of my being separate. My finiteness is not coincident with that of others; the limitations on my awareness are not the same as the limits on others; although they have their limits also. My acting or not-acting is distinguishable from those of others. My choices are made in ways which coincide or contrast with the elections of others.

Existentially we are separate from yet related to others. Subjectively we experience this as apartness. We are sometimes keenly aware of the fact that no other shares our awareness just as we ourselves know it. There is a poignancy to the sense of our uniqueness that gives added depth to our contingency and our concern. Still we recognize ourselves as a part of all men, even as we are separate.

Finding himself apart from his fellows, man experiences the existential anxiety of isolation and loneliness. Isolation is potential in the human condition and is the ultimate threat to each person. Out of this experience of separateness arises the relative existential anxiety of loneliness.

THE DREAD OF ESTRANGEMENT

When the anxiety of loneliness and isolation close in too confiningly, the person may find them too great to be borne. The experience of dread is the product of the inability to confront and incorporate his essential apartness. Ironically, the very ways in which he makes this attempt bring about his eventual experience of solitariness. This is beautifully and frighteningly illustrated in Beckett's play, *Krapp's Last Tape* (1957). Krapp is portrayed as a man who in his youth was self-consciously hungry for relationships —often chiefly sexual—but who seemed unable to endure his aloneness. At some point he began what became an enveloping library of sound recordings on tape. Into these he would speak his experiences and thoughts, trying—it would seem—to win toward greater realization of his own being and of his relations with others. Now, an old man, he lives solely in the static world of his taped self and its memories. He is a shocking derelict that is scarcely human, who lost his potential for genuine relationship in his effort to overthrow the reality of his separateness.

Krapp plays an old tape for a while, then plugs in his microphone to make the only sort of contact left to him, a new recording:

> Just been listening to that stupid bastard I took myself for thirty years ago, hard to believe I was ever as bad as that. Thank God that's all done with anyway. (Pause.) The eyes she had! (Broods, realizes he is recording silence, switches off, broods. Finally.) Everything there, everything, all the— (Realizes this is not being recorded, switches on.) Everything there, everything on this old muckball, all the light and dark and famine and feasting of . . . (hesitates) . . . the ages! (In a shout.) Yes! (Pause.) . . . . (Broods. Realizes. Switches off. Consults envelope.) Pah! (Crumples it and throws it away. Broods. Switches on.) Nothing to say, not a squeak. What's a year now? The sour cud and the iron stool. (Pause.) . . . . Crawled out once or twice, before the summer was cold. Sat shivering in the park, drowned in dreams and burning to be gone. Not a soul. (Pause.) Last fancies. (Vehemently.) Keep 'em under! (Pause.) Scalded the eyes out of me reading *Effie* again, a page a day, with tears again. Effie . . . (Pause.) Could have been happy with her, up there on the Baltic, and the pines, and the dunes. (Pause.) Could I? (Pause.) And she? (Pause.) Pah! . . . . (Beckett, 1957, pp. 24–25)

Estrangement is the experience of being imprisoned in glass, seeing the world in which others move but forever blocked from joining them, pantomiming communication but never really speaking with another person. Fleeing from our apartness, we may try to deny it through seeking to be just like another person, denying any points of difference, trying to "crawl into his skin." This is the passive route, which uses submission to seem to overcome apartness. It is not infrequently part of the dynamic pattern in homosexuality. It may be an element in the compulsively seductive person (of either sex) who has to win everyone's approval. This response of dread starts by negating the person himself—estrangement intrapersonally—and ends with a negation of any genuine relationship with others—estrangement interpersonally. The superficially opposite pattern of domination reduces to the same underlying sequence of intrapersonal estrangement to interpersonal alienation. Indeed, it is not uncommon in working with both members of a marital couple to discover that each believes himself the submissive victim of the other's domination.

Our culture's heavy emphasis on mechanistic values has an inevitable effect of spreading the disease of auto-utilization. By this I refer to the widespread tendency to think of one's "worth" as a quantity demonstrated by his visible accomplishments. Moreover, such accomplishments are usually prizes of competitive striving. The result, of course, is that a large group must go headlong into feelings of being of limited or no worth. This then heightens intrapersonal estrangement and the feelings, "Who would want an also-ran?" (The obvious answer, "Another also-ran, of which there are a great number," will only bring the scornful, "Do you think I'd settle for an also-ran?")

Parents whose love is given conditionally ("If you're a good boy . . ." "I'm so happy when you do better than the other children . . .") teach this form of auto-utilization.

A CASE EXAMPLE

Ralph is a scientist who works for a large research and development firm. He has progressed well up to a level just below that at which he would have charge of major projects and task forces of a number of other scientific workers. Although several times given the opportunity to advance further, he has declined (usually heading the promotion off indirectly before it was formally tendered). He explains this by saying, "I'd rather do the real scientific job myself. Let somebody else push papers and people around. I'm doing what I like to do and can do well."

Ralph came to therapy because of conflict with his wife and because he was finding it increasingly difficult to work sustainedly and at what he felt was his optimum level of effectiveness. He proved an unusually facile analytic subject after a first period of detached impersonal resistance. His self-image emerged early as that of a little boy who had to hide his feelings to keep from being taken advantage of and who had to produce intellectually because this seemed his only area of competence and he had no value except as he was competent.

During the first year of the analytic work, Ralph's apartness from others became the focus of our attention. His wife, feeling at once tyrannized and rejected, left him, and Ralph—

to his own surprise—found himself extremely broken up and in severe anxiety. Now long-standing, preconscious feelings of being completely unloved and unlovable came through. The conviction that his parents had rejected him for younger siblings was explicit. His deep belief that any relationship he had must ultimately end also emerged.

Ralph provides an excellent example of a person whose feelings of *Self*-worth are dependent on his being an efficient nonperson. His fear of his own feelings was such that he had to cripple his natural responsiveness. Although this was a repression born of dread of being isolated, it acted—as is so often the case—to estrange him from his wife and thus to increase his actual loneliness.

Conclusion

MULTIPLE DYNAMIC SEQUENCES

Ralph provides an excellent illustration of a point I made earlier and to which I want to return now. It is often the case that careful analysis of one dynamic sequence will, if successful, lead us to a second such sequence. Thus, in Ralph's case, once the main work had been done in paring away the resistances so that he could confront his existential apartness, a second sequence was disclosed. This had to do with Ralph's deep-lying death fears and feelings of powerlessness at the hands of fate and other forces greater than he.

Although an effective man in many aspects of his life, Ralph seemed to have the inner conviction that his successes were largely flukes and that eventually the test would come which he would miserably fail and thus be exposed. Especially did he feel this foreboding and impotency with women. Now his underlying rage with women erupted, and the dual motivations of his conflict with his wife became more evident. She had seemed to him to grant or withdraw her affection and concern in an unpredictable and selfish fashion. It was only after much analytic and some ontogogic work that Ralph came to see how his making himself into an impotent object and judging his own worth solely by achievements made him vulnerable without making possible the genuine engagement that could have eased his relation with his wife.

The notes on Ralph above are purposely oriented to bring out the two phases of his existential neurosis. The striking thing is the extent to which these phases are discriminable throughout a wide range of topics, concerns, and incidents. It should be made explicit also that during the first phase I heard frequently about Ralph's feelings of guilt, his fear of meaninglessness, and his sense of powerlessness, just as in the second phase we dealt with all aspects also. The distinguishing point is that there was a clustering around the matter of his loneliness, his estrangement from others, his fear of ultimate solitariness during the first period. It was reflected also in the tendency for such matters to be more centrally in phase with the dominant emotional theme (see Chapter 7) during this time. Later the same characterizations were true of the matter of powerlessness. During this second phase, the topic of Ralph's feeling of isolation did not disappear from our sessions, but it clearly was less frequently the emotional focus of his concern.

With the wisdom of hindsight I can see how these same polarizing influences are reflected in other aspects: his refusal to advance in his work is clearly an expression of his fear of further isolation and his underlying feelings of impotency. Similarly, isolated himself, he could not give his wife the genuine relationship she needed, and her leaving him served to confirm his anticipation of ultimate solitariness. As the focus of Ralph's concerns moved to his feelings of impotency, it was soon clear how much he felt himself the pawn of chance. Neither his attainments nor his failures seemed to him to be due to his own doings. Clearly Ralph felt the awful anxiety of being subject to fate without having any hope of changing things. He was adrift in a dangerous world without friends or refuge. His subjective experience of terror was at times nearly overwhelming.

A LOOK AT OURSELVES

I have indicated some of the gross aspects of my hypothesis about the existential neuroses. It awaits further development to warrant extensive amplification. Other therapists may find it commends itself to them sufficiently for them to want to make their own observations on these points. There are, in addition, several other aspects that may be pointed out.

Just as our patients tend to be preoccupied at various times with one or another of these areas of being, so we, as therapists, show similar centerings. Some therapists seem to be particularly astute at picking up the clues to the sense of estrangement from others, and they have found a variety of effective ways of educing this dread and of aiding the patient in working through it. Others are more sensitized to the feeling of powerlessness and show a similar kind of unconscious specialization. I think it likely also that certain of our methods are better equipped to deal with one or another of these, just as some of our theories certainly emphasize one or another. The methods of group therapy and sensitivity training are apt to be most influential in exposing and aiding the working through of the dread of estrangement and to a lesser extent the sense of blame. On the other hand it seems likely that Rogerian client-centered therapy is particularly suited to aid the patient who experiences oppressive feelings of powerlessness. Adlerian therapy, one might hypothesize, would be better adapted to deal with the dread of absurdity. These are, of course, speculative points that await more adequate research investigation. Clearly, we are implying an ideal for psychotherapy and human relations training: encouraging a working-through in each area for a genuine return to the underlying existential anxieties and then incorporation of these into authentic being in the world.

19 — *Ontogogy: in support of courage.* ▲— *Freeing from the Self and the response of faith*

As previous pages have repeatedly noted, much of our thinking in psychology has been dominated by either of two antihumanistic models of man: Clinical and personality psychology have continually employed the neurotic as the key point of reference; while experimental psychology has built its structures on the foundation of "the black box" or the white rat (in either instance a matter of treating the person as an object, not a subject). Inevitably such models do much to constrain our understanding of the full potential range of human experience. In writing within the humanistic perspective, I find, again and again, that I am still the prisoner of my own training and experience and have not freed myself as fully as I would like from these same models. However in this and the next chapter (as well as in Chapters 22 and 23), I am attempting to deal with the emergent or affirmative aspects of the human experience.

Central to the conception of ontogogy (which will be described in greater detail in subsequent paragraphs) is the conviction that the basic conditions of being human are, in themselves, neither fear-evoking nor health-inducing. They are simply the dimensions in which we have our being and within which we evolve our individual or communal ways of being in the world. Thus my intent is not to demonstrate how to make the best of the unfortunate facts that we are limited, must take action, are constantly exercising choice, and are apart from yet with others. Rather, I hope to illustrate how we may more fully capitalize upon the facts that we are able to be without having all knowledge or all power, that we may act, that choice is ours, and that we have relation with others while yet being individual.

Ontogogy

Ontogogy is a frame of reference for thinking about the "emergent end of the scale," the positive or healthy processes involved as one seeks to realize upon more of what is potential in his life (Kelman, 1953). Ontogogy is not a therapeutic procedure as such. We will offer procedural suggestions at some points, but these will most often be of the order, "This seems to be helpful to some of my patients and me when we're working in this area. You may find it useful or suggestive." Most explicitly, I do not know *the best* way to help people in this exciting but highly individual work of realizing their own being. I do find that with time, thought, and much experimentation I seem to be able to be of more help now than I was several years ago. Not the least of the influences which have contributed to that gain have been my continued efforts to free myself of my inauthenticities and to realize my own being more completely.

Any person who seeks greater authenticity for himself or who wants to help someone else toward it will gain much from the exercise of trying to think about life and human experience in nonoppositional and possibility-opening terms (Barrett, 1956, pp. 117 ff.). By nonoppositional, I mean freed of either–or, healthy–pathological, good–bad, authentic–inauthentic, resistance–growthful and similar dichotomies. To be sure, we have used these in these pages and will continue to do so. Nevertheless they are genuinely hobbling, causing our thinking to move haltingly and within a restricted sphere. To think in terms of choices among multiple courses, any of which may bring its own fulfillments and disappointments, no one of which is in itself right or better, but any of which may be a vehicle to one's own purpose and further choices, to try to think in such terms is a creative exercise. It can also be a sobering experience, illuminating just how constrained one's thinking really is.

THE ONTOGOGIC FRAME OF REFERENCE

This chapter and the next focus on the process to which we have given the name, "ontogogy," intending "a leading out into being." Ontogogy consists of those understandings and procedures by which a therapist (counselor, consultant) seeks to support the intent of a person (patient, client) to realize more fully the potentials of his being. Ontogogy supplements and overlaps with analytic psychotherapy, which is concerned with the dissolution of those processes the person employs to protect himself from seemingly intolerable anxiety but which maintain him in the non-being of inauthentic living. Ontogogy seeks to foster greater realization of being, where analytic therapy seeks to overcome constricted realization of being.

Ontogogy is a support to the patient's courage in meeting existential anxiety and the actualities of his life.

Figure II provides a schematic representation of the processes with which we are concerned here. In the figure the person's potential for being is represented as an arrow(*1*) tending toward actualization (*2*). However, the path to actualization is blocked because of the existential anxiety involved (*3*). The person tries to find ways (*4*) to gain actuality without enduring the anxiety, but this breeds neurotic anxiety (*5*). At this point the choice is made between the response of courage and the response of dread. In the response of courage (*6*) the person accepts and incorporates existential anxiety and thus is freed to actualize his being (*2*). In the response of dread (*7*) the person "escapes" into inauthenticity or non-being (*8*), which means loss of potential.

Analytic psychotherapy as I am conceiving it is directed toward reducing the resistances that grow out of the dread and thus reversing the response of dread (*7*). This is an essential task, but in my view it is not enough. It returns the person very often to a state of anxiety which is akin to that which first impelled him to flee into non-being. Ontogogy is directed toward helping the person recognize and accept the existential anxiety so that he can make the response of courage (*6*).

Some seem to argue that there does not need to be this two-stage process in therapy. They seem to say that one can go directly from the inauthentic, neurotic resolution (*8*) to the authentic (*2*).

FIGURE II *The Existential Confrontation*

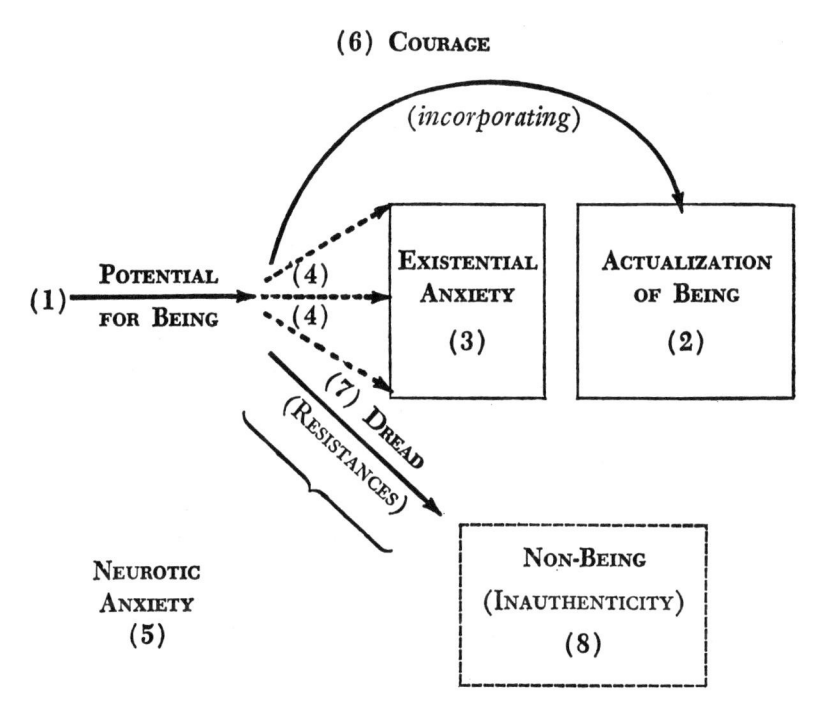

(6) COURAGE

(incorporating)

(1) → POTENTIAL FOR BEING — (4) → EXISTENTIAL ANXIETY (3) → ACTUALIZATION OF BEING (2)

(4) ...

(7) DREAD
(RESISTANCES)

NEUROTIC ANXIETY (5)

NON-BEING (INAUTHENTICITY) (8)

I do not believe this is so. I think the resolution of the inauthenticities and the resulting need to reconfront and incorporate existential anxiety are essential to genuine and lasting therapeutic results and personal realization.

PLAN OF PRESENTATION

In this chapter and the next I have the pleasant task of trying to set forth my first efforts to evolve consultative aids for the person who has attained a degree of authenticity through the resolution of his resistances and transferences and who wants to go further in the realization of his being. I will be reporting not upon a well worked out system of procedures for this purpose, but rather upon explorations and speculations from which a more refined conceptual system and procedure may eventually evolve. This is an area of genuine satisfaction and intellectual excitement, for it is one in which the unknown far outweighs the known, and it is an area of great promise for eventual contributions to human experience.

When we have gained a measure of authentic perspective on our being, we come to recognize that the *Self* may act as an encumbering monstrosity which we drag around with us but which limits our realization of true ontologic freedom. A primary undertaking of ontogogy is to reduce the bondage of the I-process to the *Me* or *Self*. This is the goal of emancipation as I described it in Chapter 15. In the following pages we will first study further this process of winning free from the *Self*.

The main body of these chapters will be devoted to studies of each of the areas of authenticity as these are derived from confrontations of the forms of existential anxiety. Picking up from the survey of the responses of dread in Chapters 17 and 18, I will elaborate on the nature of the existential needs for rootedness, identity, meaningfulness, and relatedness. The ontogogic work which aids the person seeking to make the response of courage is largely that of confronting the actuality of his being in the world. Once we have dealt with the process of confrontation, we will be ready to examine the authentic response that becomes possible when we express our courage. The authentic response is that way in which man participates in and is a part of all Being. Its characteristics are faith, commitment, creativity, and love. These are the attributes of transcendent being also. Table IV summarizes the work and hoped-for products of the response of courage.

Finally, I will offer some speculations and observations about the expressions of authentic being typically found in the person who is attaining to the actualization of his potential. These will be by way of supplementing the observations already reported in Chapter 16. For such expressions we will suggest the name "ontologic options" to convey that these are choices resident in our very being but which have no quality of mandatory "right" answers.

As I have so often, let me make explicit once again that this subdivision of the processes of authenticity into the four areas deriving from the four forms of existential anxiety (or from the four existential givens of awareness) is a heuristic convention. We need to be aware continually that this particular plan of subdividing what is essentially a unity is offered because it has proven helpful to therapeutic and ontogogic purposes and procedures, but it is not a

TABLE IV
Courage and Authentic Response

EXISTENTIAL GIVEN	Finiteness	Action potential	Choice		Separateness
CONFRONTATION	Contingency	Responsibility	Autonomy		Apartness
EXISTENTIAL ANXIETY	Fate and death	Guilt and condemnation	Emptiness and meaninglessness		Loneliness and isolation
COURAGE (EXISTENTIAL NEED)	Rootedness	Identity	Meaningfulness		Relatedness
AUTHENTIC RESPONSE	Faith	Commitment	Creativity		Love
ONTOLOGIC OPTIONS (EXAMPLES)	Limits and endings	Participation	Conflict		Devotion

statement that the ultimate nature of being is so subdivided. An important implication of this recognition is that we will expect and frequently find extensive overlapping and interweaving among the four areas.

Emancipation from the Self

Throughout this part of the book I have been developing recognition of the pervasiveness of the false equation of the *I-process* and the *Self* and of the ways in which that false equation encumbers our being. In describing the concept of *emancipation* in Chapter 15 I proposed that this key stage in the attainment of authenticity was that of dissolving this false equation.

Now we are ready to inquire into what may be the process by which this emancipation, this freeing from the *Self*, may be facilitated.

DEVELOPING COMMITMENT TO THE CONCEPT OF EMANCIPATION

The first part of the process by which the *I-process* may win free of the entangling *Self*[1] is concerned with the therapist's own acceptance of the concept and ideal of genuine emancipation. There are really two aspects of this matter. First, the therapist must arrive at some appreciation of what is intended by the notion of freeing one's being from the *Self*. Second, it must be seen that this is not simply a matter of the therapist having an abstract understanding of the philosophical construct. The therapist who would genuinely participate with his patient in the seeking for greater authenticity must do just that, participate with his patient. This means that the therapist will have gained some glimpse of the realm of greater authenticity and will himself be committed to the life pilgrimage toward that attainment. In so committing himself, he will have a more inclusive grasp of the meaning of emancipation, and this will guide his sensitivity and his skills.

Accordingly, I will enlarge on some of the meanings and significances of emancipation from the *Self*. To be candid, I think

---
[1] I am continuing to set the *I*, the *I-process*, the *Me*, and the *Self* in italics to try to aid the reader's discrimination of what is intended. Our language makes the communication task awkward because it is so replete with phrasings that falsely equate the subject and the object, the process and the substance.

that the truly emancipated person who lives in *I-process* terms is a very different sort of person than most of us, is somewhat difficult for us to communicate with and rather frightening to know. I do not know anyone who has achieved such full emancipation, but I do know people who have progressed toward it sufficiently for the extrapolation to seem warranted to me. Such emancipated people have a truer perception of the human circumstance, a deeper participation in life, and a greater realization of the human potential. The *Self*, I believe, has been a necessary aid to survival in a deficiency-oriented, human society, but I believe also that the day is dawning when we may be ready to let the importance of the *Self* drop away like an outworn suit of clothes while we emerge into a newer celebration of our being. Religion and philosophy have told us in various ways "You must lose your life in order to find it." The injunctions to "self-less-ness" are sometimes similarly recognitions, I think, of the point here being made (although, to be sure, they are often enough urgings to an inauthentic altruism). Those who have sought awareness of man's being in varied contexts seem often to have reached similar conclusions.

What would it mean to be freed of the *Self*? It would mean living fully in each moment, dwelling on the "razor's edge" of Now. This is such a basically unfamiliar concept that it is easily dismissed too lightly. Most of us, most of the time, act in the present moment with part of our awareness hostage to the future and part captive in the past. We worry about how we will look to ourselves and to others (the current cult of "the image"); we fear what will be revealed about our basic nature; we hope to win future advantage...

To be freed of the *Self* would be to meet our lives with "new innocence" (Maslow, 1962a), to choose in terms of the intrinsic properties of the alternatives, to enter into dialogue with another person without pretense and with genuine contact with him. It would mean a keener edge to experience, an intensified involvement, more acute feelings whether happy or sad (but not more mood extremes), more detachment from the trivial and popular, more risking in all of life.

DEVELOPING THE PATIENT'S AWARENESS OF EMANCIPATED BEING

The second step in the ontogogy of emancipation is to aid the patient in his awareness and appreciation of this way of being. This is most definitely not simply a matter of cognitive teaching. It is a process that begins early in the analytic phase as we demonstrate the resistances that ensnare the person's awareness and choice. While this work is progressing we begin to move toward more direct attention to the manner in which the subject–object split within the person tends to perpetuate the bondage of the *I*. Then we come to a phase in which we question more explicitly the use of the *Self* as a criterion for life decisions. Finally we may arrive at a stage in which some explicit discussion of the concept of emancipation is appropriate.

Much of our traditional psychotherapeutic attitude has been directed toward helping the person achieve greater self-consistency. We call to his attention conflicts and discrepancies in his self-percepts, we highlight ways in which he has served contrasting values, and in general convey implicitly, if not explicitly, the message that one should be more unitary, consistent, and dependable if he is to be healthy emotionally. The concept of emancipation here advanced would raise serious question as to the appropriateness of this valuing of consistency. This question is particularly pertinent when we assume an adequate analytic job has been done in the first phase of therapy, so that the person is relatively free of the distortions of the resistances and transferences.

Indeed, the contention may be advanced that consistency, when valued in itself, is a resistance to authentic being. This is not merely a matter of the person's environment being inconsistent although that is so, but that observation deals only with the reactive aspects of the matter. More importantly, *Self*-consistency ultimately intends a static and object-like conception of the human experience. Authentic being means meeting each situation with fresh awareness (which certainly includes awareness of similar past experiences) and with fresh ability to choose in terms of the intrinsic qualities of the alternatives in the situation and the creativity of the *I-process*.

> Ned, who had made good progress in his analytic work, took a two months' business assignment away from his home. In the distant city where he was working he was quite lonely until he made the acquaintance of an attractive secretary in one of the offices. She invited him to spend several week-ends with her, and Ned was greatly tempted. He refused, explain-

ing to me, "I really would have enjoyed staying with her, and she wouldn't have made any trouble, but I just never have felt comfortable doing that sort of thing." I silently noted a certain smug satisfaction in Ned's account and particularly in his assuring me of his consistency in resisting such temptations.

Then I raised a question regarding this basis for Ned's decision, "You have never done that sort of thing in the past, you say. What's that got to do with now?"

Now the point in the example is not that the therapist is concerned to teach Ned to be unfaithful or even more liberal in his sexual behavior. Rather, the point is to deal with Ned's use of his *Self*, of the past, as a basis for determining a here-and-now decision rather than authentically meeting the situation in the present.[2]

Bert had gradually worked through many of the roots of his obsessive fears that he might be homosexual. The resistance aspects had been disclosed and resolved in several important ways. Still from time to time such thoughts would recur. One day he told me, "As we came out of the restaurant, Bob and I were laughing together, and I really felt close to him in a way I never used to be able to feel. It was a good feeling, and then I had to go and ruin it with this old homosexual thing. It was like I heard someone saying, 'Look at the way you put your arm around Bob. See! You're really a queer underneath.' It makes me mad to keep going back to that."

I spoke almost sharply, "Well, if you're not a queer underneath, what are you *underneath*?" I emphasized the word "underneath" especially.

"Well, I don't know. Heterosexual, I guess."

"What makes you think that?"

"Well, I've never done anything homosexual since I've been an adult. Say, what are you driving at, anyway? You know all this!"

---

[2] It will be evident that this is the sort of challenge that can easily be misunderstood as an encouragement to promiscuity. Many laymen and not a few professionals look to psychotherapy as a license to impulse gratification in a way that is equally inauthentic. In working with Ned in this example I needed to be alert to the possibility that such an interpretation of my intervention would maintain the inauthenticity of not dealing with the givenness of the situation but again seeking an outside (extrinsic) criterion for choice.

"I want to know what you mean by 'underneath.' What would it mean to be or not to be a 'queer' or anything else 'underneath'?"

"Why, sort of basically or ... or ..."

"In your genes?"

"Uh, no, I don't think so. You know, I don't really know. Aren't some people basically homosexual and some heterosexual?"

"Perhaps a very, very few have constitutional and physical conditions that might make their sex inclinations confused. But they're usually easily recognized by the physical abnormalities. You have any physical abnormalities?"

"No, of course not. Well, now I don't know what I mean."

"I think you meant in part, 'Maybe I don't have to take responsibility for all my choices. Maybe some mysterious thing basically in me makes some of the choices.'"

"Yeah, I suppose so. It seems like I've used that fear at times to keep myself busy, if you know what I mean."

"What do you mean?"

"Well, I mean like when I left Bob at the restaurant, I was kind of sad for all the times I've been afraid to let go and have fun when I was out in any public place. Then all of a sudden this thought about being a homosexual came in, and I got kind of mad about that and forgot about the sadness."

"So you lost the chance to just be there feeling your feelings in the situation because of this idea you were something or other underneath or basically."

"That's right. Damn it, there's the same old pattern again."

Now it needs to be made explicit that in the work with Ned and with Bert I had to choose whether to focus on the more directly resistive aspects of their associations or on the opportunities to begin loosening the identification with the *Self*. These two examples are cited because they illustrate the latter choice. Earlier in the work with both men, I would have chosen to focus more on the resistance. It will also be useful to note that no attempt is made to teach the basic point about the *Self* in full at any one time. Rather, through repeated, but distributed, pointing out of the effects of the concern with *Self* the therapist helps the patient to loosen the bond and begin to meet his life more authentically on an *I-process* basis.

SUMMARY

The foregoing suggestions are by no means enough to produce or even to help another person achieve emancipation from the false equation of the *I* and the *Self*. Hopefully, they can help in preparing the way for such a freeing. My own experience in working toward such a goal for myself and in aiding those of my patients who move in that direction is far too limited for me to try to be more inclusive or definitive at this point. Certainly, all else I will say about ontogogic aids will also contribute toward emancipation.

Contingency and Faith

The sense of being subject to fate and under threat of death may make one feel like a condemned felon hopelessly awaiting his execution or may be the stuff of which one makes his identification with all life and all being. In an ultimate sense no metaphor is involved in this statement. We are here dealing with the very issues from which emerge the despised assassin and the martyred saint.[3]

THE EXISTENTIAL NEED FOR ROOTEDNESS

From the fact of our finiteness comes the awareness of being subject to contingency. Our very lives are always in jeopardy, and dimly at least we are always aware of this. Cut off from the world in the subject-object split, we feel alone and terrified. Only as we rediscover our being in the whole of being, our essential oneness with all of life, do we achieve the roots that permit us to face contingency with open awareness. This is an important point that will warrant repetition in another phrasing to make evident the significance to the work of ontogogy: Contingency is so overwhelming in its immensity and its personal significance to each of us that we cannot

---

[3] The implicit allusion to recent history is intentional. John Kennedy seemed to demonstrate his deep sense of having roots in the human situation. The world-wide reaction to his death portrayed how much he was so perceived by people of all walks of life and of all cultural and national backgrounds. Lee Oswald could serve almost as a prototype of the man without roots and without faith. His childhood family life was unsteady, his associations were transitory, and his one focus of trying to find his own ground (Marxism) proved an illusion and eventually rejected him.

sustain open awareness of it by ourselves. When we meet the existential anxiety of fate and death with dread we experience the overwhelming powerlessness that has been described in Chapter 18. When we discover our rootedness in all being—and are thus no longer alone—we are able to open our awareness to our finiteness.

COURAGE: ROOTEDNESS

On the other hand, the response that accepts the anxiety of fate and death recognizes the need that each of us has for rootedness. The awareness of contingency cuts man loose from his feeling of oneness with the eternal qualities of existence and gives rise to his need for a feeling of being grounded in existence in a sustaining fashion. Rootedness then becomes the means whereby man replaces his biological, pre-awareness ties with his human connectedness to all life. "Living is a process of continuous birth" (Fromm, 1959, p. 156). But this birth is not into disconnectedness but into a more aware tie. "From being passively rooted in nature and in the womb, man becomes one again—but this time actively and creatively with all life" (p. 157). Rootedness is a somewhat difficult concept to grasp at times because we are apt to think in overly concrete terms. As with all of the needs, it is interrelated with each of the others and stands most clearly in complementary relationship to the need for relatedness, which arises from man's experience of apartness. The person who has achieved rootedness shows in his being an awareness of his kinship to all experience, to all life, to all men. The parallel state of relatedness has more to do with particular relationships among men.

THE RESPONSE OF FAITH

Poised in the apparent chaos of raw contingency, finding no solid footing on any side, discovering all "realities" to be only probabilities, if I am aware and am aware only of contingency, then—quite literally—I will die or go mad. It does not seem likely that such a confrontation is endurable. The analogy is compelling to what we are told would be the fate of a human body exposed to interstellar space: it would explode from the inner pressures uncontained by balancing outer pressures.

But, I have said, the anxiety attendant upon contingency, the existential anxiety of fate and death, may be incorporated and a rootedness achieved that makes for greater authenticity in being. How is this possible? The answer is what I have chosen to term "the response of faith." Let me try to make clear what is intended.

Life presents us with the challenges of the existential givens. From these flow the subjective experiences and the existential anxieties that are the focus of our concern as therapists. We are initially drawn into the problem in our roles as therapists because our patients reacted or responded with dread and so became lost in inauthentic ways of living, which compounded their anxiety and reduced their actuality. There are those, however, who have not responded to life with dread, and all of us show a measure of courage in our responses. What form does this response take? In the case of the anxiety of fate and death with the attendant experience of contingency, the response of faith is that which is authentic.

Faith, as I use it here, is intrinsic faith. It is objectless faith. It is the *I* affirming its own being. It is a confronting of the infinitude of contingency with the declaration, "I am I. This is my starting place. This is my certainty, though there be no other."

This language is necessarily dramatic, but it is not metaphoric. The drama is the very drama of the human condition. It is the Promethean struggle that must be played out anew by each person who seeks to find his own being. The response of faith is man-the-creature daring to become man-the-creator, and to create his own being.

> Dora had been frightened most of her life. Her mother was a bitter, disappointed woman, who was probably nearly or actually psychotic during most of Dora's childhood. Her father was a weak, ineffectual, semiskilled worker who had once dreamed of a scholarly career but had missed out on one opportunity after another. He was completely passive with his wife. Dora was victimized in one way or another by each parent. Her mother was capable of literal cruelty at times. Her father offered Dora a furtive love which he quickly withdrew whenever conflict with the mother threatened.
>
> In therapy, Dora was docile, earnest, and unable to tolerate much psychic pain. Basically she felt futile and impotent. Her life had never shown her much to hope for, and the few hopes she had risked had often been dashed by circumstances. Certainly I, her therapist, frequently found myself wearily ready to end what seemed a meagerly promising venture. Then

Dora's shaky marriage collapsed completely as her husband wandered off.

For three sessions Dora explored the very depths of hell. Therapy had been effective enough that many of her illusions (resistances) about herself and her life no longer provided even temporary cushioning from the harsh realities she confronted. She was well into middle age, not very attractive, not well educated or trained for any truly stimulating work. For three sessions Dora considered suicide and psychosis much as one might try to choose which apartment to take. There was no dissembling in this selecting. Then she told me, "I'm so very sorry I'll never have children. I always wanted to be a mother. (She cried quietly now for several minutes.) And I'm sorry Eddie and I couldn't make a go of it. At least I'd like to have been with somebody. (Again the silent weeping.) But that's the way it is. Now, I'm going to find out what I can do."

And with that Dora began coming out of hell and out of the regrets. She entered training to become a medical technician, and some time later left therapy far from a completely actualized person but with a new dignity which she still has whenever I see her—as I do when she visits me once or twice a year.

No words can convey the feeling I experienced as Dora rounded some deep corner in her life and began to affirm herself in the face of the contingency that had dealt with her so terribly. She knew she was making a new gamble and could well lose again. She knew, much better than most of us, how all one's efforts could be overturned. But she found within her the courage to make the response of faith.

Ontologic Options Relating to Limits and Endings

> Must every love relation be for all time? When will you be ready to die? How much security in terms of material things do you really want? If you are a parent, at what age would you like to relinquish your close tie to your child?

These and similar questions may evoke one's feelings about limits and endings, an area in which our being provides us with great choice but which often we treat as though it was beyond our influence. At least in our culture, we tend to make many limits and endings impositions upon us from the outside.

Ontologic Options. I will propose here that we think of the various possibilities which are available as options we may or may not choose to exercise. Since we are examining such possibilities in the light of what is existentially given, we may term them "ontologic options."

Imagine a culture in which it was generally accepted that the appropriate way for one's life to end was by choice. When one felt that he might be ready for death, he would make an appointment with a counselor who would help him review the situation in broad perspective. If, after such a review, the person felt that he was indeed ready to die, the counselor would aid him in making appropriate arrangements to take care of any dependents, disposing of other responsibilities, and selecting and carrying through a method of dying which preserved dignity and reduced unhappiness or suffering for all concerned.

In such a culture, the average person would feel quite different about death, I would think, than does the average person in our culture. Since usually the coming of death would be known and planned for, the sense of helplessness before fate might be appreciably less. I would hazard that there would be a much better safety record with a most noticeable contrast in the frequency of automobile accidents. Exhibitionistic and vengeful suicides, elaborate and vulgar funerals, and ritualistic but meaningless mourning customs would be practically unknown.

It is hard for us, in our culture, to conceive of death as anything but an imposition and an unhappy event. We regard the Japanese tradition of hara-kiri as bizarre and the Scandinavian higher suicide rate as evidence of some strange moral degeneracy. We sugarcoat all limits and endings and especially death, dreading even to say the word and preferring euphemisms such as "passed away," "crossed over," "gone to sleep." Euthanasia is strictly punished, and medical science exerts itself to perform obscene miracles of prolonging vegetative, suffering life in burned out shells of what were once people. I think each of us has the right to choose to live or to die. It is a great presumption to feel that this ultimate right can be removed by law or public opinion.

Those who have a metaphysical conviction that the afterlife is very similar to that we know now are no exception to this generalization. They, in effect, negate the fact of death and thus demonstrate the terrible negative regard with which they hold it.

It is sometimes argued that this is a built-in, instinctual response, that "self-preservation is the first law of nature." This is manifestly not so. If there were such a first law, we would behave quite differently than we do. The present international situation, the prevalence of cigarette smoking, the speed of our motor cars—these are but a few of the many indications that the so-called "first law" is more honored in the breach than in practice. Indeed, those of us who work intensively with our patients come to know that there are many clues to what Freud called a "death instinct."[4]

Life is, period. It is not a matter of instinct; it is a matter of fact. Death is, just is, period. Again, not a matter of instinct, but of fact. We have no phenomenological evidence on what death means, only external observation. All our evidence is inferential. I am aware that a number of people are beginning to find respect for a new concept of immortality, but that is beside the issue here.[5] Ontologically and phenomenologically we can say little or nothing about the death of one's own being but much about the anticipation of that death.

There are other options of limits and endings. A familiar form occurs when patients know that they are drawing toward the close of therapy and we see a resurgence of symptoms. When the patient with whom I have been working intensively shows this, I treat those symptoms seriously because it shows he has not dealt with the ontologic options regarding limits and endings, and this suggests that there is still authenticity training which he needs. Of course I am not able to work this intensively with a number of patients for reasons of limitations in their readiness for it or in my ability to help them in such a thoroughgoing undertaking. In those instances a resurgence of symptoms at termination is a subject for interpretation and moderate reassurance, and very often can be handled within the space of several interviews at the most.

I find it useful to think about the process of living as that of a creative, artistic enterprise, not unlike the painting of a picture. If

---

[4] I don't think the death instinct a useful concept. It seems to me simply an attempt to plug a gap in psychoanalytic theory that was occasioned by the postulation of the "life instinct" in the first place. Instincts as built-in mechanisms seem to me to do much violence to the dignity of the human being and to the observed facts of human experience.

[5] I refer particularly to the intriguing ideas of Aldous Huxley (1954a, b) in this regard, and to Ducasse (1961).

we use this analogy in the present instance, we will see readily that the artist who hesitated to put an end to his picture, who created a masterpiece but then added canvas to canvas again and again and kept painting, would in time destroy his picture. Saying it differently, a part of artistry is knowing when to stop. Part of artistry is knowing what to include and what not to include. Part of artistry is knowing where the frame goes around the picture, where the edge of the canvas is. Those who engage in photography will know how important it is in composing adequate pictures to frame them properly, to know the limits, to set the limits by choice and not by chance. So it is with life; there are many opportunities for limits that can give artistry, grace, dignity, meaning to our living. If we are authentically in our lives, we use the opportunity to set limits esthetically and vitally. Of course many of us—and I certainly include myself among these—are not so creative. We are fearful of limits because we feel if we do not take all we can now, we may never get any more. In this fashion we can spoil so much that could be rich in our lives. The most exquisitely prepared meal can be ruined if we insist on gorging ourselves. The finest wine is enjoyed best when we limit our intake of it.

20 — Ontogogy: in support of courage   B — The responses of commitment, creativity, and love

As a person frees himself of the crippling effects of his resistances to authentic being and begins to reduce his wasteful efforts to construct and maintain a *Self*, he is readying for a more creative adventure in living. This adventure is that awaiting the person who goes to meet the givens of being in an affirmative way, and it is in contrast to flight from those givens into the existential neuroses. In the previous chapter we inquired into the courageous response to confronting contingency. Now we are ready to examine the responses of courage to confronting responsibility, autonomy, and apartness.

Responsibility and Commitment

The exercise of my potential to take action affects what will be present in the stream of my awareness. What is in the stream of my awareness makes an emotional difference to me. The experiencing of this emotional difference we call responsibility. Responsibility is the subjective correlate of the existential given of the ability to take action. Thus it leads to the existential anxiety of guilt and condemnation. I am not indifferent but concerned about my actions and their consequences. I recognize that my doing and not doing are importantly involved and that I must take the responsibility for such doing and not doing. Guilt and condemnation certainly evoke anxiety, but they are the expressions too of the fact that I live my life rather than being lived by it. In my acceptance of the anxiety of guilt and condemnation I affirm my identity.

THE EXISTENTIAL NEED FOR IDENTITY

In Fromm's view, "this need for a sense of identity is so vital and imperative that man could not remain sane if he did not find some way of satisfying it" (1959, p. 157). The sense of identity is the sense of "being there" in one's own life. It is the direct intuition of one's own presence in the be-ing. It is to be contrasted with the inference of one's presence that comes from *Self*-observation. Identity is not derived from seeing my body or from remembering what I have done or said or felt. To be sure, a great many people are ensnarled in this inverted and retrospective sort of identity substitute. This is, of course, the basis of the confusion of the *Self* and the *I*. When we fear to accept the burden of responsibility and guilt, we may try to abdicate the identity of being subject in our lives. Then we live the distortion of being objects, and the dread and neurotic anxiety of blame color our experience.

This point is so important that I want to restate it in other words in the hope of communicating it more fully. Rollo May makes the first of his six ontological principles (1959b, p. 5), "every living being is centered in itself, and an attack on this center is an attack on the life itself." Identity is, I believe, the form of such ontologic centeredness in which the person is directly aware of his own being and expresses that awareness through what I have called the *I-process*. Such identity is not the thinking or feeling or the talking or doing substantively but the *I* who is thinking, feeling, talking, and doing.

When the person finds his concern about guilt and responsibility for his actions (broadly conceived) mounting too high, then he may seek to preserve his center through the adoption of that distorted form of identity which is focused on the *Me* or *Self*. It is as though the person says, "I cannot stand the anxiety of being responsible for what happens in my life, so I will concentrate only on what happens to me, what life does to me."

COURAGE: IDENTITY

A unique achievement of the human experience is the creation of a personal identity (Erikson, 1959). To know that I am and that I am uniquely I is a psychological phenomenon of crucial importance in each person's experience. It is frequently pointed out that the human animal is the only one that seems to have an awareness of his own being, and this may well be so. However, what we here designate as the experience of identity is something further than the accumulated and even the systematized perceptions of one's *Self* which constitute that *Self* as described in Chapter 11. Here we are referring to the directly intuited *I-process*. Identity is not demonstrable objectively but is experienced in the very process of being. Identity is not definable substantively but is expressed through our awareness and choices.

Man can be defined as the animal that can say "I," that can be aware of himself as a separate entity. . . . Because he is not lived, but lives, because he has lost the original unity with nature, has to make decisions, is aware of himself and of his neighbor as different persons, he must be able to sense himself as the subject of his actions. . . . The infant, still feeling one with mother, cannot yet say "I," nor has he any need for it. Only after he has conceived of the outer world as being separate and different from himself does he come to awareness of himself as a distinct being, and one of the last words he learns to use is "I," in reference to himself (Fromm, 1959, p. 157).

. . . . .

Elaine hadn't believed that any man would really want to marry her. All through high school she had no dates. She was fatter than usual and had been given very little help in learning to dress and make up attractively. These certainly limited her appeal for the boys. But probably most limiting was her negative attitude about herself, which came out as a constant demand for reassurance. It was as though Elaine had only one way of trying to win approval or affection: to so belittle herself that the other person felt called upon to "make up the difference."

In her church group Elaine met a rather timid young man, and they began to date occasionally the second year after Elaine graduated from high school. Eventually he proposed, and Elaine accepted, although without the joy one might have expected. Joy would have been too dangerous. As she told me later, Elaine felt that "He couldn't be very good if he wanted me. So I knew I had to take him because I wouldn't have any other chances. So why be excited about that? Besides, if I got my hopes up, it would have only hurt more when the whole thing collapsed." And collapse it did. Shortly after the first child was born, Elaine's husband arranged a small settlement, encouraged her to get a divorce, and moved to another part of the country.

Elaine came to me about a year later. She was negative, mocking, bitter, and filled with self-hatred. In a way she entered therapy to prove that it too would disappoint her. She was very much on the go at first in social clubs and religious groups, but as these failed to yield a dependable new man, Elaine became a frequent visitor to bars, and by the time we had been working six months she was a rather heavy drinker and promiscuous sexually. In a largely unconscious way, she was bitterly proud of her degradation. She was saying to her ex-husband (although he was not around) and to the world, "See how I've been mistreated. See how badly I've been hurt, how low I've sunk."

Elaine, like so many of us, had given up being the subject of her life to escape guilt and responsibility. As the object, she could insist on how poorly she was treated and call on others to treat her better. Hidden from her conscious awareness was her responsibility for doing better for herself. What Elaine dared not see was that she was adding to her guilt and responsibility by her flight from them. Her drinking and sexual adventures were enactments of her guilt, were enactments of being done to, were relatively joyless and usually sources of bitter rather than happy memories. Joy is really only possible for the person who is the subject in his own life, for joy is a quality of awareness in being, is a here-and-now experience. When a person is, like Elaine, entrapped in being only the object in her life, then awareness looks always backward at what has happened, and thus it is always too late for joy.

THE RESPONSE OF COMMITMENT

Elaine illustrates the dread-inspired flight from responsibility that the analytic work seeks to arrest and turn back. However, it is essential to full emergence into authentic being that the person go beyond the denial implicit in such a flight and affirmatively take a stand for that which he is. So many of our patients find it difficult or threatening to say what they did out of their own choices, to state their allegiances. They are much more voluble about what they deny, what they fear, what they hate.

Commitment is, in paraphrase, the statement, "This I am; this I believe; this I do. I am the being, the believing, the doing." Commitment is not the place in which one stands, the tenet one believes, or the act one does, however. Commitment is not a subscription to something external to the person's own life, no matter how worthwhile. Commitment, as we are using the term here, is not to world peace, nor to the prevention of juvenile delinquency, nor to mental health, nor even to one's own future as such. Commitment is an awareness, an attitude, a clear and feelingful recognition of being fully present in the moment, making the choices of the moment, and standing by the consequences of those choices whether anticipated or not. Commitment is "playing for keeps" rather than vainly pleading for "slips (to) go over," as do small children in their games of marbles.

When a person is attaining to the response of commitment, genuine knowledge of what he is doing will reveal in many instances that he is concurrently taking part in some of the more familiar foci of concern. For one person this may be a social action group, for another an artistic endeavor, for still a third reading and thinking in an area of intellectual-personal interest. The form is not the significant thing. The point is that this *participation* is a consequence of genuine committedness in living rather than a cause or evidence of it. We will discuss this matter further later in this section.

DISPLAYING THE PATIENT'S RESPONSIBILITY

Authentic commitment is possible to the person who genuinely accepts responsibility in his life. Before most of our patients can achieve such commitment they must deal with several obstacles. First, for many, is the resistance to acknowledging guilt in any way. Our customary analytic techniques usually are adequate to help the patient past this block. Next is the general confusion of guilt and blame. This has much social reinforcement and may not always be sufficiently dealt with by analytic method, and so may require re-educative attempts also. I have already discussed the confusion of guilt and blame in another context (pages 82, 118) and will not review that matter here. It is important to recognize how blame may sometimes be used as a resistance to genuine acceptance of responsibility. This is illustrated in the case of Harry, where I can also demonstrate how the re-education is carried on.

Harry was very guilty and ashamed this Tuesday morning, as he was from time to time after he'd had a drinking bout over the weekend. "So, I did it again! Tied one on, swung my weight around the house, had Leah and the kids terrified. Oh, I'm the big man all right. Just let me get a snoot full and . . ."

I interrupted him, "You really sound pretty enthusiastic when you get going on cussing yourself out."

"Well, hell, I'm just no damned good. I'm to blame for every lousy thing that's wrong with my family. Why Leah puts up with an eight ball like me is . . ."

"You're just no good, huh?"

"That's right. I never was any count. My father told me I made mother sick with worry. If I was any good, I'd . . . I'd . . ."

"Well, there's really nothing to feel badly about, is there?"

"What do you mean?"

"Well, you're no good and you never have been any good. So plainly it's not your responsibility. Somebody else messed you up: God or your parents, but you don't have to carry the load."

"What? I'm taking the blame, aren't I? What do you want?"

"Sure, you're taking the blame and dodging the responsibility."

"It's the same thing."

"Is it? I don't think so. I've heard you take the blame a dozen times, and all I can see that it does is pay a little emotional bill for your drunk. Then the next time you can't deal with things you can get drunk again and pay the bill with blaming yourself and do it all over. You've never taken responsibility for yourself, only blame."

"Well, what's the difference?"

"Just this: If you took responsibility for the feeling you had before you started to drink, if you took responsibility for starting to drink, if you took responsibility for the way you treat Leah and the kids when you're loaded—instead of blaming it on the alcohol . . . If you took it on yourself to know what you were doing at each of those points, what do you think would happen?"

"I wouldn't do it. But, hell, I don't think about it that way. I just get kind of wound up, and I figure a drink would relax me and then before I know it..."

"That's the point: 'Before you know it...' You're not taking responsibility. All you do is sing the 'Ain't I bad!' song so you can do it all over again."

"Yeah, I suppose so. Maybe I do..."

Harry did not get a sweeping insight this time, but we did get two points of importance before his awareness so that we could refer to them again and again in the future: (a) he used blame to avoid responsibility; (b) if he accepted responsibility, he would find that he was fully aware of what he was doing and probably could not slide through the dismal sequence again. In dealing with these recognitions, Harry came to make his first really sincere efforts to inquire into the sources of his needs to get drunk periodically.

It will be evident that what is accomplished here is the separation of the healthy, observing ego from the ego-alien behavior. This is the usual psychoanalytic explanation of this process, and it has much to commend it. In our orientation, however, this description in terms of subdivision of the person has serious defects. Instead, we are concerned—as illustrated in the protocol—to move the patient toward re-experiencing his wholeness, his responsibility in and for his own actions.

The Ontologic Options of Participation

Participation, as I am here using the term, refers to the freely chosen expression of one's being in action. It is set in contrast with the compulsive acting of the neurotic who does not choose but is chosen by his fears and the distortions of his resistances. It is set in contrast, further, to activism (which is also a resistance to authentic being) in which value is given to acting as an end in itself. Activism draws a fallacious inference from the fact that being is a process and reifies the process into a substitute for being. Ultimately, psychologically, activism is a flight from, rather than an expression of, responsible being.

Freed from bondage to the past through the *Self*, aware of the givens of being, the person takes responsibility for his life and expresses it through participation. Such participation is a total involvement of the person.

Sarah had had a hard life. She knew it. She told people about it without much hesitation. She told me about it in detail. And it was very true, she had had a hard life. Rescued from Middle Europe by relatives during the dark days of the Nazi violations, she came to this country as a frightened little girl who was shunted from one family of cousins to another. She was always the outsider, even after she learned English, even after she finally found a measure of stability with a vaguely related "uncle and aunt" and a grandfather who was the only person from the old life who had also made it to this country. Of her parents and brothers and sisters she never heard conclusively, but it was almost certain that they died in the pogroms. So, obviously, Sarah should be eternally grateful for her rescue, should never have any reason to complain about whatever life offered.

When Sarah came to me, she was a perennially sad, long-suffering, martyr-in-the-making. She told of her hard life and looked for the crumbs of condolences she was used to winning with the recital. She was terribly guilty for being alive when her real family was surely dead. She was terribly guilty for not having been more appreciative to those who had rescued and sheltered her. She was terribly guilty because all she could give anyone else was her sad story, her hard life.

Sarah worked as library catalog clerk. She was by far the most efficient of the four girls in the office. She was continually at war with one or another of them. Her life consisted of her work, her night school, and occasional dates. She was strongly attached to a male librarian in another office and soon was involved in a furtive, joyless affair with him. The relationship sometimes seemed to move toward marriage and then would be broken off with bitterness and recriminations on both sides. Then it would be resumed, to run the same course again.

The analytic work was extended and involved many frustrations. At length, however, Sarah began to see how she kept herself exiled by her frightened need to be excused from life's demands because of her very genuine suffering. As she worked through this again and again, she began to make certain changes in her way of living. These came about without much direct attention in the therapeutic hours but clearly as expressions of her greater presence in her current life (as contrasted with her former preoccupation with the past). First the frustrating, futile affair was ended once and for all. For a period, Sarah had several brief relationships with different men, sometimes involving sexual relations, sometimes not. Then Sarah began a more lasting relation with a man whom she eventually married. Although this was far from an ideal romance, it did give both of them important emotional satisfactions.

For our present concerns, however, the interesting change that came about had to do with Sarah's changed way of living. Throughout most of her therapy she had been taking courses in night school, endlessly pursuing a vague image of materially changing her career. Now she decided to devote time to an agency working with blind children. There she started doing the same relatively routine work that she did in her daytime job, but soon she had won a place for herself working with the children themselves. This she found tremendously gratifying. With these children, Sarah could for the first time really forget that she had had a hard life. She didn't have to draw any comparisons to do so. She simply was too busy being with them and taking part in their (and, of course, her own) growth.

Sarah's story is not the story of an impressive therapeutic change. In times of stress, she will always tend to fall back on her "hard life," as she has done from time to time when she comes back to see me during periods of upset. But Sarah is no longer the prisoner of that hard life. She has other avenues through which to express herself. She is depressed for a period and then, almost without realizing it, finds herself caught up in her home or her work with the blind children, and her mood changes. She shows her increased authenticity of being through this increased range of choice, through her willingness to continue in her commitment to her marriage even though they have had some bitter conflicts, and through her participation in the meaningful work with the children.

Participation in the instance of Sarah is evident in several ways. It includes her work with the blind children, but her participation is not the work with the blind children itself. Participation, as I am here employing the term, is a characteristic of the way Sarah lives her life, not of what she does as such. Sarah is in her life. Sarah is doing things because she is in her life, not in order to have her life. If, for example, early in her work with me, I had suggested to Sarah that she volunteer time at the agency that works with blind children she probably would have done so. She might well have been faithful and dogged in helping out. (I doubt she would have been given any work with the children themselves.) This would not have been participation.

Participation is an expression of the authentic person's commitment to his own being in the world. Participation is an expression of the authentic person's identity.

Autonomy and Creativity

Throughout his history—and doubtless before the dawn of history —man has sought meanings in his world. Socrates asked, "What is justice?" Jesus taught, "Love one another." Hitler roared, "The state above all." Many values have been proposed. To some we give willing acceptance; from some we draw away. No value can be demonstrated as ultimately true for all men in all places at all times. World does not reply to our questions. We must create our own answers. And the answers we create will be of ourselves and thus limited within the unlimitedness of world (Rogers, 1960).[1]

THE EXISTENTIAL NEED FOR MEANINGFULNESS

For the person who has not worked through his resistive centering outside of himself to confront suddenly the full silence of the world as meaningless would be for that person to be thrust into total insanity. Since most of us are raised to center outside of ourselves in some measure, I strongly suspect that most of us are in some part psychotic. I mean no play on words. I am convinced that we would have a very different human experience and that our culture would be very different were we able to meet the silence of world from our earliest days without the many myths that we use to veil that awful reality. By myths I refer to the dogmas of philos-

---
[1] The reader will recognize that I have not hesitated to propose what I have termed "existential values." I find these—rootedness, identity, creativity, relatedness—very meaningful ways of ordering my experience of my own being in the world. These values seem to me to be the best ways I can find of describing what being alive means to me—for me personally and for those who are in my personal experience of world. Yet I need to retain awareness that these are my descriptions, not uninfluenced by the nature of world, but not, clearly, discoveries about world without regard to the fact that I am the observer.

ophy and religion, to be sure, but I refer also to the other sources of dogma that fill our ears: from education, commerce, government, family, and friends. "A penny saved is a penny earned," "Cleanliness is next to godliness," "Genius is 98 percent perspiration and 2 percent inspiration," "Use our soap to get ahead in the business world," "A Scout is trustworthy, loyal . . ." "The family that prays together stays together," "Has bad breath chased love away from you?" and so on and on.

Let me be clear. Many of these admonitions point to useful values, for particular people at particular points in their lives. The virtues extolled are often worthy of recognition by certain people at certain junctures. What I am indicting is the *absolute* quality, the canonization of a value above the lives in which it is involved. Fiction has portrayed this point so well in some cases (how often does literature speak a deeper truth than any other human expression!). The terrible decimation of the native populations of Polynesia by the forces of "progress" and "religion" are not matters of fiction, however. Nor are the ghastly toll of Naziism, the vicious Crusades, the horrors of the Inquisition. The point need not be labored. Virtue exalted above human lives usually ends up destroying both the lives and the virtue itself.

COURAGE: MEANINGFULNESS

"Man can create life. . . . He alone is aware of being created and of being a creator" (Fromm, 1959, p. 153). The experience of being created, being a creature, by itself would lead to the anxiety of absurdity and meaninglessness were it not that the experience of choice opens the possibility of transcending this creaturely status. As man exercises choice he takes part in creation and overcomes his object status to become subject in his world of experience. As subject and creator man creates meaningfulness. This is a supreme achievement of man's choices: the creation of meaning where there was the threat of emptiness and the potential of absurdity.

Yet often we protest this very birthright. When a child dies in a meaningless accident, we berate God or fate. We say, "Why did it have to happen?" Whether there is a "loving God" I do not know. I do know that this accident says nothing about the matter. If a creator had made us so that nothing bad or tragic could happen, we would be but his dolls. If all contingencies were benignly prearranged, we would be solely creatures, objects, things. Again, it is the Prometheus story: we have aspired to the fire of the Gods, we pay for our freedom with our very guts. Choice is not a meaningless formality; it is our announcement of our freedom.

CONFRONTING THE PATIENT WITH CHOICE

We seem to have the popular illusion that one can withhold choice. The patient many times will profit from learning that not-to-choose is a choice just as much as is choosing. Many patients seem dimly to sense this, and the frequent fear of driving on freeways and throughways possibly has some relation to this sense of being hurried along without the possibility of stopping, and with a constant need to make choices, often without feeling ready to do so.

The patient's associations will repeatedly explicitly or implicitly depict the choices with which he is faced; indeed, one could almost focus exclusively on choices and find them occurring in great number in nearly everything the patient talks about. And just as this is so, it is equally so that a great many patients have developed ways of denying that they do have choice. They hurry along without genuinely looking at the decisions implicitly made.

> Thelma's daughter wants to date a boy of whom Thelma does not approve. The daughter, 17, insists that she can handle her own affairs and that Thelma is babying her. Thelma wants to avoid being overprotective and wants to keep her daughter's affection; yet she is frankly concerned about the reputation of the boy with whom her daughter wants to go. She tells me about this at some length, pauses and seems about to change the subject.
> Th.: So what will you do?
> Pt.: Do? What can I do?
> Th.: That's a good question, what can you do?
> Pt.: I can't do a thing; she's going to go, and that's it.
> Th.: So you decided to let her go with John?
> Pt.: I haven't decided. She's the one who has decided.
> Th.: No, you've decided too. You've chosen to let her go with John.
> Pt.: I don't see how you can say that. She's insisting.
> Th.: That's what she's doing; what you're doing is accepting her insistence.

Pt.: Well, then I won't let her go. But she'll be unhappy and make life hell for me for a while.
Th.: So you've decided to forbid her to go with John.
Pt.: Well, isn't that what you wanted? What you said I should do?
Th:. I didn't say that you should do anything. You have a choice here, but you seem to be insisting that either your daughter is making a choice or that I am.
Pt.: Well, I don't know what to do.
Th.: It is a hard choice.

And so Thelma begins to confront her choice. It should be evident that this same procedure would have been followed whether Thelma had first concluded to deny her daughter permission to go with the boy or had given the permission.

CHOICE AND RELINQUISHMENT

"Every choice is also a relinquishment," it has been said. When I decide to take action A, I concurrently decide not to take actions B, C, D, . . . This is the god-like responsibility of determining actuality. Actuality is not something we encounter. Actuality is something we participate in creating. What is real is different because I am. What does not become real is also in some measure a function of my being. This is the acceptance of relinquishment.

The existential task of relinquishment is especially important. Once the person has genuinely recognized the bondage of embeddedness in his *Self* or in culture, he may begin the work of letting go. It can hardly be overstressed how pervasive and ruthless this relinquishment may become as true *Self*-transcendence is undertaken. We do not often see people who have the courage or the will to carry through the full potential of such actualization. This may be at least in part because we, as therapists, have not gone very far along this route ourselves and because we are terrified at the awful price genuine ontologic freedom demands.

We may speculate with some degree of assuredness that genuine *Self*-transcendence would mean the relinquishment of most of the pretranscendent human relationships and activities. These would scarcely escape being part of the embeddedness of *Self*-bondage. Already, at lesser degrees of freedom, we know that a high percentage of successful therapeutic outcomes are accompanied by significant changes in relationships, marriages, vocational adjustments and selections, and styles of living. How much more is this change process apt to pervade all areas of life and profoundly affect each in more thoroughgoing *Self*-transcendence.

MOURNING

There is also mourning work to be done in every process of relinquishment. The *Self* is let go of only with some pain and regret. If there were not this pain, it would be a superficial matter at best. We have invested much in the creation of our *Selves*, much of our hopes and much of our hurts are tied in with them; to set them aside is not a casual thing. Yet once the person is fully aware of the bondage of *Self* and of the potentiality of existential freedom, he is apt to feel that he can do no other than to relinquish the *Self*. It would be like a favored but outgrown suit of clothes, sadly yielded up to the emergence of the newer being.

Deems Taylor (1937) tells the story of sitting on the floor of his nursery when a small child, weeping over a favorite toy, a red fire-engine. For weeks young Deems had carried this toy with him everywhere, even taking it to bed with him. When his mother found him weeping over the toy, she asked what was the matter.

"I'm crying about my red fire-engine".
"Why do you cry about it, Deems?"
"Because some day I won't have it."
"But, Deems, you can have it just as long as you want."
"But some day I won't want it."

This is the story of ontologic growth and relinquishment. The therapist's task is not to force the relinquishment, but to help his patient face as clearly as possible what the issues of retaining and relinquishing may be at any given point; to help the patient become clear about the resistances through which he may seek to evade confronting the choice; to help the patient accept the grief work and mourning that must be done.

THE RESPONSE OF CREATIVITY

World, we discover, has few constraints. Perhaps only the four we have called the existential givens plus the physical limitations of gravity and hunger and such. World is so open. For some that openness is the terrorizing lack of meaning and control which makes it a rainy freeway without lines. For others it is the openness of a fresh canvas awaiting the artist's brush, a keyboard potent with music, a vast mountain range to be explored. The difference seems to be that the latter group responds to the emptiness with creativity, the former see only absurdity.

Creativity means not simply the public creations of artists and artisans. It means, more importantly, the inner creativity that is potential to each person (Adkins, 1959). It refers not to the product created but to the act of creation. To the extent that one makes his choices out of his own being and with faith in being, to that extent is he creative whether or not that which he produces has been made a million times over. To the extent one patterns his choices on that which is external to his own being, one is not truly creative although the product is hailed as unique by all who see it.

THE ONTOLOGIC OPTIONS REGARDING CONFLICT

Conflict is a part of life, at least as we know it. How we deal with the fact of conflict has much to do with how we express our being. Conflict, as here conceived, includes conflict of values or impulses within one's own awareness as well as conflicts between one person and another or between one group and another. Conflict is, it would seem, the inevitable outcome of the meaninglessness of the given world. Since no ultimate value is demonstrated, differences will exist. Differences in which we participate lead to conflicts of participation.

There are many ways in which one may cope with the experience of conflict. Because of the prevalence of guilt feelings, because we have been trained to feel we should know the "right way" to do things, and because we have learned to fear that differences with others will lead to the end of relationship with them, we react to conflicts as though they had meanings implicit in themselves rather than by recognizing them as events in the process of being. One consequence is that in our culture we expend much effort in denying or disguising conflict. "It's just a matter of semantics," "When you come down to practical applications, we agree," and so on, are expressions of the need to cover our differences. We seem to have the implicit assumption that genuine and abiding differences in the way we see things are destructive and must be overcome.

More authentic being will see in conflict an expected part of the human experience, a possible source of new information or deeper understanding, a challenge to creativity. The therapist can do much to help his patient toward this perspective by the example he sets in dealing with the inevitable conflicts that will arise in the therapeutic transaction itself. Not only will the therapist want to interpret the resistance of conflict denial, but he will avail himself of opportunities for demonstrating conflict utilization.

    Greta, in the earlier phases of therapy, avoided any open differences with me. She was very skillful at this, and it was some time before I realized that she was so pleasing to work with because she was always so appreciative and accepting of whatever I might say. At length I was able to help her bring to awareness her need to be so agreeable and her almost automatic suppression of her own views if they seemed at odds with mine. There followed a period in which she began to experiment with voicing nonunderstanding and even doubts. At first she was very hesitant, and we had to spend some time on a secondary resistance of creating differences that could be easily resolved but which were designed to win my approval. By the latter stages of therapy, Greta could express differences and support them, although I still found myself tending to focus on encouraging her taking this step rather than directly exploring our conflicts. Finally, the day came when I offered an interpretation to which she objected and then I came right back with, "I still think you're trying to perform well for me by raising these objections rather than really hearing my point and evaluating it yourself."

    "You make me so mad when you say that. I'm not just a docile child anymore. I thought your interpretation was wrong, and I said so."

    "You said so with a delightful smile which invited me to applaud your independence."

    "Oh, I did not!" But her voice was uncertain now, and the smile had faded. I waited silently. "Well, suppose I did. I still disagreed with you." Still I was silent. "I'm so confused now, I don't know what I did."

    "You're confused because you don't know how to perform well by disagreeing with me while yet agreeing with me that you're doing so."

    "But I don't want to disagree with you really. You're trying to help me, and . . ."

    "And you're trying to please me. But, Greta, it's this very need to please me that can keep me from helping you. If you go to the dentist and agree that every tooth he touches is the one that hurts, he'll not be able to do you any more good than if you denied that each one was the one that hurt."

"Yes, and do you know, when I do go to the dentist I have trouble saying which one it is that hurts?"

"Whether you agree with me all the time or disagree just to please me, you're doing the same thing: Both are ways of demanding that I be right all the time and thus relieve you of responsibility for yourself."

"I don't like it when you say that."

"This time you're not being agreeable, and I think you mean it."

And so we laughed in our recognition together and Greta took another step toward discovering her own responsibility for creating meaning.

Apartness and Love

I'll be loving you always.
I'll never be lonely again.
I can't live without you.
I believe in you.

The songs that we all know, that are a part of our whole understructure of life's meaning as popularly conceived, these are the songs of love. And the motion pictures and television shows, the plays and operas, novels and stories, all center in great part about love. And what is this love, the central theme of so much of our emotional seeking? The song titles above, like so many of the other forms of expression, link love with life and death, with loneliness or relation, with the very existential conditions of man's being with which we are concerned. Yet a good case may be made that man is more lonely in our day than he has ever been, real relation is more exceptional, and lasting love seems rare indeed.

The ultimate punishment in many a penitentiary is solitary confinement. West Point cadets put an offending classmate in "coventry" (they ignore him completely). The space agencies worry about the future astronauts' reactions to being alone for extended periods. We say of an eccentric older person, "He's been alone too much." Most psychologists would agree that a human being raised in complete isolation (were this possible) would not be recognizable as human in adulthood, at least in so far as personality goes and quite probably in other ways too. It is certain that such a creature neither would be nor could become sane by any of our usual standards.

THE EXISTENTIAL NEED FOR RELATEDNESS

Even if all his physiological needs were satisfied, he [man] would experience his state of aloneness and individuation as a prison from which he had to break out in order to retain his sanity. In fact, the insane person is the one who has completely failed to establish any kind of union and is imprisoned, even if he is not behind barred windows. The necessity to unite with other living beings, to be related to them, is an imperative need on the fulfillment of which man's sanity depends. This need is behind all phenomena which constitute the whole gamut of intimate human relations, of all passions which are called love in the broadest sense of the word (Fromm, 1959, pp. 151–152).

It is a manifest fact, too easily overlooked, that man is born into and lives in interdependence. Our earliest, as well as our most recent, learnings about who we are and what our world is like are set in a human context. As we pointed out above, an overwhelming proportion of our cultural fantasy and impulse life (entertainment, the arts, literature) are concerned with the experience of love in its many forms. When this focus is broadened to include sexual experience and all other forms of relationships, the preponderance is so massive as to be beyond comment.

Man has evolved many forms of relationships: acquaintance, friend, intimate; companion, opponent, bystander; family, social group, formal and informal groupings, cities and nations; lover, spouse, parent, and child; member, officer, outsider. There are ways of relating with all degrees of intimacy, with varying amounts of formality, with wide-ranging or narrow substantive focus, with relatively complete or relatively restricted personal involvement, and so on.

It is my belief, however, that the array of ways of relating is most complete in the more impersonal, detached, and segmented part of the spectrum, at least in our culture. Conversely, I think our ways of relating fully, warmly, personally, and intimately are restricted and insufficient, and I think they are in the process of change. I believe that we are in a transitional stage from which may emerge newer and fuller ways of relating intimately. To illustrate this contention, I would point to the decreasing adequacy of family and marriage, of church, of small community, of clubs and lodges, of lasting adult relations that are truly intimate. On the positive side we may note the increase in the use of various therapeutic forms—individual and group—to provide direct relationship gratification, the growth of sensitivity training and other "adult-education" ventures that are not principally content centered, the development of "prayer cells" in churches, the many informal, semi- or quasi-therapeutic groups (sometimes focused around dance, folk music, a discussion topic, body awareness training).

With Dr. Robert Tannenbaum, I have experimented with a design for sensitivity training (Tannenbaum and Bugental, 1963; Bugental and Tannenbaum, 1963) that involves the use of three relationship patterns: pairings, small groups, and a large group. The training impact was very appreciable, and we found ourselves thinking about its meaning.

> It is intriguing to speculate on the archaic roots of the participants' enthusiastic and involved response to the Dyads-Clans-Tribe design. As we have suggested by the terms we have used, we feel that the design may be congruent with basic (primitive) human-relationship patterns. Man forms alliances of many kinds, but—except in quite recent times—his most emotionally-meaningful ties have been those linking him with one other person (buddy, spouse), a small in-group (family, gang), and a larger (but still quite limited) grouping which included other in-groups (village). It seems reasonable to consider that this common and centuries-old human experience subtly permeates much of our thinking and feeling about relationships and doubtlessly affects our behavior and our very language. If these speculations are well founded, the Dyads-Clans-Tribe design should make possible an even more impactful and abiding learning and emotional growth in sensitivity training (Tannenbaum and Bugental, 1963, p. 3).

COURAGE: RELATEDNESS

Man seeks relationship with man as a way of dealing with the fact of apartness and giving expression to his being a part of life. Separateness in itself has no emotional tone, but when experienced only in its lonely aspects it leads to the experience of loneliness. Relatedness is the concurrent need of man to give an answer to his condition of separateness.

THE RESPONSE OF LOVE

"Love, the answer to the problem of human existence," is the title of a section in Erich Fromm's *The Art of Loving* (1956, p. 7). While I might take issue with calling human existence a "problem," I do not debate the central significance of love. To be sure, in making this agreement, I am—as is Fromm—speaking of existential love and not the moon-June love of popular song and movie, which is often antithetical to genuine love.

Existential love is an expression of one's whole being in relation to all Being. Existential love is—in its most transcendent form—participation in all Being, participation so complete that the subject-object dichotomy is obliterated and the essential unity of The All is revealed. Clearly, in such transcendent love, faith, commitment, and creativity are ultimately expressed.

In speaking of transcendent love we are characterizing an ultimate realization of the human potential, a point at which apartness is absorbed into wholeness. Most of our concern, however, is with love as a response to the experience of apartness, as a confronting and incorporating of the existential anxiety of loneliness and isolation. This brings our attention to a realm of more familiar experience. Here we may speak of actualizing love. Actualizing love is the "I-Thou" relation which Buber (1958) has characterized so well. It is the affirmation of one's own being in relation to another. Perhaps, in the terms we have been employing, it is the relation of *I-process* to *I-process*. In such a relation the beingness of each is recognized without the conditions or qualifications that would be involved in a *Self-Self* relation. In the latter, what one was or did would be crucial to the maintenance of love. Then, love would be constricting and demanding. This is the point that Rose learned too late.

> Rose had made excellent progress in the analytic phase of her therapy but still had difficulty effecting genuine and lasting relations with men. In early middle age, she looked back on the four years of a youthful marriage with sad regret. It had been a poor match, impulsively made and foredoomed by differences in background and life interests, she felt. Then

experiences in group therapy combined with her evolving analytic work to bring about a real reconfrontation of herself. She called for a special appointment and came in with a long dream written out and obvious intense feelings.

"Last night I reread some letters Jerry wrote to me when he was in the navy, and we were separated. I hadn't looked at them since I read them the first time. They were so . . . (she paused and broke into sobs) . . . so loving and tender. I was always saying "No" to him and he was always so forgiving. . . . For the first time I realized what I'd done. My whole life was my job, my career, my plans for the future. . . . It was the only way I could have any power in the universe, the only place I could prove I was worth anything. . . . I was afraid to be warm with him. . . ."

And so the story poured out. Rose had felt such an urgency to prove herself in her career, had been so afraid "to be like other people" (to be a housewife; for now she knew she'd always felt inadequate as a woman). Rose talked on with increasing tempo and a strong sense of urgency. I interrupted her. "Rose, slow down. You're rushing so fast to say everything just as you were rushing to prove yourself when you were with Jerry."

She stopped talking and cried in gasping sobs. When she started again, her voice was less tense. "I was an egomaniac. I was so frightened. . . . Jerry just wanted to love me and have me love him. . . ."

"Your fear made you kill something warm and loving. You are mourning for having killed that love," I told her.

"I was just so unloving, so ungiving, so unrelenting . . . and all he wanted was warmth, just some return from me. . . . And I kept refusing." For a while she went on in this vein. She was blaming herself heavily. I came in several times to reinforce the interpretation of her guilt and responsibility but not the blame. Partially I was able to put over the distinction by linking the responsibility to her fear of her inadequacy.

As the first flurry of self-accusation passed, I pointed out, "You seem surprised that Jerry could have loved you when you acted like you did."

"That's right. Why, he just loved *me!*" The shock of this recognition brought her half up into a sitting position.

"He just loved you," I told her, "But you're still thinking in terms of earning love because you're so surprised that his love lasted when you were so bitchy."

"Yes, I am." Her voice had a flat sound of deep recognition. She talked about this several minutes and then began to shake and pull her sweater around her. "I'm cold. It's like there's a draft on me. I'm so cold all of a sudden."

"You're feeling how cold you were to Jerry."

"I guess so. And I loved him so."

"That's the first time you've said that you loved him."

The sobs burst out with renewed force. "That's what I wanted to say. Oh, I wanted to say that. That's what I wanted to tell him and to tell you. I did love him. That's why I'll never see him when he's in town. I'm afraid I can't keep detached."

"So your fear meant that you had to try to kill your love as well as Jerry's."

"Yes! Oh, yes. But I did love him. And he loved me...."

Now she sighed heavily, stopped shivering. The hour was over.

THE ONTOLOGIC OPTION OF DEVOTION

As with each of the areas of ontogogic concern, there are numerous options that may be possible to the person attaining to greater authenticity in the area of his courageous response to apartness. I want to talk about devotion because it is an option that is in some apparent contrast to much that we have dealt with and, indeed, may be an option that the unwary therapist will regard as inauthentic or neurotic.

By devotion I mean the aware decision to orient one's being as fully as may be possible toward the expression of some value experienced as centrally significant to one's being. Such devotion is not to be appreciated in terms of the external expressions it may manifest; although it does seem that it is sometimes possible to say of certain patterns of behavior that they seem inconsistent with authentic devotion as it is here conceived. Authentic devotion may be—and probably does—lie back of the work of such men as Gandhi, Schweitzer, Freud, and others. I would like to rule out such people as Hitler, Napoleon, and other despots, but I am not sure it is possible. Almost certainly such devotion characterized many of the saints (not in the formal sense) of religious and political history, especially Mohammed, Christ, the Buddha.

But perhaps we confuse the issue by trying to use historical figures to clarify the concept. Devotion, as I am proposing we understand it, is not a matter of doing good works or operating on a grand scale or clearly leading a historical movement. Devotion is a choice to focus one's being in a certain way, to bring one's faith, commitment, creativity, and love into coordination with a particular value and purpose. It is not a subordinating to that value and purpose but an identification with it in which neither the value nor one's being is subordinated.

In point of fact, I have not had a patient who exercised the option of devotion in the way I am describing it. I think that this sort of dedication is quite unusual in our culture, and I am sure that I have not always understood the potential for such a choice when it may have appeared in my patients. Yet, I am convinced that a psychology of authentic being must provide for the extreme instance of the person who with real awareness chooses to focus himself in a total fashion. I am afraid that we have too often been unwitting instruments for conformity training and have treated the tentative gestures toward this kind of devotion as neurotic without recognizing that they need not be. We need to have a conceptual system that—while it may recognize the distortive in a monolithic orientation—protects the creative potential of a Beethoven, an Eleanor Roosevelt, a Van Gogh, a Thomas Wolfe, and their fellows.[2]

A VALUE IN SOLITUDE

We must not leave the discussion of relatedness without at least brief recognition that there is a real value possible in the experience of solitude. To be sure, it may be a flight from the anxiety of aloneness, but it need not be so in all cases. Jesus went into the wilderness for forty days and used this solitude for discovery of his mission. Other mystics and seers have had similar periods of withdrawal from contact with others. Admiral Byrd (1956) writes of his choice to undergo a period of utter aloneness. A troubled person goes off

---

[2] Leon Saul is one of the few writers in this area to give serious and repeated concern to this issue. His extension of the surgeon's motto, *Primum non nocere*, first of all, do no harm, is a creative contribution in its own right. "It is not the analyst's job to tamper with talent," says Saul. "In fact, if he sees infantile components in it, it is his job to leave them alone." (1958, pp. 164–166).

by himself to gain new perspective. Creative people in various walks of life have used a time alone as a way of finding meaning or purpose. Frightened people may flee into compulsive gregariousness. The group may tyrannize as well as facilitate.

CONCLUSION

When we have the opportunity to work with a person who is emerging into new realization of his personhood, we are given the privilege of discovering new meanings in the as yet little developed realm of ontogogy. Yet there remains one further contribution we can make to our former-patient-now-companion's emergence; we can let go of him.

We stand with our patient as he opens his eyes more and more to the blinding light of contingency. We help with the constant focusing and restructuring of awareness that is growth. We try to be alert to help in the resolution of lingering resistances. And then the time comes for us to stand out of the way. It is the exceptional therapist who can genuinely and readily let go of the person with whom he has made the journey from the depths of human despair to the far reaches of human potential without some mourning. The therapist needs to examine his own perceptions and motivations most acutely, for he is apt to find his awareness affected by threat, competition, jealousy, and guilt. Threat comes from the increasing authenticity with which the person is confronting that which the therapist may still find evoking great anxiety in himself. Competition may come from the therapist's own hungering for the greater authenticity that he sees his former patient attaining. Jealousy is certain to be potential, for the truly effective therapist will surely find more than one of his patients who outdistances him, at least in some aspects. Guilt will lie in the recognition that there have been ways in which the therapist has misinterpreted his patient's movement at times, has blocked rather than facilitated his growth on occasion, and has not always been all that his new companion's progress required.

The therapist must know that that day will come, if he has been successful, when his former patient will relinquish him, just as he has so much else. Then the therapist must face his own aloneness while knowing his own fulfillment.

PART FOUR *The human frontier*

As I have recognized all along the importance of the therapeutic relation, it is appropriate now to inquire into the person who is the therapist, as I do in *Chapter 21*. There are addictive or neurotic gratifications to being a therapist just as there are creative and synergic fulfillments. The mature therapist is dedicated but not self-sacrificing. Rather he is life-fulfilling in a way that facilitates concurrent growth in his patient. Immaturity in the therapist may be rationalized by many names, but essentially it is a failure of genuine encounter and mutual respect, in which the patient is exploited covertly by the therapist's needs. The therapist must accept the guilt his profession entails. When he does so in an authentic way, he is uniquely fortunate in his opportunity to know the human experience.

As we draw to a close of our ventures along the human frontier, we begin to set out beyond that border land. In *Chapter 22* I will describe some observations on the kinds of living shown by my patients who have won a measure of authenticity. Here, as in Chapters 15, 16, 19, and 20, I hope to implement my determination to find methods of thinking and talking about our human experience that are not rooted in pathology or predicated on a view of man-as-an-object. The reader will recognize that I have, as yet, been but incompletely successful in this attempt.

I am continuingly fascinated by the ranges beyond the frontier of our knowledge. What man may become when he can free himself of his resistances to authenticity, what truly actualizing being would be like, how a society of such persons would conduct itself—these are the questions about which *Chapter 23* speculates. We may be certain that we are at a very primitive stage in man's evolution. There is great encouragement in the convergences of the physical and behavioral sciences, of the humanistic sciences and the humanities, and of the Eastern and Western orientations to the nature of man. Still, we are but begun on discovering the new world of human potential. Much that we now take for granted as limiting the human experience must certainly be dissolved in time. The possibilities of discovering new realms of authentic being are surely as great as those that lie between us and our primitive forebears.

In this final section, my purpose will be somewhat different from what it has been in preceding parts of the book. Now we want to adopt a broader perspective, to concern ourselves less with technical and conceptual precision and more with the broad meanings implicit in the existential-humanistic orientation to the human experience of being and emergence. For this reason I will often approach the same phenomena with which I have dealt in a systematic way in earlier chapters from a less structured and more subjective angle. It is my hope that in this way we can gain a deeper awareness of the limitless expanse at and beyond the human frontier.

21—The person who is the therapist

It is a familiar observation that the psychotherapist is the latest descendant of a line which traces back to prehistory. The psychotherapist's predecessors are the medicine man, the sorcerer, the priest, the family doctor. In every age man has needed to have someone to turn to for help in contending with the awful unknownness of his fate. Inevitably, invariably, the one turned to has been invested by himself and by others with supranormal vision and potency. This has usually been both his greatest reward and his most terrifying burden. Certainly this is true for the psychotherapist today.

It can hardly be debated that there is a selective process, operating at both conscious and unconscious levels, which determines those of us who will come into the field of psychotherapeutic practice. We bear no mark of the caul, nor do we often experience a "call"; yet just as surely do we find ourselves making those choices in our development that lead us to this work. By no means do I imply that this is altogether a bad thing; nor do I mean to reassure that it is altogether a good thing either. For the moment let it rest that a great many psychotherapists, the present writer included, have sought through becoming psychotherapists to deal with their own anxieties, both existential and neurotic.[1]

---
[1] Indeed, let me append to this observation that one of the most frequent incentives to becoming identified with the existential viewpoint is the hope thereby to forestall existential anxiety, in other words, to deny the very viewpoint with which one affiliates.

361

Gratifications in Being a Therapist

THERAPEUTIC ADDICTION

Anyone who gets deeply involved in the practice of intensive psychotherapy is in grave risk of becoming "hooked." Exceptions to that generalization would be few indeed. I doubt that mescaline, marihuana, opium, or heroin can lastingly give the gratifications to the user that the practice of intensive psychotherapy makes available.

Now, what are these gratifications of being a psychotherapist?

ONE-WAY INTIMACY

Allen Wheelis (1958) has described what he feels is a powerful selective factor operating in determining who will become a psychoanalyst. This is a hunger for closeness, a great desire for affective intimacy, and a great fear of it. The practice of psychotherapy makes possible a kind of one-way closeness of great intimacy, quite frequently with more affective expression than is to be found in any other relationship, not excluding the marriage relationship (Warkentin, 1963). Yet it is in many ways "safer" to the therapist, in that he is supported by his ethics and training in withholding himself from the commingling which is potential. How beautifully, then, this practice fits the needs of those with a great affect hunger, a great desire for intimacy, and a great fear of affect in intimacy.

OMNIPOTENCE

Second, the practice of intensive psychotherapy provides rich nourishment for one's omnipotence and omniscience strivings. Many of us who feel frightened and impotent in living in general find in the practice of therapy a kind of splendid calm, which we and the patient conspire together to believe is the benign influence of our perspective.

Therapist's Love. I would like to comment at greater length on a frequent, special instance of the omnipotence striving being acted out in the therapeutic relation. This is the myth of the curative effect of the therapist's love. A great many therapists at one time or another seem to pass through a phase where they become convinced that ample doses of unquestioning, undemanding love from the therapist for the patient is the curative agent which can produce profound changes. This seems to come about because many patients are emotionally deprived people who seek the kind of concern from their therapists that they feel they never received from their parents. The response of the patient to seeming to gain that caring from the therapist is often dramatic and pervasive, for a period. Only when the therapist has worked with a truly dependent personality over a period of years does he begin to recognize, if he is wise, that while the patient may indeed achieve remarkable reorganizations of his life through the benign influence of the therapist's love, these are all fragilely hung on the relationship. The patient resists with frightening ruthlessness any attempt by the therapist to reduce that dependence. It is not unusual for the work of months and years, all the hard-won gains in life effectiveness the patient and therapist have worked out, to be brought crashing down in a relatively short space of time when the therapist begins to try to free the patient of his dependence upon the sustenance of the therapist's concern.

> Kathryn came to therapy because of tremendous depressive episodes that brought her several times to the brink of suicide and that seemed to be linked with her husband's drinking bouts. She found in me a person who gave her great warmth and acceptance. Her mother had been a rejecting household drudge who had evidently been afraid of close relationships and had been able to give only in terms of endless hours of work. Kathryn was a gifted woman of superior intelligence with tremendous ability to do a capable job in her semitechnical profession. When first seen, she was on the verge of being dismissed from her work because of the erratic quality of her performance. In eighteen months of therapy she effected a divorce from her husband, gained an advance in her position, was functioning at a level superior to any she had ever in her life known for an extended period. Her therapeutic sessions were characterized by exploration of very deep, primitive material, a great deal of emotional intensity, and her professions of great gratitude toward me.
> Periodically throughout this period, though, when some life crisis would occur, Kathryn would call me day and night, and repeatedly. Distraught, disorganized, in danger of upsetting all the great improvements in her life, in lengthy tele-

phone calls she made many, many bids for reassurance of my concern for and belief in her. The length and frequency of the phone calls would increase for a time, then the crisis would pass, and she would seemingly knit together and perform well again.

At length, when she achieved a degree of stability, though still punctuated with these crisis episodes, I began to withdraw some of my support, to insist that Kathryn limit the length and frequency of her phone calls. A tremendous battle ensued. Seemingly blind to her own interests, Kathryn jeopardized her position, began drinking heavily, and insisted on the need for more frequent contacts with me. Now she became badgering and demanding. She called for more and more evidences of closeness. She made threats upon her own life and eventually became threatening toward me. Wherever I had set limits, Kathryn was compelled to test, to try to overthrow those limits.

We can talk of Kathryn as a pseudo-neurotic schizophrenic, and this is probably accurate. We can speak of her tremendous passive-hostile character structure, which was unanalyzed or insufficiently analyzed, and this is probably true. We have only touched one half of the story when we characterize Kathryn in this fashion. My own neurotic needs are portrayed in my placing the main reliance on the curative effect of my concern. In a sense, I presented Kathryn with a world different from the world of contingency, choice, and tragedy. I presented her with what seemed to be a world of certainties, though those certainties hinged on me, the person. Together we created a symbiosis of the most malignant type. It could only end in the destruction of both of us if allowed to run its course. Kathryn's reality sense was adequate to present her unverbalized cues that the relationship could not continue and continue to be more and more supportive as she needed it to be. Thus she had to make more and more demands to try to quiet those cues and to reassure herself that this indeed was *the* unique relationship. On my part, committed to a course based on unstinted giving, I found myself called upon to give more and more until my own limits were severely threatened.

Let me be clear, I am not devaluing the significance, even the essential quality, of the therapist's concern for his patient. Psychotherapy is an intimate relationship. It does involve the feelings of both participants, but when this becomes an infantile acting-out then it is no longer psychotherapy; it is a *folie à deux*.

CONTINGENCY MASTERY

A third important gratification in the practice of psychotherapy is the opportunity the therapist has for a vicarious and seemingly safe way of dealing with contingency, with the basic realities of life. I have heard therapists say they found themselves using the patient as a guide dog to go through the mine field of certain threats first in order to reassure themselves that it can be negotiated. I respect the therapists who recognize this. Nearly all therapists do this in some measure, all too often without such candid recognition. We live in anxiety; we seek to become more self-trusting; we never achieve this fully. When, with full recognition of the patient's needs, we can encourage him to confront that which breeds anxiety within ourselves, we are heavily invested in the outcome.

MASCULINE TENDERNESS

A fourth gratification in being a therapist is that it provides an opportunity to give tenderness, compassion, and love within a structure in which one's masculinity is not questioned. A great many who are drawn into this field have fears of emotions, fears that they represent weakness and perhaps effeminacy within us. Often these fears are completely unconscious, and we may even be counterphobic in being overly expressive of our emotions. We document with research and learned papers the healthfulness of emotional expression and the disasters attendent upon emotional inhibition. And in the therapeutic hour, secure in our masculinity of being doctors and healers, we can dispense tenderness and love without arousing our own anxieties.[2]

REBELLIOUSNESS

A fifth, very frequent gratification in the practice of psychotherapy is that it gives us an opportunity to attack authority and tradition while armored in all the prerogatives of our own authoritative position. We have studied and observed how the needless inhibi-

---

[2] Jourard, in an exceedingly provocative paper on "Some lethal aspects of the male role" (1962), has elaborated important significances of this observation.

tions of society complicate the lives of all of us: the taboos about sexual talk and actions; the guilts about ambivalence toward parents, spouses, and others; the shame of death wishes and other hostile impulses. These, we have learned, are part of the influences that have made our patients suffer and—though we seldom verbalize this to the patients or to ourselves—have made us suffer. With the authority of being a therapist, we can strike back at these influences. Notice how often we psychotherapists, particularly in our earlier years of practice, become great users of the four-letter words (Feldman, 1955). Notice how often we are flagrant in our verbal expressions of sexual and hostile impulses. It seems quite clear that this is an acting-out, a counterphobic kind of behavior which represents the celebration of the license of being therapists. Thus we pay back society, hit back at authority. It is not a matter of chance, for example, that most therapists tend to be political and social liberals. We would like to think that this is chiefly because we have had an opportunity to see the crippling effect of social ills, and I am certain this is one significant reason. On the other hand, the person who is in some revolt against what he feels is social injustice may find in the practice of psychotherapy a relatively safe way to express his rebellion.

I have listed some of the ways in which the practice of intensive psychotherapy can provide powerful and unique gratifications to the therapist. It is inevitable that those of us who are most in need of these kinds of gratifications will be drawn to this practice. I want to make it clear that I do not feel these neurotic sorts of gratifications are by any means the only satisfactions in this work. I do think that these neurotic gratifications are much more frequently present than we generally recognize, that they are seldom completely removed by personal therapeutic experience, and that we have a responsibility to try to remain aware of their operation in our daily practice.

Synergic Gratifications

Having listed some important aspects of the practice of psychotherapy that provide addictive or neurotic gratifications, I would like to describe now some creative gratifications that are also realized in our work. Maslow's (1962a) term, "synergy" best delineates the common property these have. In a truly synergic relation that which most contributes to the fulfillment of one of the participants is most fulfilling of the other also. It should be evident that I do not hold with the view that the psychotherapist has no needs seeking satisfaction in his work. On the contrary, the therapist must find important fulfillment if he is to be able to mobilize his total resources for the task, as he must frequently do. Some of the incentives to his doing so seem to be the following.

PARTICIPATION

To the psychotherapist is offered the opportunity to participate with unique immediacy in the business of life itself. In psychotherapeutic practice one deals daily with the life *and* death of human personality and potential. I mean no play on words, and the melodrama implicit in this characterization is that of the human experience itself. As the therapist accompanies his patient in his efforts to confront the minor and the great issues of his life, to contend with the ever-present unknownness of choices and their consequences, to meet and live with the multiple emotional seekings and stresses of human relationships—as the psychotherapist visits the heights of elation and self-affirmation, the depths of confusion and madness, the brink of suicide, the bleakness of relinquishment, and on and on—then the therapist must know the limitedness of his gifts and how privileged his situation in viewing the human condition.

PERSONAL GROWTH

A good therapeutic relation is growth-inducing in both participants. Growth potential is infinite, and the therapist who is an authentic participant in his work with his patient has repeated stimulation and opportunity to increase his realization of his own potential. In a climate in which genuineness is requisite and yet always sought anew, that which is false and self-defeating in the therapist himself must ever and again be illuminated for the inauthentic self-deception it is. The therapist who has come to love the realization of human potential—and I am convinced this is a distinguishing characteristic of the dedicated therapist—will be continually renewed in his own growth (Whitaker and Malone, 1953).

PSYCHOLOGICAL PROCESSES

A high proportion of psychologist-psychotherapists entered their parent discipline of psychology because, among other reasons, of a fascination with psychological processes which may be likened to that some people show with mechanics, others with color and form in the arts, and still others with mathematics and quantitative processes. There is no other opportunity in all the world like that of intensive psychotherapy for a person with this orientation to immerse himself in the working of psychological processes in their natural condition. All our familiar psychological topics of learning, motivation, attitudes, emotions, attention, remembering, perception, and so on—all of these are displayed in endless variation and exquisite detail.

PATIENTS' GROWTH

Most patients who come to the psychotherapist show improvement. The doubters to the contrary, the psychotherapeutic experience is generally one in which there is a gain in human effectiveness and satisfaction (although, albeit, not the magical one frequently initially expected). It is for the therapist, once he has adjusted his own sights to realistic dimensions, a deeply meaningful experience to have participated in his patient's emergence. There are, of course, the failures, the disappointments, the questionable outcomes. However, with experience, constant self-development, and much learning just to wait, the proportion of favorable outcomes increases; the pervasiveness of the changes becomes more evident. It is, then, an enriching feeling to have been an intimate participant in this growth.

Maturity of the Psychotherapist

I want to talk now about some observations on what it means to be a mature psychotherapist. In one sense I am going to be describing a goal never fully attained. In another sense I am going to be describing what it means to be a mature person generally. Here, however, we are particularly concerned with the person who is the psychotherapist and so will dwell especially on that aspect. As a preliminary, we will talk about some pseudo-maturity patterns.

Pseudo-Maturity Patterns

PONTIFICATING

First, we can recognize a group of therapist behaviors that are rather clearly those of the immature personality. These include the therapist who pontificates, speaking as though the infallible intermediary between God and the patient: pronouncing judgments, giving instructions, and acting-out a certainty that is the therapist's own resistance to contingency. Whatever the patient says is the occasion for the therapist to give a lecturette. These sorts of behaviors are sometimes useful in short-term counseling and in handling emergency situations; and some use of very unequivocal pronouncements may be made by mature therapists. What is indicted here is someone who relies almost solely on this way of participating.

ACTING-OUT GIVING

A more frequent sign of pseudo-maturity, one in which the therapist's own needs are more covert and unconscious, is that form of acting-out giving by the therapist which is actually a substitute for his genuine presence in the interview. The therapists who are caught up in the delusion of the curative power of unstinting love, which was described above, would be primary examples of this type of acting-out. Genuine presence with the patient, encounter and engagement with him, seldom will be expressed through continual and unilateral giving by the therapist. Perhaps that word "unilateral" needs emphasis. The therapist who genuinely engages with his patient demands bilateral exchange, not on a "bargaining basis" but on a basis of a mutual respect, a demand which the therapist who is acting-out in his giving could not afford to risk.

ENACTED OPENNESS

A variation of this same pattern of acting-out giving as a substitute for genuine presence occurs in the kind of enacted openness which is really exhibitionism on the therapist's part. I had a patient who went to a psychotherapist who in the second session undressed himself completely as a demonstration of his openness and lack of pretense to the patient. This is clearly an acting-out designed to allay the therapist's fears of his own secretiveness and possibly to stimulate the patient to similar exhibitionism. Certainly a kind of enacted openness, which masks the lack of real presence, is often performed by therapists who are caught in the subject–object split and who treat themselves as things to be observed and manipulated for their patients' welfare, at least as they see it. They are very like the kind of martyr-mother who has so little belief in her own worth that she misuses herself, seemingly for the child's benefit. Such therapists and parents really teach a kind of alienation and a lack of presence that is highly pathogenic.

When working as a therapist to therapists, I often can get a useful clue as to the nature of the acting-out giving which is a substitute for genuine presence when the therapist is able to be giving only in his in-office life, while his extra-office life is often characterized by great loneliness and isolation. More than one therapist who is tremendously warm and giving in his relations with his patients is distant, awkward, and ungiving in relations with his children, his wife, and his colleagues.

SUBMERGENCE IN A THEORY

Another sort of pseudo-maturity that is often somewhat subtle and difficult to recognize is that in which a theory or system displaces the person of the therapist. Such a therapist becomes, as it were, an embodiment of a particular viewpoint, rather than a person in his own right. This can be true, and I think I have recognized it, in psychoanalytic, Adlerian, Rogerian, and existentially oriented therapists. "A good theory is the most practical thing," it is said, but a good theory is a tremendously effective way of avoiding contingency. Existential theory, let me assure you, is magnificent in its seeming power to offset existential reality. Writing a book or giving speeches about a theory often can be a good way to avoid being a person while wearing the mask of the theory.

ENCOURAGEMENT OF IMPULSIVITY

A final kind of pseudo-maturity pattern has already been alluded to in speaking of the gratifications of being a therapist, but needs to be mentioned again here: the encouragement of the patient in his acting-out impulsivity and overthrow of the superego. This attempt to free the patient to be that which he "naturally" is by raising no question of responsibility about the patient's impulses is an all too frequent type of therapeutic pseudo-maturity.

Genuine Maturity in the Therapist

RECOGNITION OF LIMITED KNOWLEDGE

Probably one of the first evidences of genuine maturing in the therapist comes when he expresses and evidences his acceptance of the fact that he has but limited knowledge of his patient. Since we, as therapists, get to know our patients so much more thoroughly than we know any other human beings in our lives, we often feel that we really know them fully. This is a myth; this is our omniscience fantasy being enacted. Those who have had an intensive psychotherapeutic experience will recognize how great the area is that they have never been able to transmit to their therapists, how much of their living the therapists knew little about as contrasted to the relatively smaller area in which the therapists truly understood fully.

I am speaking here of the best relationships between therapists and patients, even when continued over several years. As therapists we never know all about our patients, only some aspects. These may be terribly important aspects and certainly significant to know, but we need to recognize they are but a part of what could conceivably be known about our patients.

SELECTIVE PARTICIPATION

A second mark of the maturing therapist is his selective use of his own participation. This is to say he is able so to modulate when and how he intervenes that his participation is maximally effective in a restricted area. The maturing therapist speaks sparingly, but with precision. A very common fault of the tyro-therapist is that he talks too much or too little or at the wrong time.

GENUINE ENCOUNTER

A third characteristic of the maturing therapist is his willingness genuinely to encounter his patient. This does not mean a kind of exhibitionism or display of himself. It does mean a willingness to "be there" with his patient, to confront his patient directly when appropriate, to take responsibility for his (the therapist's) own thinking, judgments, feelings, and to be authentic in his own person with the patient. All too often therapists who believe in this sort of authenticity portray in their own manner an avoidance of authenticity that can but present a contradictory message to the patient. Sidney Jourard (1964) has the idea that one of the main things which has a curative effect in the therapeutic relationship is the therapist's serving as a model of authenticity for the patient.

Therapist Authenticity. In the therapist's handling of limits and endings we have a clear example of one of the ways in which a therapist may not be authentic. The therapist who is repeatedly careless about starting appointments on time or terminating sessions on time or who, on the other hand, is too punctilious about time-limits demonstrates this. So does the therapist who cannot sort out when to make a statement in a declarative, simple, direct fashion and when to phrase it in conditional language. Far too many therapists seem to me to talk with the kinds of qualified phrasing more appropriate to the *Journal of Experimental Psychology* than to the needs of the therapeutic hour. They are apt to say to the patient, "It seems like you may be projecting the attitude that you apparently had toward your father onto me," rather than telling the patient directly, "You're reacting to me as you did to your father." The use of many qualifiers, the use of the third person instead of the first, the statement of an interpretation as a possibility rather than a clear perception (when it is that) may be indications of this same avoidance of presence. Again, the therapist who excuses a patient from paying for a missed appointment because the patient forgot or was held up in traffic is not being authentic in his relation with the patient but is acting-out his own need to give and probably to suffer. The therapist who cannot admit his mistakes but always has some explanation for them is another example.

EVOLVING CONCEPTS

A further evidence of growing maturity in the therapist is that he has an evolving set of constructions about himself, his world, the nature of psychotherapy, and what he means by the concept of personality. I am mistrustful of the therapist who believes he has reached final answers on any of these points. Recognition of the dynamic quality of knowledge, of the continuing learning experience of therapeutic work, demands that one be changing if one be dedicated and aware.

THERAPEUTIC GUILT

I have reserved for the last one of the most difficult aspects of therapeutic maturity, the acceptance of the guilt of being a therapist. Certainly all that has been said about the neurotic gratifications of being a therapist and about the kinds of patterns found in pseudo-maturity as a therapist will have indicated already that there is inevitably a load of guilt in being a therapist. I will not re-elaborate on these points. The point is this: there is a guilt for our failure to be all that we can be as therapists to these people who come and give us their lives and their trust.

> The other day I saw Jack again for the first time in five years. I first saw Jack eleven years ago; that was for vocational guidance. He came back a year later because he was having trouble with his marriage, and I was able to be of some help in patching up a shaky relationship. Seven years ago when he came to me the marriage had collapsed at last, and he was readjusting his life to a new pattern of living. At that time we attempted intensive psychotherapy, and I saw him for several years. I think Jack was helped by the experience. However, I put it in this somewhat tentative fashion because I can see so many ways today that he could have been helped so much more.
>
> I look at Jack in my office today, and I see a man with the gray coming in at his temples. I see in him also virtually a boy of twenty-nine as I first saw him eleven years ago. The prime years of his early maturity are embraced by our relationship. As I look at Jack, I think of Louis whom I am currently seeing and who is about the age Jack was when he first came to me. Louis is going to have a much fuller life than Jack has had because I am so much more able to meet him and to help him in becoming himself. To look at Jack is to look at my own guiltiness for not having been all that Jack needed. I comfort myself that I served him with sincerity with the best of my skill at that time. I comfort myself that many another therapist might have done no more for him than I did, but this does not give Jack back his lost years.

This is a story of the therapist's guilt. If I am to be a growing, evolving person, each old patient I see again is an accusation; each patient of former years will be in some measure someone who trusted me and whom I failed by today's standards. If I become despondent or self-punitive, I am acting out a neurotic type of guilt; but if I recognize the legitimate responsibility I had in this matter I am revitalized in my own growth.

Continued Guilt. But there is yet one further way in which this guilt operates. When I recognize that I am continuing to try to grow, to increase my awareness, skill, competence in effectively being in the relationship with my patients, then I must look at my patients today and know that each one of them is getting less than I hope I will be giving his successor five years hence. There is guilt in this too.

You may protest, "This all sounds very masochistic and self-punishing. It's just the way things are. There's no need to expend guilt and regret it." In one sense you are very right; in another you are very wrong. Yes, this is the way things are, but the fact that a condition is so does not mean necessarily that it is unladen with emotional significance. It is so that I can only do so much for my patients now and that that seldom is all I potentially can do, even today. On the other hand, if the sense of guilt becomes an interference with my effective use of myself rather than part of a heightened sensitivity, then it is clearly becoming a neurotic guilt and an attempt to forestall other anxiety. The kind of guilt I am trying to characterize here is not forestalling of anxiety, nor yet laden with additional anxiety. It is an emotional fact of being.

CONCLUSION

I want to conclude by saying very briefly what it means to me to be a psychotherapist. I feel like one of the more fortunate people. The men and women who come to see me entrust me with that which is most deeply meaningful in all their experience. They offer me the awesome privilege of participating in the very essence of their lives. When I am most authentic, I am most humble in my appreciation of this opportunity.

As I started this, I called attention to the lineage from which we psychotherapists take our vocation: medicine man, wizard, priest, and family doctor. This is a proud line, and we may be proud to be part of it. These are the bearers of man's hope and man's faith. These are the personifications of man's courage and creativity in confronting the immensity of the unknown. We are for our brief time hoisted on the shoulders of our fellows that we may catch some glimpse of the yet untouched reaches of what it means to be truly man.

22 — Psychotherapy and emergent man

We need a new Manhattan Project, this time in the human sciences. We are approaching a crisis in the human experience, and we need much more inquiry, speculation, theorizing, and technique development. I propose that we employ a large number of intelligent people, educated in the whole spectrum of disciplines having to do with human experience, and put them to work. Since we need primary data on the meaning of being human, we will want to get a broad sampling of subjects, men and women of all ages and backgrounds (though perhaps it will be well to increase the proportion of the educated, intelligent, successful and articulate), some who are highly successful, many just average, and some completely unsuccessful by whatever criteria. As to methodology, let us have our investigators do several things. First they must simply listen to people talking as candidly as they can about their lives in great detail through many, many hours. Second, the investigators should try with whatever theories and techniques now exist to help the subjects make changes in their lives. In that way there can be a beginning on testing what is effectual and what is not. Third, the investigators should be asked to formulate theories, develop new methods, try to persuade each other (so that their ideas can be refined by interaction with those with similar experiences).

Now, from this new Manhattan Project, from this tremendous and utterly unique inquiry into what it means to be a person, we will expect that, slowly at first and then with gathering momentum, changes in the human experience will occur. There is no way of predicting the direction of these changes but that they will occur can hardly be doubted.

Of course, this tremendous project is already under way. Never before in the history of man have so many intelligent, trained observers been concentrating on the individual human experience of so many different people. Estimates are hazardous, but surely there are in this country alone thirty thousand psychologists, psychiatrists, psychoanalysts, social workers, ministers, and others who devote a major portion of their time to individual psychotherapy. They probably see a half-million people a year or more. Then there must be another sixty thousand such workers who devote part time to such work. They are joined by at least a hundred and forty thousand lawyers, probation and parole officers, teachers, and counselors, who also spend some time in trying to understand the individual's experience of his life, to help him make it different. Do they see a million more people? The numbers, of course, are very unimportant. What is important is that so much attention is for the first time being given to understanding and influencing individual human experience and behavior.

The results are beginning to be seen. No theory of personality that was recognized in 1945 is generally supported intact in 1965. Indeed, all theories are undergoing such rapid change and development that it is almost impossible to point to just what position any one holds beyond the writing of a particular author at a particular date. Every psychotherapist is his own Freud today. Psychotherapists are increasingly finding themselves drawn to work out their own formulations about personality, about what produces change, about the meanings of behavior and experience. This leads to the despair or derision of the orderly minded, but in an evolutionary perspective it is a highly fertile and promising state of affairs (Murphy, 1958).

Change is coming, change is occurring, change in the very center of the human experience, change in the very conception of what it means to be a man, to be alive, to *be* at all. Already the effects of this tremendous enterprise are being importantly felt in religion, in education, in the arts, in child-rearing, in literature. There are modest evidences of the wave reaching to politics, commerce and industry, the military, international relations. And the wave that is now spreading is really only a forerunner from the earlier stages of the investigations. The waves that will follow will be so much greater that the presently visible changes, pervasive as they are, will be seen to be but ripples. In the simplest terms, I think our whole conception of human life is in the process of being completely revised. Since from that conception ultimately flows all else that we know, I think the whole experience of life is under revision as well.

Some have questioned whether society can afford the "luxury" of individual psychotherapy. I am convinced that society cannot afford the wastefulness of being without individual psychotherapy. For individual psychotherapy may be the best method we have yet been able to devise for studying how well human efforts can meet human needs and for evoking the forces that will make for corrections in the direction of better coordination of the two.

I want to talk about some of the gains that are seen in patients who have a successful existential-analytic course. My intent here will be to convey a general feeling or impression of the kinds of outcomes hoped for and actually seen, rather than to catalog in any systematic fashion the various forms of successful outcomes from therapy. The latter task was better performed in Chapter 16. In the present discussion I will once more draw attention to the need for a more constructive (ontogogic) orientation that can move away from the deficit or reparative perspective that has so long dominated our thinking about personality.

. . . . .

The man who is speaking first came into my office on a rainy day well over four years ago. I remember that it *was* raining because *he* so obviously did not seem to know it. I remember clearly how he sat in my big patient's chair giving me a confused, tortured account as the rain water drained from his thinning hair, completed taking the press out of his rumpled suit, and made dark spots on his surprisingly well shined brown shoes. I was very aware of how wet he was; I'm not sure he even knew it had been raining. He had reached that far, bitter juncture in human experience where he didn't *care* enough to come in out of the rain.

Today the sun is playing in and out of scudding spring clouds as Bill talks to me. Not in the chair anymore but on the couch at whose head I sit, Bill speaks to me for the 412th time, my clipboard notes tell me. And it is certainly over the hundred mark for his participation in our therapy group. So much has happened in those five hundred plus times we have been together. We have fought and laughed and wept together. Bill has discovered me to be his father, his first sergeant, his old teacher, and he has found me out, too, as his boyhood pal, his foxhole buddy, and his self he will never be. But lately Bill has been coming to see me as me, and I like that.

Listen to what Bill is saying now:

"Yesterday, I had a case of the jitters again. I don't know why. It just came on while I was eating lunch. I was sitting alone for a few minutes while my friend went to get a coffee refill, and I was thinking about vacation coming, and then I felt that old, cold hand on my guts, and..."

This is a sad story from one who's been so long in psychotherapy. An inexplicable attack of anxiety! Surely something must be wrong. Or, on the other hand, is that what I'm supposed to think? I'll interrupt Bill.

I: "This all has a familiar ring to it."
Bill: "How do you mean?"
I: "You were alone and thinking about free time coming, eh?"
Bill: "Yeah, about vacation . . . Oh hell! Of course! Everytime I don't have someone laying the road out for me, it hits again, doesn't it? You know, I felt that begin when they posted the vacation schedules and . . ."

That is pretty much where Bill is right now. He has got a good idea of the patterns his anxieties follow, and he is getting quicker all the time about spotting their effects. What once would have taken us hours and hours to work through can now be disclosed in as brief an interchange as that we just had.

You see, Bill had a father who made things too simple for him. Bill was told when and how, as well as what, to do at every juncture of his life, from the time he was born until the time he left home, weeping and swearing, at 2:00 a.m. one week and three days after he graduated from college. Where Bill's father left off, the army took up six days later. It was not until Bill was out of the service and into graduate school that he had to begin choosing his own course of action. And, of course, he did not really do so then. What he did was to increase his skill in getting faculty members, older friends, and others to take up the reins. Then Bill married, and seven months later on a rainy afternoon he stumbled into my office.

But Bill is saying something now that he has had to do a lot of hard work to be able to express so succinctly:

"In one way I'm scared stiff of this vacation, and yet at the same time, I'm really looking forward to it. For one thing I want to use the time to get to know my girl friend, Janet, a whole lot better and to find out if she's really what I want. And, I want to . . ."

When Bill found out he was going to be a father himself, his whole shaky world fell apart. Not that any of a number of other possible jolts might not have done the trick. But for Bill, a father was someone who knew just how the world should go and what a person should do. In short, a father was something Bill was seeking, not something he had any thought of becoming. Beth, Bill's wife at the time, was so much a child herself that she got panicked by Bill's panic and took off for her parents' home and security. They never really tried to get together again. Nowadays, Bill sees the youngster regularly and with pleasure, but he's encouraged Beth to let the child make his stronger attachment to the new stepfather. Now, Janet is another cup of tea, as Bill himself recognizes.

"So she said she liked me a lot and enjoyed going out with me but she just wondered where I was going and, sort of kiddingly, if my intentions were serious. And, of course, that's just the point . . ."

And that is the point, as Bill knows so clearly now. He has worked through his old dependent way of living so many times, and he knows rather thoroughly how it came about. But what now? Where is he going? What does he stand for? What does he want? Who is he really? These are the questions Bill and his therapy—and his therapist—must now confront.

Symptom Psychology and Emergence Psychology

As we have seen in earlier pages, psychology and psychotherapy have been preoccupied with symptoms and pathology. We therapists have been most comfortable and voluble in dealing with and in describing what is wrong in a personality and what may be done to correct it. We have so many terms, theories, technologies of trouble. But all this proficiency and all this profusion have brought us to confront a new problem: what positive guidance can we offer the person who is no longer materially affected by deficiencies of adjustment but wants help to make the most of himself? This is, of course, the mission of ontogogy, as I have described it. In our discussion of actualization in Chapter 16 I illustrated some of the attainments of analytic therapy and goals of ontogogy. In discussing ontogogy in Chapter 19, I carried this further. Now in trying to extrapolate, we once again look at this issue of bringing support to the constructive phase of the work of helping a person realize his being.

As I indicated, this is a new problem, in a way. For much of the history of psychotherapy we assumed that if we but helped our patients clear away the influences which handicapped them, they would spontaneously put their healthiness to good and satisfying use. Indeed, if a patient completed therapy and still felt any need for further help, it would be suggested that he had an unworked-through transference or residual conflicts or an unanalyzed character problem or some other technical-sounding thing which simply meant the patient should have more of the same therapy he had had up to this point.

Now, of course, this was and is certainly true in some instances. In fact, I think I could defend the thesis that one could spend a lifetime in successful psychotherapy. By that I mean that one could continually find further problems and concerns to work on no matter how long or thoroughly he had worked in his therapy up to any given time. Only the dianetics people, in their naivete, speak of achieving "clears."

But the fact that therapy could be interminable does not by any means demonstrate that it should be. Indeed, most of us would feel that undue prolongation of therapy may be a disorder of patient and therapist alike. Nevertheless, there is a significant contribution to be made to people like Bill by a consultant—I am purposely avoiding such terms as "therapist" and "counselor" here—by a consultant who can aid Bill in learning to actualize his potential more fully and satisfyingly.

THE ONTOGOGIC MODEL

Let us illustrate this point by a simple analogy. If I were an economic consultant and Bill came to me because his personal finances were in chaos, I could certainly help him get his accounts in order, his bank balance reconciled, his indebtedness planned for. In this way I could help him get current and out of difficulty. Further, I might help him work out a budget realistically related to his income so that he would not have the same difficulties again. All this would be useful and worthwhile for Bill and for society. But Bill might well say at this point, "Yes, you've helped me to get my affairs in order, and I'm not apt to go in debt again, but I need a further type of counsel from you. I can see that, now my finances aren't so jumbled, I'm going to have a modest sum to invest. How about helping me learn to select profitable ways of investing?"

Within the psychological realm this is exactly what Bill is asking implicitly. Listen to him.

> For some reason I woke up early yesterday morning. I don't know why, but anyway I'm glad I did. It must have been about 5:30 or 6:00, and the birds were terrifically busy. The air was so full of sunlight and bird-sounds, and I just felt kind of fresh and ready and . . . And inside me someplace it still feels like that—full of the new morning. Oh, I have other feelings too, like the jitters I told you about. But still I feel kind of eager to have my day and to try out what I'm about.

We psychologists have arrived at the point at which we must go beyond our exclusive preoccupation with psychological deficit and try to explore the whole new realm of psychological abundance. It is probably a tribute to our evolving effectiveness in psychology and psychotherapy that we have reached a stage where it may pay diminishing returns and we have need of new concepts and new tools. I, personally, am excited by the prospect of venturing into a whole new area of human experience, an area which I strongly suspect may contain greater potentials for revolutionizing all we know of daily living and being than any of the discoveries of the physical sciences.

POSITIVE PRODUCTS OF THERAPY

I want to describe four observations about the attributes of being psychologically healthy, of truly realizing one's being, of emerging as a man. For ease in reference, I will call these: presence, valuing the full emotional range, artistry in living, and dynamic awareness of being.

These four, it will be recognized, are drawn from a contrasting angle to those characteristics of the life-actualizing person that we reviewed in Chapter 16. The present four are intended to provide us with a general sense of emergent being more than with specific technical observations.

It is my hope that in this way you will be aided to share with me the sense of fascination in exploring the human potential. These are very modest explorations, to be sure, but they are first steps that may give us a starting point for further extrapolations later in the next chapter. At this point we are still securely founded on observations of actual people. Later we will cast off for wider horizons.

PRESENCE

I have already described the significance existentialists assign to this term, but let me restate it to make evident the particular coloring which I here want to emphasize. Presence is the quality of immediate awareness in which one knows directly his own being in relation to his situation. By "knows directly" we mean to indicate an implicit awareness, an intuition, as contrasted with a reflexive observation. In terms we have developed earlier, we are speaking of *I-process* awareness as opposed to *Self* awareness. Presence is "being there" (*dasein*) in the purest sense. But I am getting ahead of the story. Let us pause a moment and listen to Ed. Ed, an intelligent man in his middle years, effective in his profession, is oppressed by a sense of emptiness and loneliness that his professional accomplishments and his family cannot offset. He is talking now about a recognition that is increasingly occupying his thoughts in recent weeks:

> You get so busy that you don't notice how the children are growing, and it's a surprise to wake up and find they're growing up, not little kids any more. And the time's just gone. Sometimes it's kind of frightening, but it doesn't last long because there's too much to do.

Do you understand him? What is he saying? Well, he is lamenting the way his children are growing up, and he is not having a real relationship with them. Whose children? Who is not having a relation? Now listen to what he said again:

> You get so busy that you don't notice how the children are growing, and it's a surprise to wake up and find they're growing up, not little kids any more. And the time's just gone. Sometimes it's kind of frightening, but it doesn't last long because there's too much to do.

The astonishing thing about this statement is that here is a man talking about his own deepest emotional longings and fears and yet he does not explicitly refer to himself once! Instead he talks about "you" and "it" and otherwise so phrases his description of his experience that it is impersonal and we must infer that it is Ed himself he tells us about and that it really matters very much to Ed.

A mere coincidence, you say. A trick of language, a style of speech. No! I do not think so. This man, and so very many of us, show in this fashion our loss of genuine awareness, our alienation from our being, our impotency in our own lives.

ALIENATION

Hold on a minute. I want to be quite clear. I do not maintain that if we but teach him to speak in the first person he will become more genuine and thus regain presence in living. He did not lose his presence because of the way he spoke. Rather his alienation is reflected in his speech.

And what is this alienation? It is the very thing of which Ed is complaining in the segment I quoted: he is lost to himself and his family in his work. He feels unable to meet the passage of time in an autonomous way, and he accepts the narcotic of work to ease the fear his sense of loss would otherwise arouse.

Listen to Ed's words, not in terms of the ideas they convey on the surface, but listen to them in terms of the kind of picture of himself and his world they most literally imply. "You get so busy . . ." he says. Clearly the "you" is himself, but equally clearly Ed does not feel at one with himself but rather tends to look at himself much as would another person. This detachment becomes even more apparent as Ed says "It's a surprise to wake up and find they're growing up . . ." Ed speaks as though the surprise were occurring someplace else and he had just happened to notice it. And so we could go on taking apart this simple everyday statement to show how it portrays Ed's feeling of being only another object in the world, how it dramatizes his sense of impotency to change the influences of forces external to him—the passage of time, the effects of his work. Indeed, Ed speaks of his own anxiety with the same passivity with which he regards the maturing of his children.

THE LOSS OF SUBJECTIVE PRESENCE

Is Ed exceptional? By no means. Listen to people talk at the next meeting you attend. Listen to yourself at lunch tomorrow. Note how often you substitute the third person for the first, how much you emphasize reasons and logic when dealing with your emotions, how readily you point to externals and objective facts when really characterizing your personal and subjective experience, and how readily you deny or dismiss your own feelings when arguing a point in which you are concerned.

Surely some will be protesting by now, "But time's movement is inevitable; children do grow up; work does make demands." Of course, that is right. But that is not the point. The point is not time's movement, but Ed's living time, Ed's opportunity to have his life and his experience of his children. Again, the point is not that children grow, but that Ed's children are growing, and his time of opportunity to be with them is moving past. The point is not that certain processes do go on whether we like it or not but that we so often regard our own being as such an external, immutable process as well.

And then some surely are protesting, "What does he want? Shall we ignore reality and go around acting only on our feelings all the time? You can't build a house or drive a car or run a bank without being able to keep your emotions out of things."

Well that's a moot point and one I would enjoy arguing some time. But right now it is not the point in question. The point is that Ed's alienation arises from the fact that he tries to live his own life as though he were building a house or driving a car or running a bank; in other words he tries to live his life by manipulating himself from the outside. He reminds me of the story of some primitive people who with great effort moved the large unfamiliar object the missionary had brought back from furlough. They struggled through the night to carry it a half mile from the railroad to his home so that he would be pleased and surprised when he woke up in the morning. He was surprised indeed. He was also terribly embarrassed to drive the object, a jeep he had so looked forward to using!

To put the matter at its simplest: we may question the immediate pertinence to letting our own subjective feelings importantly influence a decision about truly objective matters such as the kind of steel to use in a new bridge, but it is ridiculous and even tragic when we treat ourselves and our own lives in this same impersonal way.

RECLAIMING OUR LIVES

The emergent person is jealous of his own presence in his own life. That is to say, he seeks to know as fully as possible what it is he is doing, what is his role in bringing about the experiences he has and what the feelings are that he undergoes. We can make a hypothetical statement for such a person to contrast with Ed's statement. It would probably read something like this:

> I allowed myself to become so busy that I wasn't aware of how my children were growing. I was surprised to wake up and find they are growing up, to realize they're not little kids any more. I let my time go by. It's frightening to me that I have done so. It's frightening to me that I might do so again, but I am going to cherish my fear to help me keep alert so that I miss no more of my children's lives or of my share in them.

I trust it is apparent how much more the possibility of producing the desired change is implicit in this statement than in the alienated one quoted from Ed.

EMOTIONAL FULLNESS

We have seen in the case of Ed how he might come to value his feeling of fear that arose from recognizing how he had missed having more part in his children's growing up. The idea of valuing the entire range of our emotions from the most unpleasant to the most satisfying may seem strange to some. And yet I am convinced that the more a person is truly actualizing his being, then the more he is open to and appreciative of the entire range of his emotions.

A simple analogy may illustrate this point: If I am piloting a plane and certain gauges give me unwelcome information, such as that the wing is icing or that there is undue heat in a certain motor, I would be foolish indeed to disconnect those meters which inform me of these facts. It would be ridiculous to argue, "Well, what they tell me makes me uncomfortable; therefore I'll cut them off." I am sure the parallel that I have in mind is evident. When we suppress awareness of pain or fear or any other emotion, we run a similar risk of depriving ourselves of information essential to our well being.

Every once in a while one reads of a child born without a sense of pain. It is no surprise to learn that such an infant has a very poor life expectancy. Far from being freed from a curse, he is condemned and cursed indeed in having no proper warning system to use in self-protection. Those of us who are successful in suppressing an emotion, say our sense of fear, place ourselves in similar jeopardy. Thus the emergent Ed wisely says, "I am going to cherish my fear to help me keep alert so that I miss no more of my children's lives and my share in them."

THE ORIENTING FUNCTION OF FEELING

There is a further advantage to cherishing the entire emotional range. In one sense we can think that ultimately each of us is most motivated, not by reason, but by feelings, that what we seek is feeling a state of pleasure, of comfort, of realization or achievement, or of quiet presence. Whatever the names given to the feelings, these seem in their way more ultimate than all the reasons, all the logic that may serve us on our way to the feeling state. This is true even of the martyr who may undergo a hell of feelings in order to maintain what for him is even more important, the feeling of being faithful to himself and to that in which he believes. When we have clear awareness of all of our own feelings readily available, we are enabled to make sounder choices and follow through on those choices more dependably.

Still another healthful gain in cherishing the range of our feelings is that in this fashion our reality awareness is heightened. It can safely be said that much of the distortion of reality characteristic of neurosis is brought about by the attempt to deny or alter certain feelings the person fears to have. When he seeks to avoid the painful emotion, he often finds himself distorting what is real about himself and his world. In this way new confusion and new needs to distort are produced. Listen to Zelda, who after many hours of therapy, now has insight into this pattern:

> I can see now how it happened. I was so afraid my husband would treat me like my father did my mother. Dad was always finding fault with Mom's cooking, and I know he hurt her a lot. So I never dared show my husband how much I wanted to be a good wife and cook well. I always had to pretend it didn't matter, but pretty soon I began to lose interest in cooking and get restless and irritable around mealtimes. My husband never could understand why I got stomach trouble, but I guess it was just one thing leading to another.

And indeed that is the story. One distortion leads to another, and increasingly the sense of presence in one's own life and the feeling of vitality in one's own experience get lost.

The emergent man values a wide range of emotional potential that provides him with significant information by which to orient himself, that makes possible life decisions on which he can follow through responsibly, and that helps him to keep his awareness open and undistorted. Needless to say, too, such an emotional range gives life more color and meaning. Who would want to read a novel in which no feelings but happy ones were portrayed?

THE "COOL" OUTLOOK

Perhaps I can make my point even clearer by setting it in contrast to what we can think of as the "philosophy of cool." Evidently originating with jazz musicians and spreading through the beatnik groups, this perversion of self-discipline is now much admired among some people. The philosophy of cool devalues emotional involvement and emotional expression. It urges detachment and evenness of attitude.

> Peggy is a member of the young artists' community. They are no longer required to wear the uniform of sandals, dirty clothes, and stringy hair or straggly beards, but otherwise they are still heavily constrained to conformity in their nonconformity. But Peggy has a problem: She really likes art.

She gets excited by people and ideas. She is kinetic and expressive. As she tells me about it, "I just don't seem to have any cool at all. We get to talking about some of the new approaches to painting, and I get all wound up, and pretty soon I realize I've lost my cool. It's so maddening."

Poor Peggy suffers because she has a healthy response to what she likes! Now, of course, Peggy's problem is not her "loss of cool." It is her acceptance of such an inauthentic standard that she tries to cripple herself emotionally to gain a transitory acceptance. The analogy is inescapable to the way aristocratic parents in old China for style and social acceptance bound their infant daughters' feet and thus crippled them.

The philosophy of cool is not new. When I was an early adolescent, my ideal was a movie actor who personified the same distorted value. He would sit, meticulously placing his finger tips together, while the most horrendous news was given him. His manservant might announce something like, "I beg your pardon, sir, the house is on fire and your family has deserted you, taking with them your entire fortune." At which our hero would smile distantly and say, "Ah yes, thank you, Jarvis, and now bring in the tea, will you?" It wasn't until many years later that I saw in real life such a person. They are to be found in every mental hospital, of course. They are quite schizophrenic.

The cool philosophy is a schizophrenic philosophy. Only death is truly cool. Life is warm, even hot. Full life is expressive, dynamic, involved; not detached and distant. Emergent Man may not grow excited over the Beatles, but he will bring his whole being, including his emotions, to that in which he does choose to invest himself.

Artistry in Living

It has been said of Benjamin Franklin that he had "an infinite talent for being interrupted." Certainly such a man, who was exceptional in so many fields—scientific investigation, journalism, politics, and statesmanship, international relations, and commercial endeavors (not to mention his romantic forays)—certainly such a man needed to be able to move from one task to another without loss of efficiency. Yet I would suggest that Benjamin Franklin probably did not experience interruptions as such, but rather he saw himself moving from one thing to the next among various activities, each of which awaited his touch. A pianist changing from playing in a treble octave to playing in a bass would not feel the change was an interruption.

Perhaps the secret of a man such a Franklin is that for him his various activities were arrayed about him so that he might touch and bring to life first this and then that. Thus, much as a musician might with his instrument, so Franklin in his life could display the same sense of artistry and wholeness. We might think of it this way: Franklin could move from ambassadoring to inventing to romancing with ease because basically he was Franklin-ing all the time, because basically he was expressing his being through these various means all the time. People who have had a successful psychotherapeutic experience or those people who without this experience demonstrate richness of personal living show a kind of artistry, a type of beauty in the manner in which they arrange their lives. Typically we are impressed with such a person's ability to select, to act from choice rather than from compulsion; typically there is a sense of the harmony among the various parts of such a person's living.

It seems to me that in this way Franklin would be able to bring more of himself to bear on each of his tasks, whether the inventing or the ambassadoring, because he did not experience leaving part of himself behind with one when he turned to the other. Rather he could concentrate, focus his entire capacity on each one, as he chose to express his being through that one at any given moment.

THE CONTRIBUTION OF THE UNCONSCIOUS

This hypothesis is consonant with an observation often made of creative people: it is reported that the creative person has the capacity to work at a problem with great intensity until he hits a snag. Then he "turns it over to his unconscious" while he undertakes something else. Later when he picks up the blocked task again, he often finds that he has new insights into its solution which are clearly the product of unconscious work during the recess from conscious effort. I am confident that the creative person, the emergent personality, is one who makes rich and frequent use of the resources of both conscious and unconscious life.

"BACKING" INTO LIFE

An example to set in contrast to that of Franklin is provided by a man who had great difficulty talking to me when he began his therapy.

> I really want to be a good husband, you know . . . But I guess everyone says that, you know, and so it doesn't . . . What I mean is—You know, I wish I'd quit saying "I mean" and "You know" all the time. It sounds so stupid. And I don't want to sound stupid, but sometimes I think I am. Well, I don't really think I am, but I do kind of wonder, you know . . .

And so Richard would go on until he had just about torn himself apart with his constant need to interrupt and correct himself. We can speak of his obsessive-compulsive character defenses, but we will have only put a name to a very painful and destructive process. Whatever else might have been true of Richard, he was not stupid, but his terrible struggle within himself often reduced him to a kind of stupidity.

I have said that Franklin had an apparent capacity to be interrupted without loss of effectiveness because he probably was Franklin-ing all along and because the aspects of his life were arrayed before him like the keyboard of a musical instrument. In contrast, Richard is constantly interrupted, with an almost complete loss of effectiveness at times, because he is unable to be Richard-ing. By this awkward phrasing I mean to point to the fact that Richard is for himself only an object, a *Self*. He is so busy looking at that object and trying to make it right that there is no experience of being the subject of his life. Franklin, rather clearly, was the subject who did things in his own life. This makes the crucial difference.

Remember the old poem?

> A centipede was happy quite
> Until a frog in fun
> Said, "Pray, which leg comes after which?"
> Which raised her mind to such a pitch
> She fell distracted in a ditch
> Considering how to run.   (Craster, 1937)

Where Franklin was a musician, an artist composing an esthetic production of his life, Richard is striking only discords and producing a miserable verbal jangle.

Dynamic Awareness of Being

Richard provided us with an example of a kind of static self-awareness which can only follow haplessly along trying to correct that which has already occurred against one's desires. Were it not so tragic, it would be humorous, rather like a Dr. Seuss creature that has a whisk broom for a tail and constantly wipes out its trail wherever it goes. Many patients when they come to therapy are fearful of what they will learn about themselves, even though they may not show as extreme a pattern as did Richard. Listen, for example, to Pete.

> I have thought about coming to see you for a long time. I know I need to, but frankly I've been scared. I've read about the unconscious, and I know there are things about myself I don't know, and sometimes I don't know whether it would be good to know them. I'm afraid of what I might find, what you may tell me about myself that I don't want to know.

Listen to Nell.

> It's funny, as I lie here on the couch I listen to see if you will say anything and hope that you're going to tell me something that will help me clear things up. But just as much as I hope, I'm afraid you're going to tell me something. Every time you start to speak, I tense up. It's like I'm saying to myself, "Now he's going to let me have it. Now he's going to tell me what I've always been afraid I'd find out about myself." And I don't even know what that is!

IMPOTENCY IN BEING

Pete and Nell and many of us fear the disclosure of what is secret even from ourselves. It is as though some terrible truth would be revealed that would be devastating to accept. There is implicit in such fear the same sort of helplessness that we have heard in the other observations we have been making about our ways of being. Pete and Nell say, in effect, "When you show me what's true of me, I'll have no recourse but to accept it as lastingly so. I have no hope that I can be different whether I like what you disclose to me or not."

At first blush this seems a strange thing for a person engaged in the process of psychotherapy to say. But all too often the patient has been so thoroughly indoctrinated with the picture of himself as the pawn of forces greater than himself, that he sees psychotherapy only as an opportunity to get solace. He braces himself for grim knowledge or the need to make bitter compromises with reality. When a patient comes into his own in a successful psychotherapeutic course, he changes this concept, he changes his way of looking at himself. Listen now to Gordon.

> For such a long time I was afraid of what I would discover in therapy. I thought you'd tell me or I'd find out all sorts of bad things, frightening things about myself. Now I can see that it isn't that way at all, that I am creating myself every day. I know now that I'm not something fixed and unchangeable, and besides I've got something to say about who or what I am. It's really kind of exciting.

CREATIVITY IN BEING

Gordon has caught the essence of it, as few do. He is coming to realize that living, at its most real, is a creative process. It is an artistic process in which in some measure we choose our way of being at each moment. Psychotherapy is not a matter of discovering static, predetermined facts about oneself. Rather, truly useful, intensive psychotherapy has almost the contrary aim: it seeks to release the person from the static *Self* to realize his true freedom.

This is a difficult understanding to come by. You and I have learned to think of ourselves and other people as being thus and so: bright or stupid, friendly or unpleasant, talkative or shy, and so on. And so people are. But partly they are so because they were taught just as we were, because they feel that is the way a person should be. It does seem to simplify what might be confusing if everybody kept changing all the time.

But, then, of course, that is just what everybody does do. Everybody *is* changing all the time. Just as the physiologists tell us all cells in our bodies are replaced each seven years or so, so the psychological aspects of us are in some change at all times.

Perhaps I can make the point more clear if I move to an example from a different area. Ask the question, "What is the Mississippi River?" We may answer, "It's the greatest river in North America." True, but what *is* the Mississippi River? Is it the water that at this moment is in the river? No, just observing the way we phrased our question distinguishes the water from the river. Is it the bed in which the river flows? No, again it is not so. Just as the water which is in the river today will be gone a year hence, though the Mississippi River will still remain; just as the channel or bed of the river will be changed by the Corps of Engineers or by nature, and still the Mississippi River exists—so it is with us, with me. What am I? The essence of my being cannot be pinned to any one palpable extension of my being. I am the process of I. I am the I-ing!—the ongoingness, the essence expressed in my existence. Not with Descartes' self-as-object inferring, "I doubt; hence I think. I think; hence I am." Rather, partaking of the very process of creation, "I am that I am!"

AWAKENED AWARENESS

As we draw toward closing this chapter, let us return to Bill, about whom I told you first. Bill is putting on his coat at the end of the session, when he pauses right in the middle. For at least twenty seconds it is quiet as he looks at me so very intently. Then Bill says all I have been trying to say, and he says it very simply.

> The other day I went to visit my dad. I hadn't seen him in quite a while. I was so mad at him for so long, you know. And I was startled because I really saw him for the first time in my whole life. Do you know, he's scared. Really scared. He's chased so many people away from him, and now he's scared. And I was sorry, and I told him so. For a minute, I thought we were going to have a fight. Then he just took my hand and squeezed it. And, it may sound kind of silly, but right then we became friends for the first time. Now I'm my own man. And sometimes I'm frightened too. But I'm ready to be frightened because I'll be a lot more than that too.

23 — Beyond the human frontier

Our journeys on the human frontier thus far have always been modest explorations into the speculative areas, within sight of established psychological and psychotherapeutic positions. Most of what we have hypothesized that is original has had the founding, at least, of clinical observation or theoretical argumentation. It has been my hope that in this way what I would write would be most useful to the psychotherapist and most accessible to readers in general.

Now, as we draw to a close, I want to loose the reins on my imagining and venture much further into the *terra incognita* that lies beyond the human frontier. I want to extrapolate more boldly about where man is going and what man may become. I want clearly to set these ideas outside of the systematic thinking of previous chapters, especially those in Part Three. In those discussions I was trying to achieve a first measure of technical precision or orderliness, to set forth, at least, a vocabulary for further communication. Here, I have no such intent. Here I hope to freewheel without regard to getting others to pick up from any of these specific ideas and without any commitment to do so myself. I do hope, however, others will be encouraged to undertake their own speculations on the same basic question.

In the previous chapter I used the caption, "Emergent Man," to convey the idea of man released from captivity or constraint and emerging into fuller being. This same concept of emergence is implicit in this chapter, although I will now try to carry it much further. I am not as much interested in adding something to the human endowment as I am fascinated with the liberation of what is already potential or latent. Plato's Allegory of the Cave expresses well what I have in mind. His dwellers in the cave saw only the shadows on the wall. But in time some sought and found their way to the mouth of the cave, and some at long last emerged into the sunlight of full day and saw themselves and each other as full-bodied, colorfully alive, and mutually aware beings.

Now doubtlessly some will protest that Plato was an essentialist and the cave allegory speaks of the ideal as opposed to the existential. So it is, to my mind, with all such categories. Eventually we must transcend them, or they will strangle us. If I write of essences in an existential orientation, I am well content.

PLAN OF CHAPTER

I will divide my presentation into two phases. First, I will speculate about further levels of personal emergence. What would emergent man be like in terms of his inner life and in terms of the culture he would bring into being? How would that culture contrast with the one we know? Then I will offer a few tentative thoughts about the further meanings of the observations and speculations otherwise reported. Here my intent will be to "stretch" our thinking as far as I can at this time. We will be venturing over the border into the realm of metaphysics, but that cannot be helped. Only time will tell whether that is a more advanced or more primitive kingdom than our more familiar land of psychological science.

Further Levels of Emergence

Thus far we have talked of emergence as it is demonstrated in the lives of those who have had a successful psychotherapeutic course. But this is, perforce, a limited perspective. Indeed, we may surmise that our achievements are not apt to outrun our imaginations, while more courageous imagining may prepare the way for greater achievements.

In this section we will take the values and experiences we have found to characterize those who actualize their lives more fully and let our fancy imagine these magnified in individuals and generally shared by most people in the culture. What would the inner life of a more truly life-actualizing person be like? If most people were actualizing more of their potentials, what would their social world be like? Which institutions that we know would survive, which would be changed, what new ones might arise (Sykes, 1962)?

The Inner Life of Emergent Man

What would the inner experience of emergent man be like? Can we extrapolate from our own more liberated hours, from the perspectives glimpsed during the peak experiences, and from blendings of our reason and our fantasy to speculate on the values that would be important, the functioning of awareness that would be attained, and the forms participation would take in the truly emergent man? This will be our attempt in the following paragraphs.

AUTHENTICITY-CENTERED VALUES

For emergent man the key value is authenticity. First of all he would ask "Is it real?" meaning by "real" that which is in accord with our best understanding of the givenness of the human condition. Emergent man would simply not be interested in that which pretended vitality but was inherently a violation of actuality. Statements such as the following are such violations.

> Don't let bad breath hinder your career.
> He ought to be ashamed to feel that way.
> This lipstick will make you more lovable.
> Nice girls don't even know about such things.
> She was so brave; she didn't even cry.
> If he weren't so lazy, he'd be more successful.
> Anything worth doing at all is worth doing as well as possible.
> If you want to be a better person, you have to keep trying as hard as you can all the time.
> If you loved me, you wouldn't say that.

The list could be extended endlessly. To emergent man these views would be at least as incomprehensible as to us is the idea that the elongated necks or distorted lips of certain primitive peoples are evidences of beauty or desirability.

DECLINE OF MANY CURRENT VALUES

A great many values now compete for our allegiance. They range from the seemingly trivial to the most existential, but often there is too little recognition of their differential significance. The result is that today we live in a value anarchy. This situation is heightened by a fallacious egalitarianism that proclaims one value as valuable as the next and that is, in itself, a distortion of the value of autonomy. This distorted autonomy makes us fearful of the responsibility to be explicit about the judgments we all make privately. It leads to all sorts of dodges and devices to try to "objectify" value judgments through having rules and criteria make the decisions rather than people. A mature, life-actualizing person would certainly discard such subterfuges and accept—even demand—the birthright of his own aware choice.

Equally certainly such a person would find little meaning in such values as popularity, superficial sex appeal, having the newest, the biggest, the loudest, the shiniest, and so on, where these qualities had no intrinsic significance to that which they described. So much is easily understood, for such attractions are little valued by many today. However, when we extend the list of apparently extraneous-to-life values we come into realms more jealously retained: ambition, aggressiveness, thoughtfulness, consistency, courtesy, cleanliness, neatness, organization, efficiency, economy, simplicity, complexity, colorfulness, rapidity, certainty, generality, concreteness, practicality, and so on. All of these are often regarded by many of us as values *in themselves*. ("Why did you do that?" "Because it was the most efficient thing to do.") None of these is truly an ontologic value in itself. Each may be a valued attribute of an action or situation that is authentically important and thus lends value to the attribute. ("To save the trapped miner, we used the most efficient methods available.")

FANTASY

However, to say that authenticity would be a prime value for emergent man is not to say that he would devalue fantasy and imagination. Probably, quite to the contrary, he would see in fantasy a way of exploring possibilities, a way of building esthetically pleasing contrasts and complements to the more tangibly actual, and a way of stretching and celebrating the freedom of awareness. Fantasy, so used, is authentic, for it is used as that which it is in actuality, rather than as a substitute for unwanted actuality. It is my belief that emergent man would greatly value fantasy when used in this way, which gives to authenticity an added dimension and richness.

SUCHNESS

In one sense the only emergent value would be authenticity, but already we have illustrated the perception that authenticity has many facets. Another aspect that would be much valued would be suchness. The person who has mounted to a high mountain peak and seen spread out around him so much of the world has the opportunity to know something of suchness. If the person has climbed, rather than ridden, to that vantage point, if he can look silently without trying to identify landmarks or compute distances, then he is even more likely to know suchness. If, finally, he has wanted no conversation, has let his eyes go slightly out of focus with distance, has found his awareness of the scene somehow slipping away and returning as he let go of conscious thought about the scene, then he is most likely to have been part of suchness. And yet we cannot write the definitive specifications. Those would have to do with the silent communion of the viewer and the view, in which the difference between them is overcome and they become one.

Microcosm and Macrocosm. Suchness is not, however, only the panoramic view. The contemplation of a drop of water, a hand, a curl of dust, a single leaf—any of these or any other thing can be the doorway to the experience of suchness. The many stories of the seemingly odd actions of the Zen master often portray this fact. Similarly, a passage quoted by Suzuki makes the point even more explicitly:

> As soon as one particle of dust is raised, the great earth manifests itself there in its entirety. In one lion are revealed millions of lions, and in millions of lions is revealed one lion. Thousands and thousands of them there are indeed, but know ye just one, only one (Barrett, 1956, p. 24).

Suchness in the Event. Still we must recognize that suchness is not an exercise in the relations of the general and the particular. It is not the contemplation of a majestic panorama or an insignificant bit of dirt. Suchness is the aware opening of one's being to the givenness of all being in which the gap between one's own being and all being is transcended. Thus suchness may be the experience of an event or action. In a game of tennis when the ball comes over the net to the player, he may so experience the speeding ball, himself and his racquet, the court and net, his opponent, the light and the wind, that he returns the ball smoothly, esthetically, elegantly, and without concentrated thought. This expresses suchness also. So with a driver rounding a curve at high speed but with full awareness, with a ballet dancer leaping freely with the swell of the music, with a jazz musician improvising a chorus, and with a father and his child in play. In suchness we transcend apartness and know oneness without straining, without thought, without *Self*-consciousness.

FREEDOM OF AWARENESS

The viewer on the mountain, whom we described above, can most give himself to the view when his awareness is most open or free. Freed of bondage to a *Self*, such a person can attend totally to the experience of the moment. It is almost impossible for most of us to grasp fully just what such awareness would be like. To look out at a panorama with total awareness, with all one's awareness being devoted to the intercourse with the panorama, this is an experience few have had. Our usual awareness is so busy with concerns about the *Self*. ("I wonder just how high this peak is? Is that the Colorado River? I must remember to tell Mary about this. There's haze in the south. I might have seen further except for that. Maybe I'd better leave before it turns cold. Oh, I'm enjoying this view so much. I wonder if I could write about it. How magnificent the mountains are. Make me feel so insignificant. Maybe I should say a little prayer. Oh, there's a plane, and it's below me! . . . ") Now, I do not mean to burlesque unduly our viewer's stream of consciousness. I am sure a genuine recording for any of us would be very similar. Like a poorly tuned radio, so much is going on that it is hard to hear the main signal. Many of the other stations are sending out worthwhile broadcasts, but they "jam" the one we intend hearing. So our awareness need not be of the ostensibly petty or narrowly selfish kind, and yet it keeps us from the kind of total awareness that emergent man would have.

I have purposely used the phrase "awareness being devoted to the intercourse with the panorama" to take advantage of the graphic meaning of that term. It is important to recognize that full awareness is a kind of interpenetration with that to which we attend. This is the element of suchness that is evidenced when we overcome the separation between observer and observed. Full awareness transcends the subject–object dichotomy.

CREATIVE EMPTINESS

As much as I have said about the bondage of the *I-process* to the *Self*, I find my own awareness continually encountering further instances of how pervasive that bondage indeed is. To know my being in pure *I-process* terms, freed of the substantive qualities of the *Self*, still eludes me. Yet there is the potential for the ultimate creativeness in the very emptiness of the fact of being, in its openness to whatever we will write. Like the bird on fluid wing, we have no predetermined path nor does our passing so mark the freedom that we are then constrained. Alan Watts in a memorable sentence summarizes this well: "Where he expected to find the specific truth about himself he found freedom, but mistook it for mere nothingness" (1958, p. 154). This is the tragedy of our limited awareness, our seeking for the very categories of being that would imprison us.

This quotation from Watts is a part of a longer statement in which he makes evident the inauthentic "role-playing" in which most of us engage and the sense of being lost that can come when we try to stop the role-playing without having awareness of our more authentic being.

> Anyone who becomes conscious of role-playing will swiftly discover that just about all his attitudes are roles, that he cannot find out what he is genuinely, and is therefore at a loss what to do to express himself sincerely. Thereupon he is self-conscious and blocked in his relationships, finding himself in the double-bind predicament where every road is closed. This leaves him in a state of complete paralysis if he persists in thinking that there is some "right" course of action and some

particular set of feelings which constitute his real self. Where he expected to find the specific truth about himself he found freedom, but mistook it for mere nothingness. For human freedom does indeed comprise an order, yet because it is the nonlinear order of *li* and of the Tao, it cannot be classified; it cannot be identified with any particular role. Therefore at this point of the double bind he must wait, and see what happens of itself, spontaneously. He will find that the sensation that every road is barred abruptly switches into the sensation that every road is open. He can play all roles, just as in Hindu mythology the true self is pictured as the godhead acting all the parts of the multitude of finite creatures (Watts, 1958, 153–154).

CONSTRUING OUR EXPERIENCE

A person is not a thing. An event is not a thing. We have falsely assumed that the essential natures of persons, events, and things were the same. In Chapter 11 I demonstrated that a person is best understood in his essential being if we think of the *I-process*. The *I-process* stands for the *I*, for the pure subject of being. Things are objects. The *I-process*, when authentically regarded, is never an object. An event, similarly, is not truly an object or a thing. An event is a relation between objects or between the *I-process* and an object (thing) or between two or more *I-processes* (persons).

So understood, it will be recognized that events have only relationship qualities and not absolute, inherent, or intrinsic qualities. The nature of an event lies in the subjects and objects it relates, not in the event itself. A frequent demonstration of this that every clinical worker in the humanistic areas knows is that experienced when first one and then the other partner in a marital couple is seen.

> Mary Jane described the dispute with Darryl with the utmost sincerity and great feelings of hurt and disappointment. She tried her best to be fair, recognized how she may have overreacted, and ended with a bitter question, "I thought he loved me; yet if he did, how could he treat me that way?" Listening to her the counselor could not help but wonder at Darryl's blindness and cruelty.
>
> The next day Darryl told of the same dispute. At least, so the counselor reminded himself, it was supposed to be the same dispute. Darryl's account showed how with loving patience he had tried to forestall the unhappiness, how he had

exercised great self-control because of his love for Mary Jane, and how, finally, he had struck back only because of excessive provocation. He asked, "If she loved me, how could she act that way?"

It will not do to think that Darryl or Mary Jane is lying or even that they are chiefly self-deceived. There may be some element of falsehood in their accounts, but it is trivial. There probably are appreciable amounts of resistive distortion in both of their perceptions, but these do not explain the differences fully. We must recognize that events are not things. What happened in the dispute between Mary Jane and Darryl does not truly exist in the abstract. What happened is what Mary Jane said and what Darryl said. If we work with them analytically and reduce their resistances, we will learn new accounts of what happened. These new accounts will also be "true." (See the discussion of explanations on pages 228 to 231.)

We construe the meanings of events out of who we are and what the objects involved in the event are. Those meanings then change as we change. This is the creative potential of our awareness. As George A. Kelly beautifully puts it, "The key to man's destiny is his ability to reconstrue what he cannot deny."

An Emergent Society

In a society of Emergent Man the social institutions with which we are familiar—education, religion, government, business, science, the arts, entertainment, the healing arts, the military—would certainly be materially revised in every instance. I cannot think of one that would survive unchanged. This is not really surprising if we think of institutions as the instruments of common human purposes. Changes in human purposes and values should certainly then be reflected in changes in the institutional instruments. On the other hand, as an indication of the extent to which our present values and their institutional extensions tend to be oriented inauthentically, this is a shocking state of affairs.

I propose to devote several pages to speculations about the changes that seem to me most probable in a culture that was truly oriented around what we have been developing as existential values: rootedness and faith, identity and commitment, meaningfulness and creativity, and relatedness and love. These values would be expressed through the more operational values I have described in the preceding section: authenticity, free fantasy, suchness, open awareness, and creative emptiness.

GOVERNMENT AND INTERNATIONAL RELATIONS

Why have we turned over so much of our lives and our futures to those in politics and government? Why do we give them control, not only of government, but of our hopes, our being with others, our money, our thoughts, and even our lives? Is it not astounding that we let but one aspect of our lives, the relations obtaining between the groupings of people by where they live (which we call nationalities), preempt every other aspect—social, physical, spiritual, and even the preservation of our species? Of course, each side will say that the other threatens all of these. But to the extent this is true, it is true only because man has so shrunk his recognition of himself and of his world that this distortion is generally accepted.

It would be as sensible to agree that the loser in the next Olympics should commit national suicide as that the loser in the Geneva negotiations should do so. No! It would be more sensible, for at least then the nonlosers would remain. There can be no nonlosers in the way we have redefined ourselves-and-our-world. We have constricted ourselves to our political-military dimensions and forgotten that we, Man, are so much more than this.

In some part, we may have done so because we vaguely recognize that the political-military dimension is our own creation and hope thereby to persuade ourselves it can be made to do our bidding and truly serve to comprehend world. Once man hazarded everything in the name of religion. Today we largely ignore religious beliefs and nonbeliefs in deference to the political-military conceptions of life. At another time trade and commerce provided the prevailing definition. They are now often explicitly devalued. If man survives another generation or so, perhaps a particular scientific conflict might be used to nullify our fears of unknowability and subsume our being.

What has the so-called "ideological conflict" between East and West to do with the many areas of nonconflict among men East and West. With laughter and love and growing and eating and sexuality and dying and hoping and praying and fearing and fathering-and-mothering and sickening and moving and belching and thinking and scratching and reading and listening to music and fighting and defecating and dreaming and singing and . . . ?

THE FALLACY OF FEAR AS A MOTIVATION

These musings about the international situation bring us to a second area in which an emergent society would surely contrast with our own. In our public lives one of the most frequently employed devices for bringing about a measure of control is the use of fear. "Do not commit murder, or the state will murder you. Pay your taxes, or the state will put you in jail. Vote, or the rascals will take over the country. Cross only at corners, or you'll be hit by a car. Do well in school, or you'll get a low grade. Wash your face, or people won't like you. Say your prayers, or God will punish you." The list could be extended indefinitely. The point that is overlooked too often, however, is that this is a list of failures also. Murder is commonplace. Many people cheat a bit on their taxes. A minority of citizens vote regularly. Students do not use their full potentials in the schools. And so on.

Fear is a heavily relied upon means for controlling other people. Fear ultimately fails wherever it is used. The record is nearly perfect.[1] Very little in psychology has caught up with this basic observation. Whenever fear is used to try to motivate people, it fails of its specific objectives every time. To be sure people will be

---
[1] This fundamental psychological fact was first brought forcibly to my attention by an editorial by John Campbell in a science-fiction magazine, not by a psychology professor or textbook. The latter tend to talk about fear as a motivator in terms of the behavior of rats in a maze and to ignore the thousands of years of recorded history of man's experimentation in life. I do not find the study of rat behavior the problem; rather it is the willful ignoring of so much human experience.

Psychology has been so concerned to be scientifically respectable that the authentic use of fantasy has only recently begun to occur in psychological circles (for example, Baker, 1963). Much excellent extrapolation from scientific roots has long been found in the physical sciences, but psychological science-fiction has not come from psychologists very often. Perhaps we may soon reach a point at which we can let our fantasy have freer play without fearing that we will lose our footing in reality or relax our firm grips on our membership cards in the American Association for the Advancement of Science.

moved to do something by fear, but seldom to do that which the fear-invoker intends. The manifest failure of fear to affect such familiar social phenomena as cigarette smoking, the production and possible use of atomic bombs, and the reckless use of automobiles is all too evident.

The failure is not only on the broad social scale. Parents who rely on fear as a way of training their children find again and again that they have taught much beyond what they expected or intended. The child who is prevented from normal sexual experimentation by fear is the one who is most apt to engage in distorted forms of sexual expression, including, but by no means limited to, the abnormality of abstinence. The child who represses his anger toward his parents because of fear is the one who ends up rebelling and rejecting them.

FORMS OF PSEUDO-CONFRONTATION

In Chapter 17 I described how the confrontation of our ontologic givenness and the existential anxiety attendant upon it acted as a pivotal point at which we would choose whether to make the response of courage and move toward authentic being or would make the response of dread and become enmeshed in inauthenticity. Most of us, at least in some part, take the latter course. Yet we seek to return to that confrontation and to choose again in more fulfilling ways. Anxiety, however, keeps us from doing so. In this conflict we turn to forms of pseudo-confrontation, which give us the vicarious experience of dealing with life more authentically but which we know will actually prevent a full, naked, coming up against contingency, responsibility, autonomy, and apartness.

Some of the main institutions we use in this way are the various forms of entertainment (including sports), religion in its institutionalized forms, and education. Let me be quite clear: I believe there are very authentic values served by entertainment, sports, religion, and education, but I think we also use each of these as a way of seeming to confront life while yet actually avoiding doing so.

ENTERTAINMENT

Fiction may be a vehicle for creating fresh meaning in appreciation of the human experience. Fiction has conveyed more truths about psychology than have all the textbooks. But much fiction falls far short of those exalted achievements. The typical television or motion picture "drama" or paperback novel is a way to sedate one's awareness by preoccupying it with what is manifestly only a fiction—and a fiction in which the limits of contingency are reasonably well known in advance. The viewer or reader has the comforting assurance that he will not be brought genuinely to face the unknown, while he is encouraged to deal with a simulation of the unknown through identification with the characters in the fiction. Contingency is shown as an outrageous monster who is miraculously overcome by the hero; responsibility can be mocked; autonomy is traded for bland conformity and popularity; and a caricature of love is eternally triumphant over apartness. An authentic society would have little place for such deceptions, which only debase the dignity of man.

SPORTS

Many sports, especially spectator sports, seem to be very similar in their effects to entertainment. They provide controlled and safe confrontations of contingency and autonomy especially, without encouraging a genuine dealing with life.

RELIGION

It is sad to have to say that many of the same comments apply to much of institutionalized religion. With emphasis upon buildings, numbers, budgets, and "objective indices" of the church's growth, the metaphysical meanings are lost. Far from helping the participants to greater awareness of their being, such religion offers palliatives and soporifics. Sometimes there is, as in much fiction, the spicing of mild proddings of guilt or anxiety, but usually even these are softened down to avoid real existential stirrings. To be sure, a new generation of the ministry seems to be trying to inject fresh vitality, but over-all the weight of dogma, tradition, and "practical considerations" makes it difficult indeed for any but the most dedicated to win free to present a religious message that leads toward real recognition of the need to confront our being in its most fundamental dimensions.

I want to add one thought about what seems to me to be a frequent error of clergymen who recognize the shallowness of much that passes for religion. They often, it seems to me, become punishing toward their congregations, acting out a reaction formation to the general slackness. This not infrequently takes the form of an emphasis on existential dread as though it were the basic given of the human condition. These men, in all earnestness, increase feelings of powerlessness, blame, meaninglessness, and isolation.

EDUCATION

Many of the things that I have been saying about entertainment and religion are, unfortunately, applicable to much of education. Education is offered and used, all too often, as a way of seeming to overcome contingency or of apparently discovering ultimate and universal meaning. Education today, with its increasing emphasis on the pragmatic and the practical, can be misused to obscure the truer potentials for human experience. This has the effect of emphasizing such pseudo-values as efficiency, orderliness, uniformity, and so on, rather than asking, "Efficiency for what? Is orderliness the most satisfying? Can individuality be rescued from uniformity?"

What I am saying here is that too often education becomes a powerful influence toward making persons into objects, toward treating people as interchangeable units, toward increasing our alienation from ourselves and our estrangement from each other. When education has these sorts of effects it is failing in its most central function. The uneducated man, the primitive man, is the man who is most at the mercy of natural forces, economic influences, and social and traditional pressures that keep him in a reactive stance, keep him an object. Education's finest accomplishment is that it makes it possible for man to be the subject of much more of his life.

SCIENCE-ARTS

Science is so varied a phenomenon that it is not possible to characterize its authenticity as a unit. Like any social institution, it is in itself neither authentic nor inauthentic, but it is employed both ways. Individual "scientists" seek to deny contingency and to "prove" meaningfulness through their work. They are the currently fashionable descendants of the revivalists of the more fundamentalist religious sects of an earlier generation. They are clearly identifiable, often enough, by their unilateral attitudes about the nature of "reality," "facts," and "science" itself. Far from being open, inquiring, and broadly aware, they tend to be frightened, bitter, and jealously clutching to themselves the fragile shield of a certainty established only by their own protestations.[2]

Another form of science which has much of the inauthentic in it is that which is concerned to produce rather than satisfy need. An authentic society would make meaningless the efforts of those who try to create obsolescence, who plan unimportant design changes that can be magnified to seeming significance, who seek to play on human fears and hungers to induce futile expenditures.

Much of science, however, represents some of man's most authentic responses to his being in the world. The true scientist does not always fit the classical picture of the open-minded, broadly informed scholar (Taylor, 1959), but he does show a readiness to meet the ultimate unknowability of being with respect for that very fact. Authentic science is an existential adventure which recognizes that each new area opened increases the area in which we do not know geometrically while increasing the area in which we do know only arithmetically. There is no valid field of human knowledge that is not a door to infinite possibility.

While all of our present sciences certainly would prosper anew in a truly authentic culture, we might well see the development of new disciplines that might be thought of as science-arts. Where once the temple of metaphysics stood, we should see a new structure of knowledge and inquiry. The whole realm poorly lumped together under the title, extrasensory perception, would certainly deserve much more respectful mining. The meanings and potentialities of transcendence as we have been using that term have scarcely been guessed at; while the phenomenon of death has only recently begun to receive any creative attention at all (Ducasse, 1961; Feifel, 1959). We have only smatterings of understandings about sleep and dreams; yet these are but vague words for what

---

[2] Such terrified but dangerous people can often rise to important educational or administrative posts in our culture where the responsibility for judgment is so much feared. The kind of "scientist" I am describing is driven to produce many publications, to use esoteric and highly technical procedures and equipment in order to protect his fragile security. As a result he shows up well on "objective criteria" that equally frightened administrators use to avoid the danger of acting as subject and making decisions on the more authentic subjective criteria.

may well be a whole new continent of man's experience. Probably too there are immense potentials for investigation in the areas of human relationships and love.

CHANGED PLACE OF THE ARTS

I have spoken of the development of "science-arts." This hyphenated term was an attempt to convey the recognition that the two forms of human expression which we are accustomed in our society to regard as separate actually share a great deal. Emergent men would surely sense the underlying commonality that is the human seeking to explore that which is potential, to translate more of the possible into the actual, to experience in ever new ways the suchness and wholeness of all existence. The separation of the methods and products of science from those of art is artificial. The purest science is the most artistic; the most genuine art is scientifically valid. Here, again, we may look for the transcending of dichotomy as we gain in awareness.

The arts—in all their manifold forms—are essential to man's very humanity. That life is less than human in which there is no place for form, color, grace, composition, harmony, and contrast. Fantasy, melody, movement, and inspiration are the very stuff of our most authentic being. In an emergent society the science-arts would probably be the central concern of most people.

OTHER EVOLUTIONS

Let us quickly note some other areas in which change is likely. We would expect less violent conflict between people and between groups of people. Murder and war would be equally abhorred. The use of the fear motivation would certainly be unacceptable, both because of its violation of authentic values and because of its manifest failure as a means of affirmatively influencing people. There would almost certainly be a refusal by an authentic society to tolerate correctable suffering, whatever its nature. The present situation in which multitudes can starve to death while in other parts of the world food surpluses lead to wastage would be incredible in an authentic society. Perhaps another point of important difference would be decline of the emphasis on exclusive relationships, whether they be denominated as "love" or "parenthood" or however else.

Genuine feeling of community certainly is predictable when one is authentic.

We should expect there would be a lessened emphasis on the physical as opposed to the psychological in the human experience. We have a rather absurd situation at present when it is taken for granted that physical life and well-being outweighs almost any other value, even the value of comfort in one's physical being. We agree that psychological distresses may produce physical defects, but we are loath to recognize that constructive psychological forces can correct physical defects. Yet it is clear that just this does occur and can be fostered. We keep miserable, painful life in people because we fear to make choices and because we overvalue the physical. Certainly an authentic society would not tolerate this. Rather it is reasonable to predict an increase in euthenasia and in public acceptance of it. Birth control and optional abortions would certainly follow. I think there probably would be an increase in suicides, but these would be less compulsive and the results of distorted processes and more the acts of aware choice. We might likely see an increase in open differences of opinion hotly pursued but without the meaningless recourse to violence or physical force or threat as a way to resolve differences.

A Truly Open Society

Finally, we may be reasonably sure than an emergent culture would be characterized by a different implicit definition of society. Today our governments write laws with the expectation that they are solving problems for all time. Laws are written, implicitly, for eternity. This epitomizes a general myth we have about life: that it is a finite system in which science will work out all possible knowledge and government will write all needed regulations. The idea of the "wasting away of the state" is not unique to Marxism. Only a glance at the constantly increasing calendars of all legislative bodies is needed to demonstrate how fallacious is this view. Far from arriving at an ultimate body of law, we are adding to the jumbled mass of legislation at a ridiculous rate, while old, outdated codes encumber the whole process.

What has just been pointed out about laws applies to the whole of our conception of being. Authentic society would be open society. Emergent man would recognize that continually we are evolving and that no final laws will be written and no ultimate scientific discoveries will be made. Just this change in the conception of our lives would be pervasive in its influences.

Man, I have said so many times in this book, is finite in the midst of an infinite universe. Now we need to recognize as well that man partakes of that infinity.

Beyond the Human Frontier

What is man's relation to The All? This is the ultimate question of all psychology, all science, all knowledge, all life. When we capitalize The All, we suggest a parallel to the Deity, to God. I do not know whether there is a God in any of the familiar senses of that word. The All is a way of saying what is knowable in some partial way: the totality of existence. The All is a way of indicating a feeling of awe, perhaps even of reverence, before that incredible fact.

Man is a part of The All. So much is manifest. Man is at least dimly aware of The All, and perhaps man is the only creature so aware. This is speculation. But man is more than a creature, and in his sensing of The All, however dim, man is in a different relation to The All. Throughout the preceding pages I have spoken repeatedly of transcendence, of overcoming the subject–object split between ourselves and world, as well as within our own being. Transcendence must mean that man becomes Man, that Man is ultimately one with The All. I do not know very clearly what that sentence means, but I want to speculate a bit further.

THE EMERGENCE OF AWARENESS

At conception, it would seem, awareness is born. At first it is little more than protoplasmic irritability. By birth it is ready to emerge both literally and psychologically into a broader world. The protecting amniotic sac is left behind to atrophy. The new protecting membrane is the symbiosis with the mother, but by school age this too begins to be discarded. Now emerging awareness is growing within the family and more and more within the restricted social world of childhood. In late adolescence, with new wrenchings and tearings, the child emerges into new awareness and allows the child-family protective "membrane" to atrophy. Through adulthood we may trace the steadily growing realm of awareness, the periodically dropped away protective housings that are outgrown. And then, perhaps, the need for the physical, the body, is outgrown. It too can be dropped away and allowed to atrophy. I do not know. It could be so.

Our image is like that of a space ship, lifted on many boosters, which drop away and burn up stage after stage to set free the capsule carrying man in the immensity of space.

A MUSING ABOUT THE ULTIMATE MEANING OF THE RESISTANCE

My thoughts about the full emergence of awareness set the stage for me to muse about the resistance in relation to The All. I have made much of the significance of the resistance in my discussions of the human condition and of the analytic and ontogogic phases of the therapeutic work. However, we may speculate even further about the ultimate meaning of the resistance. These speculations do not at this point seem pivotal to the understanding and analysis of the resistance in most therapeutic courses; however it will be evident that they may have underlying implications which further study will show to have influences on actual therapeutic work. Only time and much further study will tell.

The resistance might be thought of as the expression of the effort of identity to resist reincorporation in the All. It is the insistence of a node of being that it is identifiable with all Being. The resistance is a "sin" against God, a sin called Man, to use an older language. This is the "original sin." This is the eating of the fruit of knowledge (of identity) which leads to the expulsion from the paradise of homogeneous all.

This is the renunciation of creaturehood as our sole destiny. The resistance is an insistence on creatorhood. It is identity demanding to partake of the Godhead. We resist to find our being. We move past resistance to take part in the creation of Being. This is the prodigal's return.

Clearly world is our creation, not God's. We create world as an expression of resistance to The All. But also as a way of taking part in the creation of The All. By world I mean all that we usually call "this life" and its contents. Somehow it is all the same, whether there are endless galaxies or just our own globe. It is all the same whether there are trillions of billions of people or just I.

Conclusion

And so I have described some of the lessons my colleagues who are my patients have been teaching me. These people are engaged in that bitterest and most terrifying conflict of all, the struggle with what is unknown within one's self. As I listen and participate with them as best I can, I am again and again deeply moved by one or another of three strong feelings.

First, and most often, I feel genuine awe at the great sturdiness of the core of hope and striving that is deep within each of us. Some people whom their acquaintances have long since written off as weak, hopeless, or cowardly are in the loneliness of their own spirits contending with such seemingly impossible odds that I wonder that they have not long since given up the struggle, that they somehow find the resources to renew the attempt day after day.

Second, I feel the thrill of adventure and discovery as my companions open to me new vistas of the functioning of human personality. In this book I have told you about these vistas.

The third of the emotions I feel is one hard to characterize clearly. Perhaps I can come closest if I speak of a feeling of reverence. It is my emotional response to my dim sensing of what it may mean to be truly a Man. So often as I listen to those who talk to me, indeed as I listen to myself, I feel a kind of rage and dismay. As I recognize what we do to ourselves and to each other—even to those we love most dearly—I want to cry out that we are still truly primitives in a jungle. Psychologically we practice such rites of mutilation and torture upon ourselves and each other.

But then a quieter mood will replace my anger, I will hear those same voices expressing their own seeking for more than the brutality, the superstitiousness, the blind lashing out of our ignorance. Then I can begin to get those hazy glimpses of the something more that is potential within us, the fantastic but real evolution that can be if only we can become what we most truly are.

I referred earlier to Plato's "Allegory of the Cave" in which he described those who dwelt in the darkness all their lives and saw only the shadows that their fellows cast in the flickering firelight. You will remember the wonder and awe and fear they experienced when they emerged into the light of the sun and saw themselves and each other for what they truly were.

I think that in some measure we have all been dwellers in the cave. As psychotherapy, social amelioration, education, reduced fear of privation, and improved communication have all contributed to the process, I cherish the hope that some may be nearing the truer light in which we may begin to see what it is to be truly human. I recognize that genuinely Emergent Man is probably yet many generations away; nevertheless, I am hopeful that we are on the verge of a qualitative—as well as a quantitative—gain toward that fuller emergence.

24—The search today

The earliest human vocation was that of nomad, and nomads we remain. We are creatures of the road, travelers always en route. It is in our deepest nature to be seekers, to look always toward the horizons of tomorrow, of what may be, of what we may become. As individuals and as a species, we are drawn forward by the mystery of the possible.

Some mistake this human orientation for striving or for attachment, both ill-regarded in our times. It is not either of these. It is, rather, the expression of qualities intrinsic to our very nature: the endless changefulness of our embodied being, the capacity to value and to discriminate among experiences, and the potential to transcend the finite actuality with visions of the infinite possible. Psychotherapy is an expression of our response to the call of the road. Psychotherapy is but one of many ways in which we women and men look for escape from the petty constraints of cramped living and for realization of the riches each of us senses latent within ourselves. Psychotherapy is a searching of the possible.

On the Nature of Existential Psychotherapy

Psychotherapy is a partnership drawing on the infinite resources of the human healing/growth process to enlarge and enrich both partners' experience of being alive. Psychotherapy, thus conceived, is a unique human endeavor. It is not a healing or a repair; thus it is not a medical activity, although physicians have made notable contributions to its development. It is not a religious practice, since it does not work from predetermined beliefs or injunctions, although its concerns often overlap with the concerns of religion. It is closer to being an art form, since it calls for sensitivity, skill, emotional involvement, discipline, and esthetic judgment; yet it is less concerned to create than to release creativity. It produces no objective product, and indeed sees the concern with productivity as a frequent source of counter-therapeutic problems.

Psychotherapy which is focused upon how the person is experiencing his/her life and which mobilizes the forces of beingness itself is without direct parallel in any other field. The therapeutic partnership has antecedents in the relationships of intimates—friends or family—but is different in important ways. Psychotherapy is two people joining forces to bring greater resources to humankind's ancient quest for living that is more subjectively authentic. As such, it is something spawned by affluence, the charge of critics who call it superficial or effete. In the forms I describe, it is neither. Affluence, the release of human energies from the grinding struggle for survival and security (Maslow's "deficiency motivation," 1968), has been linked repeatedly in history with great cultural advances. Psychotherapy is at least that.

THE PSYCHOTHERAPEUTIC PARTNERSHIP

I find it difficult to characterize the relationship which seems to be most effective for intensive psychotherapy. The difficulty has two sources: First, there are many contrasts among the relationships I have with individual clients, and these differences are most pervasive in the objective and specifiable aspects of those relationships (whether the client uses the couch, how frequent the interviews, how much talking I do). On the other hand, the commonalities in the relationships I have with those who gain the most are real and important, but extremely difficult to render explicitly. Perhaps I can convey a sense of those commonalities through some capsule characterizations of the way several people and I work together with good results.

Frank[1] complains a lot, tells me that nothing's helping, and accuses me of only caring about the fees he pays. I tell Frank he's full of shit, point out how he uses complaints to avoid really getting into himself, and express exasperation at the way he and I repeatedly get sidetracked

Louise[1] and I nearly whisper together in some interviews. We are intimate in our way of communicating, and there is more than a hint of sensual-sexual closeness in our being together. She wears, at times, quite revealing clothes, and I openly enjoy her doing so.

Carol is very demure and proper, on the other hand; superficially, it seems as though she doesn't even know I'm here. She uses the couch, goes so deeply into herself that she is in an altered state of conciousness. From time to time I make brief observations about what she is exploring, and she may or may not use these. At the end of the hour, she surfaces with a shock of reawakening.

Ken treats me as an indulgent and caring older brother. He brings problems and experiences to relate to me, and I have to be alert to point out how readily he entertains me with his achievements and sexual adventures. He accepts these reminders with small grumbles and gets down to more productive work.

Since Hal[1] is himself a psychotherapist, he and I continually get drawn into arguments about concepts and procedures. Then one or the other of us will blow the whistle on this, and we go back to sort out where we got off the track and to explore the leads thus provided.

These are people at work in intensive psychotherapy. The capsules are as much caricatures as characterizations. It is impossible to reduce to less than a hundred words an intense working relationship of hundreds of hours and tremendous ranges of ideas, emotions, and interactions. Still, it is possible to put forth some shaky generalities about the therapist's role and participation.

---

[1]The psychotherapy experiences of these people—as well as those of others—are described in detail in Bugental, 1976.

THERAPIST INVOLVEMENT

Genuine confrontation with life's anxieties, naked exposure of one's guilts and shames, authentic facing of responsibility—these do not occur in the presence of strangers or in front of familiar but uninvolved observers. Psychotherapy is not something a doctor does to a patient; psychotherapy is a no-holds-barred battle with what one fears most in his/her own deepest self. Psychotherapy is not a role-playing; it is actual encounter with that in oneself which robs life of meaning, satisfaction, and vitality. Psychotherapy cannot depend on observer accounts, even when the observer is the person most involved (the client, his/herself); psychotherapy occurs *in vivo*, in the living moment, or it does not occur at all.

All these characterizations should make it evident that the therapist needs to take her/his courage in hand and accept the role of active—if junior—partner in the venture. For myself this means that I am much more participant than formerly, involved in my partner's struggles personally (though mindful not to take them over), intervening, challenging, arguing, and feeling all emotions. Though I talk a great deal at times, I am silent much more than in a usual social conversation. I try to moderate my tendency to stand on the soapbox of experience by reminding myself—and informing my client at times—of the many pratfalls that have punctuated my course to this day.

THERAPIST ENTANGLEMENT

As this term has been used in proper psychotherapeutic circles, it is always spelled with four letters. Therapists can be *involved*, within careful limits, but they should never become *entangled* with their clients. I now believe that attitude is counter-therapeutic. Messy and unexpected entanglement—not tidy and deliberate involvement—often occurs when the partners relentlessly pursue the therapeutic search. This is an issue that troubles many practitioners, so I will discuss it more fully.

Traditional teaching about psychotherapy—and too much

practice—has been founded on a model in which the patient reported symptoms and complaints to the doctor, answered questions, provided accounts of life outside the consultation room, projected unrealistically onto the therapist, received interpretations of his/her problems (which demonstrated that they were unreal and should be given up), and then changed accordingly. This image is pure fiction; it doesn't work, and it often does a great deal of damage, if no other way than by turning people off from seeking genuine therapeutic help. In this model, the therapist remained carefully apart; he was perhaps kindly, but personally distinctly uninvolved.

I believe the only way psychotherapy can truly aid a person to making lasting and pervasive changes in the experience of being alive is by abandoning this detached, clinical model and allowing the client's way of being-in-the-world to emerge right into the therapeutic room. That means involving and entangling the therapist as well. In the traditional model the therapist worked out her/his interpretations from the patient's accounts and from one-way projections on her/him which the patient expressed in the hour. The parallel to medical practice in other times or places in striking, for in such instances the physician (male) would never actually see the body of a (woman) patient, but would rely on accounts the patient or someone else might provide. In some instances, the physician would not actually perform surgery but instruct some hireling.

The therapist who stays aloof from entanglement with his client will seldom see at first hand anything but the surface of the client's ways of relating and perceiving. As with many human patterns, the self-defeating ways of being that bring an adult to psychotherapy are complex and layered, and are only fully brought out when called into play in a living interaction.

> Belle had had a very hard childhood, seldom feeling secure or loved. As an adult, reasonably enough, she sought out people who were strong and dependable and built her relationships with them. A therapist is, by definition, strong and dependable. Belle worked well in therapy, frequently expressed immense appreciation for my interpretations and support, and began to make

significant changes in her life. Then one day I was checking over my outstanding accounts—a wise practice for a therapist—and I was startled to see how in much arrears Belle was on her account. When I talked with her about it, she was apologetic and promised to catch up promptly. Then I looked for a book I needed, and only after some time I remembered I'd lent it to Belle. About this time I realized how often it was difficult to end the hour with Belle on time, how she repeatedly had last-minute items of importance to discuss. And so it went. The pattern was suddenly clear. In half-dozen ways, Belle was winning extra privilege, additional evidences of my concern, and continually seeking more. When I began to display the pattern to her, she was repentant, then saddened and hurt, then furious and accusing.

This is a very brief account of the surface aspects of an elaborate system of resistances and transferences that Belle had developed to try to feel safe in the world but that were gradually suffocating her in their intricate webbings. Only as we became caught up in our relationship, as I became a real person in her life, could the whole tangled skein begin to unravel so we could deal with it directly. The important point to be recognized here—and another at variance with the traditional model—is that my interpretations were of limited value to the confrontation and working past of these patterns. What made the difference was our being caught up in them together, exposing their operation in our own lives right there in the therapeutic setting, and thus exploding them directly. In this way, Belle did not need to learn a lesson about a pattern and then try to change it. Instead, she experienced the pattern with the classic phrase that betokens opened inward vision, "Oh, I see! I never knew that was what I did, and yet I've always known it." *I didn't know that, but I've always known it.* The dual recognition of opened awareness. As we will see a bit later, this is the difference between abstract insight and true inner vision.

Here is the key point. Belle did not have an insight and change a neurotic pattern, replacing it with a healthy one. Belle did not have a corrective emotional experience and decide she didn't need handicapping old ways any more and so drop them. Belle didn't get rid of anything, neurotic or not. Belle didn't change herself the way one repairs a balky motor. Belle loosened her linkage to a way of being that is still available to her, that will still show up from time to time, that at times will bring her pain again, but with a difference. Belle knows that *she* is not just that way of being, that she has other possibilities, and that she ultimately is much more than that or any way of being.

Our truest nature is our contentless being. It has no habits or patterns, no neurosis or, for that matter, health. It is pure awareness, pure subjectivity. Subjectivity, bending on itself, takes on form—content, perceptions, self-creation-by-awareness—which brings the expression of our beingness into the objective plane. Therapy, by fostering the client's loosening of compulsion or identity with the objective layer, releases the creative potential of his/her underlying subjectivity. This means that the real work of psychotherapy occurs beyond words, beyond logical-verbal understanding. Thus, the descriptive-report-and-corrective-interpretation approach to therapy is foredoomed to be incomplete and stranded on the objective-verbal level. The full experiencing of engaged and entangled relating which is lived through and continually brought out into the open provides subjectivity with input beyond the objective and thus is more lasting and pervasive.

This means that the therapist will inevitable and necessarily get entangled in the client's ways of relating to significant others, that this entanglement will occur at least to some extent without either partner fully realizing it, and that it is the therapist's job to join his/her companion in keeping aware of what is happening in their relationship—not just what is wrong or distortedly transferred. Out of this continuing seeking for awareness will come some of the most profound confrontations, the most emotionally laden working through, and the most lasting therapeutic benefits. But it doesn't happen because the therapist stays clean, aseptic, and apart, but because the therapist lets himself be genuinely involved.

License or necessity? To those who protest that this means license for all sorts of acting out, the answer is that acting out is the name of the game: All therapy that is more than verbal tennis continually involves the enactment of impulses which are denied consciousness; enactment is essential to a vital encounter. As to it being a license, it is time to question what the advocates of stringent control so greatly fear. The therapist will, in some instances, take advantage of the client's needs. True, but that occurs frequently as it is. The fear of seeming to give permission for that to occur ignores the fact that it happens despite the prohibitions or rationalizations against it. The only way to protect clients' interests is to help both clients and therapists attain as authentic as possible an understanding of the meaning and consequences of what they do in the therapeutic hour. And this includes firmly insisting that everything which happens is part of the therapeutic process and must be open to description, discussion, analysis, and the sharing of responsibility for it by both partners.

The fear of transference and counter-transference acting out that pervades so much literature about psychotherapy is itself an acting out of a major transference.

RESISTANCE AND TRANSFERENCE SEEN TOGETHER

The primary work of the kind of psychotherapy I am describing is that of facilitating the client's inquiry into her/his own life and his/her efforts to bring about significant and lasting changes. Anything which intrudes upon, disrupts, or deceives that quest is a resistance and very likely a transference as well, since it is worked out in the partnership: Although conceptually there are advantages to distinguishing (p. 138)[2] these intruding processes, in actual clinical practice I no longer find that helpful. This, as I have already suggested, is because there is nearly always an interpersonal aspect to the resistance, just as there is clearly a repetitive warding-off function to the transference, and both are parts of the acting-relating repertoire of the person. Indeed, it is a valid question whether there is any part of that repertoire that does not have some resistive element.

Summary

Before leaving this statement of how I now view the processes and procedures of psychotherapy, I will make a summarizing rephrasing which sets the whole matter in the most existential form I can support.

What is a human being?

A human being is being in human form. A being is a point of awareness, is an existence in subjective space. Being is the process of existence. As such, it has "is-ness" and is eternal. Non-being is a myth, is nothing, is no thing. Being can take many forms. One of those possibilities is the human form. A human being is a being in human form, is a point of awareness, exists in subjective space, has is-ness, and in her/his beingness is timeless.

Beingness as a point of awareness has neither form nor content. But awareness includes awareness of being, and out of that comes the possibility of taking form, acquiring content. A human being is beingness taking human form and acquiring content. A human being is beingness taking human form and acquiring human content.

What I have called *I-process* is our pure beingness. The human form it takes is what I have called the *Self*. The *I-process* is awareness, exists in subjective space, is outside time. The *Self* is content, is objective, is of the nature of time. The *I-process* is perceiving; the *Self* is being perceived (read that two ways: is beingness perceived, is that which is perceived).

For beingness to take form in the objective world it must accept the limits that are objective. We cannot know the true potential of being; to know it would be to objectify it. Limits are of the objective sphere; beingness is outside limits.

The infant is pure beingness, as nearly as it can exist in the human form and the objective world. The infant must add to its form, take on content if it is to be able to survive in the objective world. The ways of being in the world the infant takes on, learns, become its *Self*.

WHAT IS THE THERAPEUTIC PROCESS?

When a human being finds that content it has taken on to be burdensome, anti-life, tending to the suffocation of beingness, the person may seek in some way to alter the situation. Many pathways for doing so are open—religion, meditation, changed life commitments, illness, criminality, violence—and one of these is psychotherapy.

Intensive psychotherapy of the kind I am describing seeks to aid the person in loosening the bonds of acquired content, of the *Self* sufficiently that new content may be added and old content may be experienced in new contexts. This is accomplished through aiding the person to discover a deeper indentity in the beingness, the *I-process*, and as a part of the same process to relinquish identification (at least in some degree) with the *Self*.

Therapies vary in the extent to which they carry out this two-sided-but-single process. Each person who is a client interacting with a person who is the therapist works out a choice about how far to take this venture and how directly to pursue it in the terms I have just used.

Emancipation from the Self. When a client chooses and the therapist supports, this process may go a long way toward reducing the identification with learned content and increasing that with the pure light of aware being. This does not mean, at least in my experience, that the *Self* totally drops away. It can mean that awareness comes to include the *Self* promptings and reactions, but a great deal more as well.

When the person has pursued this quest to the point of being largely in her/his identity as *I-process*, changes may occur that ordinary reason would deem unreal or impossible. Among these are the transmutation of emotions so that anxiety can be broken up into its constituent excitement and apprehension, for example; self-healing of psychosomatic and organic disorders, changed experience of time so that pleasant experiences are prolonged and unpleasant abbreviated subjectively, greater sense of community with all life, reduced apprehension about physical death, experiences of telepathy and clairvoyance, and others (see Bugental, 1978, pp. 120—144; Walsh, 1976).

The work of this kind of therapy involves cleaning the lamp of awareness so that the beingness of the person can be focused on concern with the real issues of life. To do this, the ways in which the learned content is distorting, pain-accumulating, and destructive must be brought out in the open not just in verbal descriptions, but in living and shared experience, and repeatedly exposed for their simultaneous expression of the power of the person (seeking, valuing, trying, persevering) and of the disruptive use that that power has come to serve (resistance to confronting and incorporating the anxieties of being).

SIGNIFICANCE OF THIS WAY OF VIEWING MATTERS

There are several immediate consequences of conceiving the nature of human beings and the process of psychotherapy in these ways. For one, the human experience is seen in simpler terms, so it is not useful to distinguish a reparative (analytic) phase as distinct from a growth (ontogogic) phase. Essentially the task in both is to aid the client in reducing identification with the *Self*, the objective sense of being, and in increasing awareness of a truer identity with pure subjectivity, with the *I-process*. To be sure, the earlier phases often emphasize the first half more, while the exploration and celebration of subjectivity tend to occur in later sessions.

The same simplification reduces the need for separately categorizing the three processes of emancipation, actualization, and transcendence.

THE PROPER FOCUS OF THERAPY

Human beings are being in human form, existences in subjective space. Our nature is awareness; awareness is solely subjective. Human beings are dwellers in subjectivity, are the very stuff of subjectivity. Centuries, even millennia, of trying to work out human affairs in purely objective terms have all too clearly failed.

All that we know, all that we do, all that we feel—all that we are is received into, interpreted in, responded to out of our subjectivities. No sophistication of machine, instrument, or artificial intelligence can replace human subjectivity as the ultimate repository of actuality and decision (Bugental, 1967, chap. 1).

The therapist who seeks to work with clients by treating them objectively compounds their problems. To be sure, many clients want exactly that kind of impersonal and overt treatment. This permits displacing the heavy responsibility of being human and fosters a kind of self-manipulation that supports the suppression of inner anxiety and anguish.

The therapist who knows clearly that his/her business is with the soul, with the subjective core of being, and not with the *Self* or the superficial content of the objective aspect, will meet his/her partner in a genuine way and foster confrontations that are liberating.

SEARCHING AND THE HEALING-GROWTH PROCESS

Concern is a uniquely human capacity. To feel concern about something is to be invested in it and its vicissitudes. When that something is a person, concern is a kind of caring that takes very seriously what that person's experience is and how it can be bettered. When that person is oneself, concern is the appropriate attention to the state of one's being and to what may affect that state for good or ill. Concern is an essential human capacity; yet a great many of us are crippled in our ability to feel concern for our own lives.

The client usually comes to psychotherapy because of her/his concern about how life is going. Nevertheless, once she/he is in therapy, that sense of concern is difficult to mobilize to serve its proper function of guiding one's examination of one's life. Clients treat themselves impersonally, with contempt or indifference, with sarcasm or criticism, or in other ways that separate their experiencing selves from their observing and concerned potentials. This is the familiar work of resistance blocking the client's experience of his/her concern to bring it to bear in life renewal.

The process of mobilizing concern and using it to guide

one's inner explorations may be thought of as a kind of searching. I want to portray how this process works in a succinct fashion, and for that reason I will offer a series of brief statements which synopsize the process (adapted from Bugental, 1978, pp. 48–60):

Ten Postulates for a Conception of Existential-Humanistic Psychotherapy

ONE: THE CLIENT'S CONCERN FOR HIS/HER LIFE PROVIDES THE ESSENTIAL DYNAMIC AND ORIENTATION FOR THE THERAPEUTIC PROCESS.

Concern, so used, has four elements that need to be present (although their amounts and balance will vary widely): (a) distress, pain, or anxiety; (b) yearning for new possibilities in life; (c) readiness to make some commitment to inner exploration; and (d) hope that change within oneself will be the way to realize the possibliities which are sensed (Bugental, 1978, p. 47). The client's genuine presence (being truly accessible and expressive) in the relationship is the means for mobilizing and focusing concern.

In all this it is important for the therapist to bear in mind that it is the *client's* concern which is primary and that no amount of good will or therapist concern can be a substitute. This means, in most instances, that the therapeutic work centers around disclosing and working through the interferences (resistances) to the client's being genuinely present and operating out of mobilized concern.

TWO: ULTIMATELY THE CAPACITY TO DEAL WITH ONE'S LIFE CONCERNS RESIDES CHIEFLY WITHIN THE PERSON HAVING THOSE CONCERNS.

This is a foundation of the perspective I am describing. In brief, it says that the concern and the capacity to do something about that concern are but two sides of the same human process. That process is expressed when a person finds pain or anxiety from some state of affairs in his/her life, and it is equally expressed in the actions and commitments which lead to a reduction of pain or anxiety—perhaps through changing the state of affairs or perhaps through responding in a different way to that state. This is a simple equation, but it represents a total recasting of the nature of the therapeutic enterprise. Reared to regard psychotherapy as parallel to medical practice—in which the ailment, the patient's pain and anxiety, and the healing treatment are generally seen as largely separable—therapists find it something of a wrench to come to see that in the psychological realm at least, they are all expressions of the same life process.

It is important to recognize, also, that the first two postulates explicitly and forcefully identify the center of the psychotherapeutic effort in the client in terms of both the locus of the matter to be dealt with and the locus of the power for dealing with it. The therapist's motivation and influence—important as they are—must be genuinely regarded as secondary.

THREE: THE CLIENT COMES TO PSYCHOTHERAPY BECAUSE HIS/HER ABILITY TO DRAW ON THIS LATENT CAPACITY IS IMPAIRED.

This sets the task of psychotherapy: to aid the client in regaining access to that which is hers/his, which already exists, but access to which is blocked—that is, the client's own power to shape and direct his/her life. Therapy does not need to add some missing ingredient, but must instead facilitate the removal or redirection of what interferes with the exercise of capacity already present.

FOUR: DEVELOPING (OR REFINING) ONE'S SKILL IN SUBJECTIVE SEARCHING IS THE PRIMARY MEANS THROUGH WHICH THE INTERFERENCES WITH THE CLIENT'S ACCESS TO HER/HIS CAPACITY CAN BE DISCLOSED AND REDIRECTED.

Today I see the core of psychotherapy to be this process of inner exploration that I call *searching*. It is indeed a search for the authentic sources of one's way of being, the underlying truth of one's existential nature and freedom. It is an exploration, and at the same time it is the ameliorating agency. The next several postulates describe this process further.

(I want to make an aside here to comment on the significance of this searching process. Much of psychology for the past half-century has been concerned with the regularities of human experience, especially the phenomenon of learning. Learning is what makes human beings able to do many important things they would not otherwise be able to achieve. But learning also makes human beings repetitive, predictable, and controllable. Searching, a companion process employed by a person when learned responses are not adequate to a situation, has to do with individuality, creativity, and what makes human beings unpredictable and thus uncontrollable. Humanistic psychology will do well to give as much attention to searching as behavioristic psychology has given to learning.)

> **FIVE: THE PERSON WHO DESCRIBES A LIFE CONCERN FULLY AND WITH PRESENCE SETS IN MOTION THE SEARCHING PROCESS.**

Searching is not an esoteric procedure; it is a natural response of a person concerned about her/his life. Unfortunately, many of our learnings about ourselves are incompatible with effective searching—for example, the injunction, "Don't think about yourself so much," or the denigration of fantasy and daydreaming. It is surprising how often a client will report having "thought and thought" about some issue; yet further inquiry soon demonstrates that most of the supposed thinking was either unproductive, circling rumination or rigid objectification of one's life in an attempt to apply abstract rules or logic. Neither, of course, is the natural searching process. That process, when released, begins with surveying and resurveying the problem, gradually including additional elements and drawing on other awarenesses that logic might not have chosen, becoming more and more free-ranging in moving into the subjective potentialities—imagery, impulse, fantasy, and similar elements.

This postulate points to the simple starting place of this

vastly productive and too little appreciated human potential. Describing one's concern as fully as possible, doing so with as much presence and involvement as possible, and maintaining a set or expectancy of discovery (in contrast to one of reporting)—these three specifications for the client's description of her/his concern are necessary and sufficient to set searching in motion.

Six: The interferences with the searching process that are displayed are identical with the disruptions of life effectiveness that concern the client.

The resistances that intrude upon the therapeutic work, as we saw in earlier pages (pp. 88 ff.), are the same influences that constitute the "neurosis" or source of the client's distress and are, as well, the ways in which the client is avoiding the anxieties of existence. This apparent chain of inauthenticity is actually but a single pattern having several points of visibility. It is this fact which gives tremendous power to the therapeutic working-through process, since it becomes possible to contact the sources of the concern directly by opening up the way the client carries out the search into her/his concerns. Failures of presence, difficulty in emotionally investing in the work, slipping into an unexpectant and dependent reporting mode—these and many other patterns display how the client is trapped in inauthentic being.

Seven: The psychotherapist facilitates the searching process by his/her attitude and involvement with the client.

The ways in which the therapist supports and participates in *the client's* searching are these:

—by maintaining and repeatedly evidencing her/his conviction of the client's capacity to deal with his/her own concern (postulate two).

—by calling for the client to bring to bear her/his greater and unrecognized latent potential to enrich the searching.

—by the therapist's interacting as a whole and present person primarily dedicated to the client's emergence; thus the thera-

pist is part of both the resistive and the emergent potentials.
—by identifying his/her own experience and its interrelations with the client's, so that the resistances are displayed and fully identified and experienced.
—by providing support during the inevitable times of despair and anguish.
—by insisting on the client's immersed presence and expectant attitude.
—in all, by taking the client and the client's search completely seriously.

EIGHT: THE FREE RANGING OF THE CLIENT'S SUBJECTIVE SEARCHING PROCESS BRINGS THE CLIENT GENUINE INNER VISION.

Inner vision is the lost sense (Bugental 1976, chap. 1) of our own being, our knowing of what is true for us. "Insight," as that term is used in many psychotherapeutic contexts—as an explanation or history of a symptom or neurotic system—is a deteriorated form of inner vision. Insight of that kind is powerless (Freud is said to have remarked, "Insight alone is not enough"). Inner vision is itself a change or healing process.

What is too seldom recognized is that one person, such as a therapist, can no more give another person inner vision (or true insight) than he/she can give another a dream. This is a point that psychotherapists often mistake when they focus their attention on finding explanations (the "whodunit" school of therapy). Inner vision is a private and unique subjective experience. I will talk more about it in a few pages.

NINE: A RELATION OF GENUINE MUTUAL RESPECT AND CARING IS THE IDEAL MEDIUM IN WHICH THE SEARCHING PROCESS AND THE DISCLOSURE AND WORKING-THROUGH OF RESISTANCES CAN OCCUR.

Mutual respect and caring mean involvement and personal—not solely professional—participation with each other. Although the roles are not the same, they are not distinguished by one being the subjective actor and the other being the objective observer or even objective observer-participant. Those models carried over from physical science, and already being seriously questioned there, are inappropriate in this work. Mutual respect and caring occur between persons, not roles; roles are important and deserving of allegiance, but they are only part of the story. Since I have elaborated on this above, I will not say any more now.

TEN: FOLLOWING THROUGH THE SEARCHING PROCESS WILL BRING THE PERSON TO AN ENLARGED SENSE OF HIS/HER OWN IDENTITY AND POWER IN LIFE.

The chief outcome of this process is a changed experience of life, not the solution of problems or the elimination of symptoms. When, as is not infrequently the case, problems remain, they are experienced differently because they are set in a broader context and the person sees them from a stance of greater choice and power. I will talk more about the changed experience of being immediately below.

One final observation about the outcomes of carrying the searching process forward. It is likely that there is no limit to what may be brought out through liberated searching. Certainly, it leads rather surely to creativity and expanded views of oneself and one's life-world. When this path is followed even further, the person comes to a point of relinquishing identification with the *Self* (pp. 209-210) or ego.

SUMMARY

These ten postulates provide a skeleton on which rest the living processes of intensive psychotherapy. The characterizations of these postulates have been exceedingly brief, of course, but taken in the context of the earlier portions of the book, they compose an evolved and productive way of describing and thinking about the mobilization of human possibilities to enrich human lives. Now it will be helpful to look further at the outcomes toward which this process works.

The Goal: An Expanding Sense of One's Own Being

How big is a human being? By what measuring stick can we take the person's dimension? In what fashion may we assess the size of human experience, human aspiration, human potentiality? Clearly, the only valid parameters are those that interrelate human potential, vision, and actuality. Here clinical workers, humane thinkers, and our everyday inner awareness converge: We do not begin to fulfill our possibilities. We dream beyond our attainment, to be sure, but our unrealized potential may well equal or exceed our dreams. How big is a human being? As big as the person's intent when it is vitalized by committed effort; as big as the person's aspiration when it is liberated from the chains and cobwebs of false learnings and distorting fears. ◆

I have come to believe more and more that the goal of intensive psychotherapy is helping the client gain a fresh perception of human (and his/her own) potential, a vista which forever shows the person that life offers possibilities far beyond what she/he has ever realized and that the chief obstacles to making those possibilities actualities are self-imposed. It is this changed view of one's own being that is the most profound and lasting contribution psychotherapy—or any other change influence—can make.

What about symptoms? I do not think that symptom removal is a frequent and lasting result of psychotherapy of any kind, although symptom suppression and substitution is familiar enough. I do not think that life reorganization often occurs directly as a result of therapeutic work on the troubling or disorganized parts of living, although changes in work, marriage, relationships, or affiliations certainly frequently occur—often with some improvement in satisfaction, but almost as often with the old patterns reasserting themselves after a time. I do not think that basic character structure (whatever that may be) is fundamentally altered by even the most thorough-going psychotherapeutic course, although a client may live with those character qualities differently.

What is the difference? It is a difference in the place or basis from which one lives. Always what we feel, think, say, and do are at least in some part derivatives of how we see ourselves and our world. When we see ourselves as weak, as the helpless victims of forces stronger than we are, we meet life differently than when we operate from a sense of immense possibilities open to us and with a confidence in our own powers to make our experiencing more accord with our deeper seeking. Thus we move beyond being fixed and static and become *more than*—more than our "personalities" or our immediate experiences.

>Kate[1] came to therapy because she felt constricted and unable to live and work as she wished and felt possible. Therapy disclosed her tendency to see any immediate state of emotional affairs as the way it would always be, as the end of all pain or all joy forever more. Today, some years after leaving therapy, Kate still tends to see her emotional experiences as ultimate, but there is a difference. Kate may suddenly burst out laughing, "I'm doing it again! I'm convinced that it's never going to be different . . . and though I know that's not really so, it still feels that way." Kate knows deep depressions and elated highs, as she always did, but today she also sooner or later recognizes that these are not her essential being and that they will change. Thus Kate can work much more effectively, relate much more satisfyingly, and realize much more of her very real potential.

>And so it goes. Louise still is inclined to be uncomfortable or anxious when people may disapprove of her. She is unusually sensitive to others' inner experiencing, and she is impelled to try to take care of their needs, sometimes even before they are aware of them. Yet she can recognize these feelings in herself now, and she can choose not to carry them into action. She can even enjoy being at odds with others at times and asserting her own needs in competition with someone else's. Still, her sensitivity and caring for others is a profoundly rich attribute that she retains and that those who know her value deeply but that also causes her pain and anxiety at times.

The Necessity of the Self. We learn ways of being-in-the-world very early. They are continually challenged and amended and reinforced by our experiences, but the core sifts out and becomes durable and persistent. It is well that this is so, for otherwise our lives and relationships would be chaotic. When we find we want to change our ways of being, there is no dressing room where we can strip and try on a new personality. We always operate from within our way of being-in-the-world, our ego structure. But while we cannot remove it, we can certainly enlarge it, gain a perspective on it that reduces its iron grip, that lets us add ways of being, and that—in some instances when the person persists in the searching process long enough—may eventually allow the person to move psychologically and spiritually within his way of being.

To my mind, this is the meaning of the spiritual quest to overcome the *Self* or ego: When one becomes sufficiently aware of one's learned ways of being-in-the-world to be able at any important juncture to recognize the limiting effects of that way of being and to step beyond them, then the ego is, for all practical purposes, dissolved, and the *Self* is transcended (in Gunther's happy recognition, "trance ended," (1971).

The development of a vista on human—and one's own—being that opens possibility in this way is not a one-time affair. One cannot "take therapy" and then have new vision and go ahead on a transcendent plane. It is, rather, a life-long enterprise. Psychotherapy, if one is fortunate, can open that perspective and help to demonstrate it in the only terms that will deeply and lastingly persuade—intense personal and subjective recognition. But psychotherapy provides only a starting point, although that can be enough. If my client emerges from our work together with a quiet but abiding sense that her/his being is an opening and expanding universe into which he/she may grow and with the parallel assurance that the limits on that growth are ones she/he can gradually go beyond, then I am immensely pleased with our work together. We have done our job, and we have done it well.

Working-through—a dubious idea. An implication of what I am saying is that the psychoanalytic notion of "working-through" (or in other perspectives, "discharging," "clearing," "curing," or "reversing") neurotic patterns so that they no longer exist is an inaccurate description of what happens in therapy (or psychoanalysis or any other form). These terms arise from a mechanistic conception of human beings in which a defective part could be identified, repaired or replaced, and the person would then be factory fresh. I just don't think that occurs. We are all that we have ever been, but we can be more than we have ever been also.

The Primacy of the Subjective

The procedures and outcomes of psychotherapy have their locus in the subjective experiencing of the client, not in any external or objective setting. Therapy is initiated by the subjective sense of concern; it principally employs the subjective process of searching to do its work; the therapist must be subjectively involved and not remain an objective observer; the disclosure of subjective resistances is one of the key ameliorative tasks; and the outcomes most typical and most desirable are changes in the subjective experience of being.

In our time the undoubted values of objectivity have been inflated as though they were the only values. That distortion has cost humans dearly, and if its governance in the political and economic spheres is not balanced soon by some more humanistic and subjective perspective, it may cost our species its very being. The subjective-objective issue is no mere academic quibble; it profoundly affects our lives in many ways.

Psychotherapy needs to aid the person in reclaiming his/her subjective sovereignty, to foster the client's development of the skills and potentials of her/his subjective nature, and to open the possibilities of subjective transformation. In no area is this charge more practically and yet pervasively important than in distinguishing between the truly subjective power of inner vision and the simulation of that power which is too often called "insight" in therapeutic circles.

Insight vs. Inner Vision

The therapist and client meet most truly and—if wise—engage most surely in their work on the subjective plane. This means they must follow the pathways of concern rather than those of logic. This means they must respect the imcompleteness of any moment in order to keep faith with the completeness that is beyond expression. This means they must accept into their intercourse the mythic, the fantastic, the dreaming, and the poetic. The stuff of the subjective real is pre-verbal, is beyond verbal, is ultimately inexpressible in all its fullness.

> Imagine yourself waking in the morning from a rich, many dimensioned, and deeply involving dream. Struggling toward consciousness, you sense so much that preceded and ornamented the part of the dream which is still most vivid, but as you try to capture those images you realize they are falling away into irretrievable forgetting. Now, still drugged with sleep, you rouse your companion and begin telling the dream, hoping to preserve it by putting it into words. But there is so much that eludes the grasp of language; images that were so vital now twist and fragment; connections that seemed so significant drop apart. What you are able to convey is such a paltry and disorted residue of the once mind-filling imagery. Finally, if later you should hear your companion telling someone else of your dream—no matter how caringly and with what faithful attention to what you had reported—then you look on the mutilated remains of what once was so vital and rich.
>
> Insight, rightly understood, is a product of inner sight, inner vision. It is not to be captured in words. Those who equate a verbal account of inner sight with the inward vision itself make the familiar semantic error of mistaking the map for the territory. What can be said about an inner sight is always less than the sight itself and is always relatively impotent in bringing about true life changes, especially when compared with the power of one's own liberating inward realization. . . .
>
> Rightly understood, insight is like a dream. It is inner sight, seeing a vision within one's own being. Another's insight is irrevocably someone else's; it can never be one's own, and one's own can never be that other person's. The therapist who tries to

give her or his client insight is attempting to be the eyes of a blind person—blind to the therapist's vision, but not blind within the client's own self. Such a therapist presumes too much, does not recognize or respect the ultimate autonomy of each person, is more apt to interfere with the client's inner vision than to facilitate it. (Bugental, 1978, pp. 56-57)

Ontogogy and the Human Circumstance

WHAT SHALL WE CALL OUR WORK?

What's in a name (or categorization)? A great deal. A rose might smell as sweet if it were called a weed, but it might get smelled much less often. A substance having mood-affecting qualities had the misfortune to become known as a narcotic rather than as an benign alternative to alcohol or tobacco, and that categorization has led to struggles, injuries, lives permanently damaged, and deaths. Psychological efforts to aid people to live more fully originally under the banner of the church were preempted in the last century by medicine—in part because of the largely irrelevant academic background and economic necessity of the most outstanding contributor, Sigmund Freud. Freud himself originally wanted an academic career, did not like the practice of medicine, and came to favor non-medical preparation for the work of psychoanalysis (Jones, 1957).

I think of my work as "evocation" (a calling forth) or as "ontogogy" (leading out into greater beingness). But these are simply my own private terms and have no general currency. I no longer see my work as a form of treatment of a patient or as a curative or restorative effort. This is not a form of medical practice; it is psychological in the truest sense—having to do with the psyche or soul or spirit of human beings. The small revival of interest in inspiritedness (Jourard, 1964; Bugental, 1978) may point toward a coming rehabilitation of the ancient recognition of the deeper core of human beings.

In earlier pages (p. 15) I used *ontogogy* to distinguish efforts to increase the realization of the healthy potentials of persons who had—usually through the analytic phase—freed themselves of many of their neurotic constraints on being. That distinction no longer seems useful to me, as I'll describe below. Instead, I have dropped the division into phases and think of ontogogy as a quality characterizing the entire span of my work with a client-partner.

Once I saw the analytic phase as needed to roll back the resistances and restore the person's basic emotional health before she/he might go on to try to attain more than usual realization of life's potentials. I knew, of course, that we never free ourselves totally of the resistive patterns, but it seemed likely that by materially reducing them, one would be more ready to assimilate new learnings of a higher order.

I think now that one's ways of being-in-the-world are at once resistances and expressions of health or strength. I think that one does not get "rid of" resistances, but so enlarges one's sense of one's own being that the resistances lose their compelling power—at least in some degree. I think that the work of exposing and working through resistance is part of the process of expanding one's sense of identity—maybe is the core of it. Thus, it is not possible to separate the analytic from the re-educative (ontogogic). The *Self* is the sum of one's ways of being-in-the-world—not just as actually perceived by the person, but as perceivable by her/him. As one gains awareness that the *Self*, the ways of being-in-the-world, are tools, are available to being bypassed or experienced but not yielded to, then one is beginning to be emancipated from the *Self*. There is now the possibility of actualizing other potentials not previously accessible. Thus the old way of being, the old *Self*-world is transcended. I don't think this is a state many people—if any—remain in for any length of time. I think that for most of us at least, we work toward it in our several ways (therapy, meditation, spiritual disciplines), achieve it for intervals ranging from a few seconds to several days, lose it, retain some sense of the vision we have had, seek for it anew, feel hopeless and doubt our potential or our vision (the same thing), and then find it again unexpectedly or lose it and fall away into the familiar *Self* and world.

THE EXISTENTIAL CONDITIONS OF BEING

Human beings are beings being human. Our being is pure subjectivity and thus contentless, formless awareness. As beingness is expressed on the objective plane, it takes on structure, and we accept the human circumstance. Arising from the encounter of subjectivity with objective constraint, the conditions of conscious (in contrast to, existentially aware) living may be conceptualized in various ways. In earlier chapters (pp. 285-321), I described a way of doing so, and I will now comment on that and supplement it.

In general, I have found that the chief values of the conceptual grid of existential givens, confrontations, anxieties, and related experiences have been two: *First*, in a valued colleague's happy phrase, "we are rescued from chaos without being put into a box." The existentially inclined therapist needs always to be open to the infinite variety of human life and to avoid the inviting traps that extensively derived categorizations offer. Yet it can increase our sensitivity to give thought to the main issues we humans must face and the main paths we've followed in doing so. *Second*, scholars and researchers find it useful to work with constructs such as these to try to deepen and extend our understanding of the human experience. Sabath (1978) has made an imaginative and productive development of the core dynamic sequence (pp. 286-290). Thauberger and his associates (1979; Thauberger & Cleland, 1979, undated; Thauberger & Davis, undated; Thauberger & Sydiaha, 1979; Thauberger & Sydiaha-Symor, 1979; Thauberger, Thauberger, & Cleland, 1977) have developed a number of scales that seek to measure ontological characteristics and to relate them to the predicted patterns of confrontation. While I find it hard to identify the psychotherapeutic phenomena I have described with the objective scales and scores, I am intrigued by their work and hopeful that greater convergence of the clinical and the experimental approaches may be possible because of such efforts.

Changes from the earlier descriptions. It must be remembered that we are here concerned with naming constellations, after all a quite arbitrary process and not to be confused with discovering stars. Thus, we seek to find terms and relationships that most simply lend themselves to clinical observation and everyday communication. Viewed this way, it is desirable that our glossary grow and change with experience. I have made two significant changes: adding a fifth existential given, *embodiedness*, and making explicit place for existential joy. In addition, I continue to experiment with how best to group common human experiences; the reader will thus find some changes of names and locations in the descriptions below and some omissions of terms that have proved of limited value.

EMBODIEDNESS

My own observations and the suggestions of well-informed associates have led me to add a fifth dimension to the schemata, the existential given of embodiedness. As beingness is manifested on the objective plane, the physical body is its vehicle and sets its limits. Our bodies are the always-present condition of our conscious experience, so that the fact of embodiedness permeates all phases of our living.

EXISTENTIAL CONFRONTATION WITH CHANGE

Our bodies are continually emerging, evolving, growing, aging, declining, dying. Thus, they confront us with the inexorable fact of continual change, and no amount of clutching at overhanging branches can pull us from the stream that relentlessly carries us toward the waterfall. We are changing; our very nature is change, and our truest being is process, not structure. As it has been said, "Structure is the secretion of progress." The creations of our being that are unchanging are static and inevitably must be abandoned.

EXISTENTIAL ANXIETY: PAIN AND DESTRUCTION

Our bodies early introduce us to the paradigm for all negative experience that will follow. *Pain* comes as a surprise, as a dimension not anticipated, as an instrustion of the objective into the serenity and continuity of the subjective. Pain insists—if continued or extreme—on our consciousness paying attention. Severe pain—agony—pre-empts living and drowns out other awarenesses. And pain, the relative anxiety, is a forerunner of destruction, the absolute.

Destruction is irretrievable loss. It is a death of a kind, but not *the* death. Destruction is experienced when the crumpled body of our pet lies at our feet, when a scar becomes permanent, when our family moves us forever away from a best friend, when we first realize that someone close to us is truly dead, when accident or natural cause destroys possessions or possibilities.

Pain and destruction are our first teachers about existential anxiety. No shielding parents can be omnipresent enough to ward off this learning, no matter how they may defer other confrontations.

OTHER ASPECTS OF EMBODIEDNESS

Increasingly we are recognizing that physical disability is an expression of the total person, not an isolated event of the somatic system. When dread governs the individual's response to life, *illness* is more likely to occur; when the person mobilizes courage to meet the conditions of being, the experience is one of *wholeness*, which is the physical aspect of authenticity. Finally, full living calls for a quality of being in one's body and one's experiencing which—following Jourard (1964)—I find most adequately named *spiritedness* or inspiritedness (Bugental, 1967b, 1980). This is an expression of vital, aware, and courageous participation in being. Table V brings together the major elements of the existential grid as I now find if helpful to organize it.

EXISTENTIAL JOY

I said above (p. 152) that tragedy has been more suppressed than joy, and perhaps this is still true, but joy has suffered great mutilation from being confused with amusement, entertainment, and humorousness. Joy is none of these, and only distantly

Table V
Estimates of the Conditions of Being Human

CONDITIONS OF BEING	Embodied	Finite	Action-able	Autonomous	A-partness[a]
CONFRONTATIONS	Change	Contingency	Responsibility	Choice	Separate-yet-related
EXISTENTIAL ANXIETY	Pain and destruction	Fate and death	Guilt and condemnation	Emptiness and meaninglessness	Loneliness and isolation or absorption[b]
EXISTENTIAL JOY	Movement and vitality	Hope and mystery	Surgency and real-ization[c]	Beauty and ecstasy	Encounter and communion
DREAD	Illness	Powerlessness	Blame	Absurdity	Estrangement
COURAGE	Wholeness	Faith	Identity	Creativity	Love
EXISTENTIAL NEEDS AND VALUES	Spiritedness	Rootedness	Commitment	Meaningfulness	Relatedness

[a] In the sense of *a part of yet apart from*.
[b] Absorption into another with loss of one's own identity.
[c] In the sense of making real what has previously been only visualized.

related to any of them. Joy is the experience of full subjective participation—that is, without *Self*-consciousness.

It arises when one has confronted existential anxiety and incorporated the facts of being so that one can transcend the preoccupation with anxiety and dread—note *transcend*, not detour around. My use of the concept of existential joy will become clearer as we examine its forms in relation to the givens of being.

JOY AND EMBODIEDNESS

When we are fully in our healthy bodies and experiencing them, we find the existential joy of *movement*, of feeling our selves using our structures—whether in sports, in dance, in lovemaking, in walking, in restful sleep. The sense of *vitality* that emerges from this way of being is a rich one we too often link with youth; it can be known at any age when we take the responsibility and opportunity to accept and fulfill our embodiedness.

JOY AND BEING FINITE

Our finitude, so often the source of anxiety, can also give rise to the sense of *hope*. Knowing our limits, we know also that we are not the sole authors of our experience, and we can find the existential hope that is neither self-delusion nor the postponement of responsibility. Such hope is the amazing and wondersorking potential of those who somehow overcome great physical or psychological handicaps to lead richer lives than the pessimistic would have though possible: the quadraplegic who becomes head of a state department of rehabilitation, the patient given six months to live with terminal cancer who comes back ten years later with no evidence of the malignancy, the child of destructive parents and improverished environment who forges his/her way to the top of her/his chosen field.

We dwell always in the midst of *mystery*, the ultimate mystery of our being, the commonplace mysteries of love and creation, the forgotten mysteries of our own God-nature. Mystery is the source of possibility, and the promise of a more always emergent. When contingency is truly incorporated, it tells us of fate and death to be sure, but it tells us as well that we cannot know either without recognizing that each is but a partial statement of what may be. This is the joy of our finitude.

JOY AND THE ABILITY TO ACT

To be able to act (or to withhold action) gives our doing meaningfulness and uniqueness. My act bespeaks me, and when I fully accept that, my act becomes an expression of deeper layers of my being, rising from my intentionality, reaching toward my values. Thus the experience of *surgency*, of the rising fullness of aliveness. Out of this comes the wonder of *realization*—making real that which was only potential before, innovating, creating, seeing the work of one's hands or mind or spirit as existing in fact.

JOY AND AUTONOMY

One of the most neglected of human potentials—at least in our Western culture—is the esthetic, the capacity to appreciate and participate in *beauty*. Perhaps because of the over-emphasis on the rationalistic and the objective, this rich vein of being is little regarded even by those who profess humanistic values. Yet beauty is no superficial aspect of being, but the expression of the innerness finding completion in that which is outer. It is thus a special bridge between the two worlds in which human beings live. Moreover, beauty has its roots in our individuality: "There's no accounting for tastes." Those who shirk the risks of recognizing beauty merit the impoverishment of their individuality that results. Beauty does not equal prettiness; it is closer to the mathematician's elegance, is best known by the impulse to sigh, "Ah . . . ." as Koestler (1967) has said.

Ecstasy is an altered state of awareness characterized by an emotional transcendence of everyday experience and a total participation in subjective discovery-recognition. Ecstasy may be religious, spiritual, sexual, esthetic, or in any other subjective dimension. Its essence resides in the choiceful yielding to the sweep of the experience and to the—at least momentary—relinquishing of the ego or *Self*. The ecstatic experience is the choice to be choiceless and emancipated from *Self*.

JOY AND A-PARTNESS

The paradoxical human circumstance of being at once separate from all other beings and yet irrevocably related to all makes possible the experience of genuine meeting with the other that can be called true *encounter*. In encounter with another person, I discover the amazing but obvious truth that there is in the other a subjective awareness with its own world of being, and in that moment I know that I am similarly discovered. This moment of intersubjective recognition is the I-Thou experience (Buber, 1958), in which each of us confirms the beingness of the other. So simple, so seldom fully realized, so profound in its affirmation of our transcendent oneness!

In *communion*, recognition is carried the further step of experiencing that oneness in which the boundaries of self-other are momentarily dissolved. This may be simply the overwhelming sense of relationship and involvement with another; it may take the form of feeling such love for the other that that person's interests seem to equal if not supersede one's own concerns; or it may be moments of truly losing the sense of one's separate identity and finding thoughts and feelings shared without being labeled as belonging to one or the other (sometimes called telepathy). Communion brings intimations of a deeper-than-conscious level of awareness in which is manifested our essential oneness in separateness and separateness in oneness.

SUMMARY

The existential grid is a construction developed to array some of the more important human experiences into interlocking clusters with a view to helping our sensitivities be attuned to recognize the wholeness of being and the facets of experience. The clinician will not be likely to have need of the concepts during actual conversations with clients, but she/he may find them useful to reflect on (and amend and supplement) with a view to expanding his frame of reference. In this way one is helped to attend to what is happening behind the symptoms and specifics of daily experience, while avoiding esoteric systematizations that can so easily lead to losing track of actual client experience.

The reader is reminded that these are but descriptions and estimates; they are not discoveries about the true or ultimate nature of being. Each reader must use the existential grid with responsibility and autonomy.

Emergent Human Beings Revisited

In the fourteenth century, Barbara Tuchman tells us,

> Violence was official as well as individual. Torture was authorized by the Church and regularly used to uncover heresy by the Inquisition. The tortures and punishments of civil justice customarily cut off hands and ears, racked, burned, flayed, and pulled apart people's bodies. In everyday life passers by saw some criminal flogged with a knotted rope or chained upright in an iron collar. They passed corpses hanging on the gibbet and decapitated heads and quartered bodies impaled on stakes on the city walls. In every church they saw pictures of saints undergoing varieties of atrocious martyrdom—by arrows, spears, fire, cut-off breasts—usually dripping blood. The Crucifixion with its nails, spears, thorns, whips, and more dripping blood was inescapable. Blood and cruelty were ubiquitous in Christian art, indeed essential to it, for Christ became Redeemer, and the saints sanctified, only through undergoing violence at the hands of their fellow man.
>
> In village games, players with hands tied behind them competed to kill a cat nailed to a post by battering it to death with their heads, at the risk of cheeks ripped open or eyes scratched out by the frantic animal's claws. Trumpets enhanced the excitement. Or a pig enclosed in a wide pen was chased by men with clubs to the laughter of spectators as he ran squealing from the blows until beaten lifeless. Accustomed in their own lives to physical hardship and injury, medieval men and women were not necessarily repelled by the spectacle of pain, but rather enjoyed it. The citizens of Mons bought a condemned criminal from a neighboring town so that they should have the pleasure of seeing him quartered. It may be that the untender medieval infancy produced adults who valued others no more than they had been valued in their own formative years (1978, p. 134).

Do human beings change? Is human nature the same now as it has always been? Have we advanced any from the cave people, from the time of Imperial Rome and the coliseum, from the fourteenth cnetury?

There are those who bemoan human fallibility and decree that we are as bad now as ever humans were. To my mind they reveal themselves ignorant of history or prejudiced in their views. Tuchman's description of fourteenth-century village sport is eloquent in giving us a benchmark for judging the matter. And the answer is clear: Slowly and painfully, with many setbacks and far too numerous exceptions, we make our way toward realization of more of our truly humane potentialities.

It is not that there are no atrocities in our day. God knows they are all too plentiful still. Idi Amin, My Lai, Auschwitz, the Dacca racetrack—the list is dismayingly easy to compile (Wheelis, 1973). No, it is certainly not that there is no violence in our age. Man's inhumanity to man continues, as the daily paper and newscast persistently record. We are continually shocked out of any complacency we might slip into.

But that is the point: We are shocked. We no longer take outrageous violence for granted; we do not expect it, and only under exceptional instances do we take pleasure in it.

The viewers with alarm insist that since some violence persists, it is demonstrated that the potential for violence still remains in us. And they are right. But they are so very limited in their understanding of the fact they cite. It is not that we have lost the capacity to be violent, to conceive and execute outrages upon ourselves. We still have the power to act; we still have choice about our actions, but we are using our powers and choices differently.

Humankind's progress is to be traced in changes in *expectancies*, not in changes in *potentialities*. Those who misunderstand this point are at heart mechanists wanting the human machine changed so it will not be able to do evil. By nature we are neither good or evil (pp. 142–143), and that freedom is our birthright and the source of our true gains. We can do violence, but we no longer—as a people generally—expect to do so.

Our changes in expectancies are evidenced by the ethic of contribution which is now widely accepted. Imagine trying in the fourteenth century or almost any period before the last one hundred years to collect for the Red Cross, for Amnesty International, or for an anti-war campaign! Many nations today give appreciable amounts to aid less fortunate countries, an inconceivable possibility in most of human history in which weaker nations were viewed only as objects for conquest. On the individual level, the practice of contributing services to organizations serving others is widespread and makes possible many activities that would not otherwise be adding to human welfare. The list, of course, can be extended.

It misses the point entirely to protest, as do some, that there are often gains to those who contribute services or to nations that help less developed countries. The very recognition of this synergic potential is a major step in the evolution of human expectancies and in the realization of human relatedness.

Clare Graves (1966, undated) has devoted many years to studying the stages of development of individuals and cultures. He has demonstrated three phases (interspersed with others) in the evolution of the relations of persons or social groupings with one another: At the most primitive, the other is regarded as a legitimate object for conquest, enslavement, or elimination. A second level sees the other as suitable for domination and utilization (as animate objects). The third and most evolved level, recognizes the essential bond with the other and works for mutual benefit and growth. It seems obvious to me that generally we have moved beyond the first level, that the second is in many ways the dominant expectation of most people and nations today, but it is equally evident that we are beginning to move beyond that toward the third and synergic possibility.

Conclusion

I have had more than fifteen years of life since I wrote the final words to the first edition of this book. Those have been very full, very emotionally charged, very growthful years for me. I am no longer middle-aged; I am an older man (Bugental, 1976, chap. 8). My perspective on my life and work has moved along during this time. I am happy to see how much of my earlier statement still makes sense to me, but I enjoy too seeing the new territory that this time in life provides.

Human beings are, for me, the most fascinating subject matter one can study. I feel very fortunate to have had a lifetime of doing that, and I look forward to continuing that quest yet a good while. As the scene slowly changes, I find I think more often about the human condition generally, relating the experiences of individuals—myself or others—to the development of all of us. Thus I wrote just now about emerging human beings rather than about emerging individuals. It is good to feel the general in the specific and to sense the specific that expresses the general.

One conviction grows stronger for me each year: We have barely begun to explore the human possibility. We have but scratched the surface of what we may be, what we may do, what we may become. It's a fascinating search, the search we're all engaged in, knowingly or not. It's the search for authenticity, but that authenticity is not any one end state. Human authenticity is to be searching, realizing, moving on, searching and arriving, and moving on again.

References for the Enlarged Edition

BUGENTAL, J. F. T. (Ed.). *Challenges of humanistic psychology*. New York: McGraw-Hill, 1967(a).

BUGENTAL, J. F. T. Existential non-being and the need for inspiriting in psychotherapy. In P. Koestenbaum (Ed.), *Proceedings of the San Jose State College Conference on Existential Philosophy and Psychotherapy*. November 18, 1967; San Jose, CA., pp. 24-39.

BUGENTAL, J. F. T. *The search for existential identity*. San Francisco: Jossey-Bass, 1976.

BUGENTAL, J. F. T. *Psychotherapy and process: The fundamentals of an existential-humanistic approach*. Reading, Mass.: Addison-Wesley, 1978.

BUGENTAL, J. F. T. The far side of despair. *Journal of Humanistic Psychology*, 1980, *20*, 49-68.

GRAVES, C. W. Deterioration of work standards. *Harvard Business Review*, 1966, Sept–Oct, 117–126.

GRAVES C. W. *The broader meaning of the concept, the levels of human existence*. Unpublished manuscript, undated. (Available from Clare W. Graves, Department of Psychology, Union College, Schenectady, New York.)

GUNTHER, B. *What to do till the Messiah comes*. New York: Collier Books, 1971.

JONES E. *The life and work of Sigmund Freud.* (Vol. 3). New York: Basic Books, 1957.

JOURARD, S. M. *The transparent self.* New York: Van Nostrand, 1964.

KOESTLER, A. The three domains of creativity. In J. F. T. Bugental (Ed.), *Challenges of humanistic psychology.* New York: Mc-Graw-Hill, 1967, Pp. 31-40.

MASLOW, A. H. *Toward a psychology of being.* New York: Van Nostrand Reinhold, 1968.

SABATH, C. J. An existential model of authenticity: A theroretical and validating study. Unpubl. doct. dissert., California School of Professional Psychology, Los Angeles, 1978.

THAUBERGER, P. C. The avoidance of existential-ontological confrontation: A review of research. Paper presented at the meeting of the Canadian Psychological Association, Quebec City, June 1979.

THAUBERGER, P. C., & Cleland, J. F. Avoidance of ontological confrontation of loneliness and some epidemiological indices of social behavior and health. *Perceptual and Motor Skills,* 1979, *48,* 1219-1224.

THAUBERGER, P. C., & Cleland, J. F. Psychometric explorations of the relationship of an avoidance of existential-ontological confrontation to neuroticism. Unpubl. manuscript, undated. Available from Patrick C. Thauberger, Ph.D., 5425-144 'B' Avenue, Edmonton, Alberta, Canada.

THAUBERGER, P. C., & Davis, J. Some initial indices of existential confrontation in a sample of maximum security inmates. Unpubl. manuscript, undated. Available from Patrick C. Thauberger, Ph.D, Edmonton Institution, P.O. Box 2290, Edmonton, Alberta. T5J 3H7.

THAUBERGER, P. C., & Sydiaha, D. Acceptance of self and others and the existential persuasion. *Psycholoqhical Reports,* 1979, *44,* 483-488.

THAUBERGER, P. C., & Sydiaha-Symor, D. The relationship between an avoidance of existential confrontation and neuroticism: A psychometric test. *Journal of Humanistic Psychology,,* 1977, *17,* 89-91.

THAUBERGER P. C., Thauberger, E. M., & Cleland, J. F. Avoidance of the ontological confrontation of death and a phenomenological encounter with a simulated death atmosphere. *Perceptual and Motor Skills*, 1977, *45*, 171-178.

TUCHMAN, B. W. *A distant mirror: The Fourteenth Century.* New York: Knopf, 1978.

WALSH, R. N. Reflections on psychotherapy. *Journal of Transpersonal Psychology*, 1976, *8* (2), 100–111.

WHEELIS, A. *The moralist.* New York: Basic Books, 1973.

REFERENCES

Adcock, C. J. Free will and freedom. *J. gen. Psychol.*, 1961, *64*, 139–146.
Adkins, L. J. The creative factor in man. *Christ. Cent.*, 1959, *76*, 40–42.
Allport, G. W. The ego in contemporary psychology. *Psychol. Rev.*, 1943, *50*, 451–476.
Allport, G. W. *Becoming: Basic considerations for a psychology of personality.* New Haven: Yale Univ. Press, 1955.
Angel, R. W. The concept of psychic determinism. *Amer. J. Psychiat.*, 1956, *116*, 405–408.

Baker, R. A. *Psychology in the wry.* Princeton, N. J.: Van Nostrand, 1963.
Barrett, W. (Ed.) *Zen Buddhism.* (Selected writings of D. T. Suzuki) Garden City, N. Y.: Doubleday, 1956.
Beckett, S. *Krapp's last tape and other dramatic pieces.* New York: Grove Press, 1957.
Beckett, S. *Endgame.* New York: Grove Press, 1958.
Ben-Avi, A. Treatability. In Council of Psychoanalytic Psychotherapists (Ed.), *The concept of treatability.* New York: Coun. Psychoanal. Psychother., 1960, pp. 6–9.
Berne, E. *Transactional analysis in psychotherapy.* New York: Grove Press, 1961.
Berne, E. *The structure and dynamics of organizations and groups.* Philadelphia: Lippincott, 1963.
Bettelheim, B. *The informed heart.* New York: Free Press of Glencoe, 1960.

BLAKE, R. R., & RAMSEY, G. V. (Eds.) *Perception: An approach to personality.* New York: Ronald Press, 1951.
Boss, M. Anxiety, guilt, and psychotherapeutic liberation. *Rev. existen. Psychol. Psychiat.,* 1962, 2, 173–207.
BROWN, N. O. *Life against death.* New York: Random House, 1959.
BUBER, M. *I-Thou* (ed. 2). New York: Scribner's, 1958.
BUDD, W. C. Is free will really necessary? *Amer. Psychologist,* 1960, *15,* 217–218.
BUGENTAL, J. F. T. An investigation of the relationship of the conceptual matrix to the self-concept. Unpubl. doct. dissert., Ohio St. Univ., 1948.
BUGENTAL, J. F. T. Behaviors characteristic of patients progressing in psychotherapy. Paper read at Western Psychol. Assn., Fresno, Calif., April 1952. (a)
BUGENTAL, J. F. T. A method for assessing self and not-self attitudes during the therapeutic series. *J. consult. Psychol.,* 1952, *16,* 435–439. (b)
BUGENTAL, J. F. T. Existential tragedy and the psychotherapeutic process. Paper read at the Calif. St. Psychol. Assn., Los Angeles, Dec. 1962. (a) [*J. Existentialism* (in press)]
BUGENTAL, J. F. T. Five paradigms for group psychotherapy. *Psychol. Rep.,* 1962, *10,* 607–610. (b)
BUGENTAL, J. F. T. The nature of the therapeutic task in intensive psychotherapy. Unpubl. paper, 1962. (c)
BUGENTAL, J. F. T. A phenomenological hypothesis of neurotic determinants and their therapy. *Psychol. Rep.,* 1962, *10,* 527–530. (d)
BUGENTAL, J. F. T. Precognitions of a fossil. *J. humanistic Psychol.,* 1962, *2* (2), 38–46. (e)
BUGENTAL, J. F. T. Self-fragmentation as a resistance to self-actualization. *Rev. existent. Psychol. Psychiat.,* 1962, 2, 241–248. (f)
BUGENTAL, J. F. T. The existential crisis in intensive psychotherapy. *Psychotherapy* (in press).
BUGENTAL, J. F. T. Humanistic psychology: A new break-through. *Amer. Psychologist.,* 1963, *18,* 563–568. (b)
BUGENTAL, J. F. T. Investigations into the self-concept: III. Instructions for the W-A-Y experiment. *Psychol. Rep.,* 1964, *15,* 643–650. (a)
BUGENTAL, J. F. T. Psychodiagnostics and the quest for certainty. *Psychiatry,* 1964, 27, 73–77. (b)
BUGENTAL, J. F. T. The third force in psychology. (Basic postu-

lates and orientation of humanistic psychology). *J. humanistic Psychol.*, 1964, *4* (1), 19–26. (c)

BUGENTAL, J. F. T., & GUNNING, EVELYN C. Investigations into the self-concept: II: Stability of reported self-identifications. *J. clin. Psychol.*, 1955, *11*, 41–46.

BUGENTAL, J. F. T., & TANNENBAUM, R. Sensitivity training and being motivation. *J. humanistic Psychol.*, 1963, *3* (1), 76–85.

BUGENTAL, J. F. T., & ZELEN, S. L. Investigations into the self-concept: I. The W-A-Y technique. *J. Personality*, 1950, *18*, 483–498.

BUHLER, CHARLOTTE. *Values in psychotherapy.* New York: Free Press of Glencoe, 1962.

BURTON, A., & LUNDE, D. T. Bibliographic sources of existential thought. Agnews St. Hosp., Calif., 1961 (mimeographed).

BYRD, R. E. *Alone.* New York: Grosset & Dunlap, 1956.

CANTRIL, H., & BUMSTEAD, C. H. *Reflections on the human venture.* New York: New York Univ. Press, 1960.

COLBY, K. M. *A primer for psychotherapists.* New York: Ronald Press, 1951.

COOPER, L. *Aristotle on the art of poetry.* Ithaca, N.Y.: Cornell Univ. Press, 1947.

CRASTER, MRS. E. The puzzled centipede. In J. E. Brewton (Ed.) *Under the tent of the sky.* New York: Macmillan, 1937, p. 155.

DEIKMAN, A. J. Experimental meditation. *J. nerv. ment. Dis.*, 1963, *136*, 329–343.

DUCASSE, C. J. *A critical examination of the belief in a life after death.* Springfield, Ill.: Chas. A Thomas, 1961.

ELIOT, T. S. The hollow men. In *Collected poems 1909–1962.* New York: Harcourt, 1963, p. 221.

ERIKSON, E. H. *Identity and the life cycle.* New York: Internatl. Univ. Press, 1959.

FARBER, L. H. Martin Buber and psychiatry. *Psychiatry*, 1956, *19*, 109–120.

FARBER, L. H. Introduction to the William Alanson White Memorial Lectures, Fourth Series, by Martin Buber. *Psychiatry*, 1957, *20*, 95–96. (a)

FARBER, L. H. What is effective in the therapeutic process? *Amer. J. Psychoanal.*, 1957, *17*, 21–26. (b)

FARBER, L. H. The therapeutic despair. *Psychiatry*, 1958, *21*, 7–20.
FARBER, L. H. Schizophrenia and the mad psychotherapist. *Rev. existent. Psychol. Psychiat.*, 1962, *2*, 209–227.
FEIFEL, H. *The meaning of death.* New York: McGraw-Hill, 1959.
FELDMAN, J. J. The use of obscene words in the therapeutic relationship. *Amer. J. Psychoanal.*, 1955, *15*, 45–48.
FINGARETTE, H. On the relation between moral guilt and guilt in neurosis. *J. humanistic Psychol.*, 1962, *2* (2), 96–100. (a)
FINGARETTE, H. Real guilt and neurotic guilt. *J. existent. Psychiat.*, 1962, *3*, 145–158. (b)
FINGARETTE, H. *The self in transformation. (Psychoanalysis, philosophy, and the life of the spirit.)* New York: Basic Books, 1963.
FREUD, S. *The question of lay analysis.* New York: Author, 1933.
FREUD, S. *New introductory lectures on psychoanalysis.* New York: Norton, 1936.
FREUD, S. Why War? In J. Strachey (Ed.), *Sigmund Freud: Collected Papers.* Vol. 5. London: Hogarth, 1953, pp. 273–287.
FROMM, E. *Escape from freedom.* New York: Holt, Rinehart and Winston, 1941.
FROMM, E. *Man for himself.* New York: Holt, Rinehart and Winston, 1947.
FROMM, E. *The art of loving.* New York: Harper & Row, 1956.
FROMM, E. Value, psychology, and human existence. In A. H. Maslow (Ed.), *New knowledge in human values.* New York: Harper & Row, 1959, pp. 151–164.
FROMM-REICHMANN, FRIEDA. *Principles of intensive psychotherapy.* Chicago: Univ. of Chicago Press, 1950.

GALBRAITH, GEORGIE STARBUCK. White revelations. *Sat. Even. Post*, 11-27-54, p. 72.
GIBRAN, K. *The prophet.* New York: Knopf, 1955.

HAIGH, G. V. Existential guilt: neurotic and real. *Rev. existent. Psychol. Psychiat.*, 1961, *1*, 120–130.
HARTMANN, W. The free will controversy. *Amer. Psychologist*, 1961, *16*, 37–38.
HORA, T. The process of existential psychotherapy. *Existent. Inquir.*, 1959, *1* (1), 11–12.

HORA, T. Existential psychiatry and group psychotherapy. *Amer. J. Psychoanal.*, 1961, 21, 58–70. (a)
HORA, T. Transcendence and healing. *J. existent. Psychiat.*, 1961, 1, 501–511. (b)
HORA, T. Beyond self. *Psychologia*, 1962, 5, 84–87. (a)
HORA, T. The epistemology of love. *J. existent. Psychiat.*, 1962, 2, 303–312. (b)
HORA, T. Existential psychotherapy. In *Current psychiatric therapies*, 1962, II, 38–40. New York: Grune & Stratton. (c)
HORA, T. Responsibility. *Rev. existent. Psychol. Psychiat.*, 1962, 2, 259–264. (d)
HORNEY, KAREN. *Neurosis and human growth.* New York: Norton, 1950.
HUXLEY, A. *Doors of perception.* New York: Harper & Row, 1954. (a)
HUXLEY, A. *Heaven and hell.* New York: Harper & Row, 1954. (b)

JOURARD, S. M. Some lethal aspects of the male role. *J. existent. Psychiat.*, 1962, 2, 333–344.
JOURARD, S. M. *Personal adjustment: An approach through the study of the healthy personality* (ed. 2). New York: Macmillan, 1963.
JOURARD, S. M. The phenomenon of resistance in the psychotherapist. *J. existent. Psychiat.* (in press), (a)
JOURARD, S. M. *The transparent self: Self-disclosure and wellbeing.* Princeton: Van Nostrand, 1964. (b)

KAISER, H. The problem of responsibility in psychotherapy. *Psychiatry*, 1955, 18, 205–211.
KAISER, H. (Untitled posthumous book on psychotherapy.) Scheduled for 1964.
KAUFMANN, W. (Ed.) *Existentialism from Dostoevsky to Sartre.* Cleveland: Meridian-World, 1956.
KELLY, G. A. *The psychology of personal constructs.* Vols. I and II. New York: Norton, 1955.
KELLY, G. A. The abstraction of human processes. Read at the Fourteenth International Congress of Applied Psychology. Copenhagen, Denmark, Aug. 1961.
KELLY, G. A. Psychotherapy and the nature of man. Read at the Amer. Psychol. Assn., Philadelphia, Aug. 1963.
KELLY, G. A. A psychology of the optimal man. In A. Mahrer (Ed.), *Goals of psychotherapy* (in preparation).

KELMAN, H. *The process in psychoanalysis.* New York: Amer. Inst. Psychoanal., 1948.
KELMAN, H. What are constructive forces? *Amer. J. Psychoanal.*, 1953, *13*, 4–8.
KELMAN, H. The use of the analytic couch. *Amer. J. Psychoanal.*, 1954, *14*, 65–82.
KELMAN, H. Life history as therapy: Part I. Evaluation of literature. *Amer. J. Psychoanal.*, 1955, *15*, 144–162.
KELMAN, H. Life history as therapy: Part II. On being aware. *Amer. J. Psychoanal.*, 1956, *16*, 68–78. (a)
KELMAN, H. Life history as therapy: Part III: The symbolizing process. *Amer. J. Psychoanal.*, 1956, *16*, 145–166. (b)
KELMAN, H. "Kairos" and the therapeutic process. *J. existent. Psychiat.*, 1960, *1*, 233–269.
KNAPP, P. H., LEVIN, S., MCCARTER, R. H., WERMER, H., & ZETZEL, ELIZABETH. Suitability for psychoanalysis: A review of one hundred supervised analytic cases. *Psychoanal. Quart.*, 1960, *29*, 459–477.

LASKO, A. A. The existential crisis in intensive psychotherapy. Paper read at the Western Psychol. Assn., Santa Monica, Calif., April 1963.
LECKY, P. (Ed. and interpreted by F. C. Thorne) *Self-consistency: A theory of personality.* New York: Island Press, 1951.
LEWIN, K. *A dynamic theory of personality.* New York: McGraw-Hill, 1935.
LYONS, J. An annotated bibliography on phenomenology and existentialism. *Psychol. Rep.*, 1959, *5*, 613–631.
LYONS, J. A bibliographic introduction to phenomenology and existentialism. In R. MAY (Ed.), *Existential psychology.* New York: Random House, 1961, pp. 101–126.

MCCLEARY, R. A., & LAZARUS, R. S. Autonomic discriminations without awareness: An interim report. *J. Personality*, 1949, *18*, 171–179.
MAGILL, F. N., & MCGREAL, I. P. (Eds.) *Masterpieces of world philosophy.* Vol. I. New York: Salem Press, 1961, pp. 174–179.
MARZOLF, S. S. The disease concept in psychology. *Psychol. Rev.*, 1947, *54*, 211–222.
MASLOW, A. H. *Motivation and personality.* New York: Harper & Row, 1954.

MASLOW, A. H. (Ed.) *New knowledge in human values.* New York: Harper & Row, 1959.
MASLOW, A. H. *Notes toward a psychology of being.* La Jolla, Calif., Western Behavioral Sciences Inst., 1961, Report No. 7.
MASLOW, A. H. *Summer notes* . . . Del Mar, Calif.: Non-Linear Systems, Inc., 1962. (a)
MASLOW, A. H. *Toward a psychology of being.* Princeton, N. J.: Van Nostrand, 1962. (b)
MAY, R. Historical and philosophical presuppositions for understanding therapy. In O. H. MOWRER (Ed.), *Psychotherapy: Theory and practice.* New York: Ronald, 1953, pp. 9–43. (a)
MAY, R. *Man's search for himself.* New York: Norton, 1953. (b)
MAY, R. Contributions of existential psychotherapy. In R. May, E. Angel, & R. F. Ellenberger (Eds.), *Existence: A new dimension in psychiatry and psychology.* New York: Basic Books, 1958, pp. 37–92.
MAY, R. The existential approach. In S. Arieti (Ed.), *American handbook of psychiatry.* New York: Basic Books, 1959, pp. 1348–1361. (a)
MAY, R. Toward the ontological basis of psychotherapy. *Existent. Inquir.,* 1959, *1* (1), 5–7. (b)
MAY, R. Existential bases of psychotherapy. In R. MAY (Ed.) *Existential psychology.* New York: Random House, 1961, pp. 75–85. (a)
MAY, R. (Ed.) *Existential psychology.* New York: Random House, 1961. (b)
MAY, R., ANGEL, E., & ELLENBERGER, H. F. (Eds.) *Existence: A new dimension in psychiatry and psychology.* New York: Basic Books, 1958.
MENNINGER, K. *Theory of psychoanalytic technique.* New York: Basic Books, 1958.
MILLER, A. Tragedy and the common man. *Theater Arts,* 1951, *35* (3), 48–50.
MOUSTAKAS, C. E. *The self.* New York: Harper & Row, 1956.
MOUSTAKAS, C. E. Honesty, idiocy, and manipulation. *J. humanistic Psychol.,* 1962, *2* (2), 1–15.
MURPHY, G. *Personality.* New York: Harper & Row, 1947.
MURPHY, G. *Human potentialities.* New York: Basic Books, 1958.

NATIONAL TRAINING LABORATORY IN GROUP DEVELOPMENT. *Explorations in human relations training: An assessment of experience, 1947–1953.* Washington: Natl. Educ. Assn., 1953.

ORNE, M. T. On the social psychology of the psychological experiment: with particular reference to demand characteristics and their implications. *Amer. Psychologist*, 1962, *17*, 776–783.

POSTMAN, L., BRUNER, J. S., & McGINNIES, E. Personal values as selective factors in perception. *J. abnorm. social Psychol.*, 1948, *43*, 142–154.

RAIMY, V. C. The self-concept as a factor in counseling and personality organization. Unpub. Doct. dissert., Ohio St. Univ., 1943.

RAIMY, V. C. Self reference in counseling interviews. *J. consult. Psychol.*, 1948, *12*, 153–163.

RAPAPORT, D., et al. *Diagnostic psychological testing.* Vol. I. Chicago: Year Book Publishers, 1945.

REICH, W. *Character analysis.* New York: Orgone Inst. Press, 1949.

RIESMAN, D. *The lonely crowd.* New Haven: Yale Univ. Press, 1950.

RIESMAN, D. *Individualism reconsidered.* New York: Free Press of Glencoe, 1954.

ROBINSON, F. P. *Principles and procedures in student counseling.* New York: Harper & Row, 1950.

ROGERS, C. R. *Counseling and psychotherapy.* Boston: Houghton Mifflin, 1942.

ROGERS, C. R. *Client-centered therapy: Its current practice, implications, and theory.* Boston: Houghton Mifflin, 1951.

ROGERS, C. R. Some directions and end-points in therapy. In O. H. MOWRER (Ed.), *Psychotherapy: Theory and research.* New York: Ronald, 1953, pp. 44–68.

ROGERS, C. R. A theory of therapy, personality, and interpersonal relationships, as developed in the client-centered framework. In S. KOCH (Ed.), *Psychology: A study of a science: Study I. Conceptual and systematic. Vol. 3. Formulations of the person and the social context.* New York: McGraw-Hill, 1959, pp. 184–256.

ROGERS, C. R. *A therapist's view of personal goals.* Wallingford, Pa.: Pendle Hill Pamphlet 108, 1960.

ROGERS, C. R. *On becoming a person.* Boston: Houghton Mifflin, 1961. (a)

ROGERS, C. R. Two divergent trends. In R. May (Ed.), *Existential psychology.* New York: Random House, 1961, pp. 85–93. (b)

ROGERS, C. R. Toward a science of the person. Presented at Rice Univ., Houston, March, 1963.

SAUL, L. J. *Technic and practice of psychoanalysis.* Philadelphia: Lippincott, 1958.

SCHACHTEL, E. G. *Metamorphosis.* New York: Basic Books, 1959.

SCHALLER, J. P. Psychologie clinique et liberté humaine. (Clinical psychology and human liberty.) *Angelicum,* 1959, *36,* 3–25.

SCHWARTZ, E. K., & WOLF, A. The quest for certainty. *A. M. A. Arch. Neurol. Psychiat.,* 1959, *81,* 69–84.

SHAPIRO, S. B. Ego therapy in action: A case study. *Psychol. Rep.,* 1962, *11,* 821–831. (a)

SHAPIRO, S. B. A theory of ego pathology and ego therapy. *J. Psychol.* 1962, *53,* 81–90. (b)

SPENDER, S. Preludes. In *Collected poems.* New York: Random House, 1955, p. 8.

SPIEGEL, J. P. The social roles of doctor and patient in psychoanalysis and psychotherapy. *Psychiatry,* 1954, *17,* 369–376.

STEVENSON, B. E. (Ed.) *Home book of verse.* New York: Holt, Rinehart & Winston, 1918.

SYKES, G. *The hidden remnant.* New York: Harper & Row, 1962.

SZASZ, T. S. The myth of mental illness. *Amer. Psychologist,* 1960, *15,* 113–118.

SZASZ, T. S. *The myth of mental illness.* New York: Harper & Row, 1961.

TANNENBAUM, R., & BUGENTAL, J. F. T. Dyads, clans, and tribe: A new design for sensitivity training. *N. T. L. Hum. Rel. Trng. News,* 1963, 7 (1), 1–3.

TAYLOR, D. *Of men and music.* New York: Simon & Schuster, 1937.

TAYLOR, D. W. Education for research in psychology. *Amer. Psychologist,* 1959, *14,* 167–179.

TILLICH, P. *The courage to be.* New Haven: Yale Univ. Press, 1952.

VAN DUSEN, W. Existential analysis: The English Literature. *Existent. Inquir.,* 1959, *1* (1), 16–30.

WALDHORN, H. F. Assessment of analyzability: Technical and theoretical observations. *Psychoanal. Quart.*, 1960, *29*, 478–506.
WARKENTIN, J. The therapist's significant other. *Ann. Psychother.*, 1963, *4* (1), 54–59.
WATERS, R. H. Mechanomorphism: A new term for an old mode of thought. *Psychol. Rev.*, 1948, *55*, 139–142.
WATTS, A. W. *Nature, man and woman.* New York: Pantheon, 1958.
WATTS, A. W. *Psychotherapy East and West.* New York: Pantheon, 1961.
WHEELIS, A. *The quest for identity.* New York: Norton, 1958.
WHEELIS, A. To be a god. *Commentary*, 1963, *36* (2), 125–134.
WHITAKER, C. A., and MALONE, T. P. *The roots of psychotherapy.* New York: Blakiston, 1953.
WINN, R. B. *A concise dictionary of existentialism.* New York: Philosophical Library, 1960.
WOLBERG, L. R. *The technique of psychotherapy.* New York: Grune & Stratton, 1954.
WOLFENSBERGER, W. The free will controversy. *Amer. Psychologist*, 1961, *16*, 36–37.
WYLIE, RUTH C. *The self concept.* Lincoln: Univ. of Nebr. Press, 1961.

INDEXES

INDEX OF NAMES

Adkins, L. J., 348
Allport, G. W., 200, 202
Aristotle, 154, 160

Baker, R. A., 405 fn.
Beckett, S., 306–308, 310–311
Ben-Avi, A., 56
Berne, E., 211
Bettelheim, B., 134
Bolgar, Hedda, 90 fn.
Bonner, H., 10
Boss, M., 89 fn., 173
Brown, N. O., 43
Bruner, J. S., 234
Buber, M., 353
Buhler, Charlotte, 10, 284 fn.
Burton, A., 14 fn.
Byrd, R. E., 356

Campbell, J., 405 fn.
Colby, K. M., 67

Ducasse, C. J., 332 fn., 409

Eliot, T. S., 202
Erikson, E., 335

Farber, L. H., 52, 249, 284 fn.
Feifel, H., 409
Feldman, J. J., 366
Fingarette, H., 173, 212 fn.
Franklin, B., 389–390

Freud, S., 16, 43, 63, 74, 88, 92, 93, 145, 193, 200, 232, 355
Fromm, E., 10, 29, 284, 285 fn., 328, 335, 336, 344, 353
Fromm-Reichman, Frieda, 68

Galbraith, Georgie Starbuck, 289
Gibran, K., 165

Haigh, G. V., 301
Hollingworth, Leta, 187 fn.
Hora, T., 71, 72, 89 fn., 99, 100–102, 243, 250–251, 277–278, 284 fn.
Horney, Karen, 168, 212, 267
Huxley, A., 48, 205 fn., 251, 332 fn.

Jourard, S. M., 10, 249, 284 fn., 365 fn., 372

Kaiser, H., 72, 88–89 fn.
Kelly, G. A., 284 fn., 403
Kelman, H., 66, 68, 71, 317
Kierkegaard, S., 249
Knapp, P. H., 56

Lasko, A. A., 180 fn., 205 fn., 277
Lazarus, R. S., 234
Lecky, P., 210
Lee, Dorothy, 10
Lewin, K., 18
Lunde, D. T., 14 fn.
Lyons, S., 14 fn.

McCleary, R. A., 234
McGinnies, E., 234
Malone, T. P., 367
Maslow, A. H., 1, 10, 50, 73, 183, 185, 213–214, 246, 251, 254, 263, 264–266, 286, 323, 367
May, R., 10, 27, 71, 89 fn., 217 fn., 232, 261, 275, 284 fn., 335
Menninger, K., 68, 72, 111
Miller, A., 152, 154
Moustakas, C. E., 10, 30, 162, 249
Murphy, G., 202, 377

Orne, M. T., 206

Plato, 396, 414–415
Polybius of Megalopolis, 81
Postman, L., 234

Raimy, V. C., 205, 209–210
Reich, W., 77, 88 fn., 101
Reisman, D., 198, 210
Rogers, C. R., 10, 68, 71, 89, 107–108, 246, 254, 284 fn., 343

Saul, L. J., 68, 111–112, 356 fn.
Schachtel, E., G., 10, 299

Schwartz, E. K., 74, 171
Shapiro, S. B., 211
Shoben, E. J., Jr., 10
Spender, S., 203
Spiegel, J. P., 55
Suzuki, D. T., 279, 399
Szasz, T. S., 54

Tannenbaum, R., 352
Taylor, D., 347
Taylor, D. W., 409
Tillich, P., 26, 40, 164, 171, 284–285, 294

Van Dusen, W., 14 fn.

Waldborn, H. F., 56
Warkentin, J., 362
Waters, R. H., 1, 210
Watts, A. W., 401–402
Wheelis, A., 20, 362
Whitaker, C. A., 367
Winn, R. B., 26 fn.
Wolberg, L. R., 58, 68
Wolf, A., 74, 171
Wylie, Ruth, 249

INDEX OF SUBJECTS

Absurd, the, 28
Absurdity, dread of, 287, 293, 306–309
Action potential, 37–38, 285, 287, 321
Action-derivation sequence, 208–209
Actualization, 263–276, 318–319
   and appreciation of suchness, 272–274
   and centeredness, 275
   and changing nature of concern, 266–268
   clinical observations, 266–276
   and courage, 26
   and happiness, 272
   implications of *I–Self* distinction for, 213–214
   and intensified participation, 270–272
   Maslow's findings, 264–266
   nature of, 266–276
   and selective commitment, 268–270
   and the *Self*, 213–214
   and the subject–object split, 275
   and wholeness of experience, 274–275
Adaptation, 33
Adjustment, 33
Aesthetic living, 272–274, 389–392
Alienation, 260–262, 293, 384–385
All, The, 412–414
   awareness and, 221
Alliance, therapeutic, 85–87
Aloneness, 28–29

Analytic perspective, 16
Anxiety, 24, 94–97, 171, 287
   see also Existential anxiety
Apartness, 39, 350–357
   confrontation of, 287, 293, 308–310, 321
Art of Loving, The, 353
Artistry in living, *see* Aesthetic living
Arts, authenticity of, 408–410
Authenticity, 102–103
   attributes of, 45, 285, 287
   and emergent man, 397–400
   forfeiting of, 43–45, 162–163
   nature of, 33–35
   as primary existential value, 31–33
Autonomy, 38–39, 343–350
   confrontation of, 287, 293, 305–306, 321
Auto-utilization, 312
   see also Subject–object split
Awareness, 12
   alterations of, 231
   aspects of, 237–239
   being and, 283, 288, 392–394
   causality and, 228–230
   constraints on, 231–234
   and construction of "world," 97–99, 219
   evolution of, 220–222, 412–413
   expansion of, 239–244, 394, 400–401
   fallacious view of, 223–224
   feelingfulness as a part of, 219–220

givens of, *see* Existential givens
inaccuracy of model of, 224–228, 259
lack of training and, 233–234
learned inhibitions and, 232–233
memory and, 224
nature of, 219–234
ontogogic aids and, 235–244
open, 400–401
preconscious exploration of, 242–243
problem solving and, 226–228
realistic view of, 222–228
resistance and, 232
teaching new concept of, 236–237
and The All, 221
varied experiences of, 231

Being
active vs. reactive, 255–257
definition of, 27, 282–283, 288
dynamic awareness of, 392–394
existence and, 27, 282–283, 319
and non-being, 27, 287
Being-motivation, 183, 286
Blame, 87, 118
confusion of guilt and, 303–304
dread of, 287, 293, 302–304

Causality, 228–230, 259
Centeredness, 275
Choice, 12, 23, 38–39, 119, 171, 195–196, 209, 285, 287, 321
confronting the patient with, 345–346
magic and, 196–197
morality and, 197
relinquishment and, 346–347
responsibility of, 196–197
Commitment, 268–270, 287, 321, 334–343
Concern, 266–268
Condemnation
anxiety of, *see* Existential anxiety, of condemnation
threat of, 37–38
Conditioning, 209

Confirmation, 29
Conflict, ontological options of, 321, 348–350
Confrontation, 283–284, 287, 289, 293, 318–319, 321
pseudo-confrontation and, 406–408
Congruence, 107–109
Consciousness and awareness, 217 fn.
Contingency, 22, 36–37, 327–333, 365
confrontation of, 287, 293, 295–297, 321
potential of, 297–298
"Cool" philosophy, 94–95 fn., 388–389
Core dynamic sequence, 286–290
Couch, use of, 66–67
Courage, 26, 102, 287, 321
Courage to Be, The, 26, 285
Creative emptiness, 401–402
Creativity, 28, 287, 321, 343–350, 393–394, 401–403
Crisis, *see* Existential crisis
Culture, *see* Resistance, derived from culture, *and* Emergent society

Death
conceptions of, 27, 294, 331–332
dread of, 292–300
threat of, 36–37
see also Existential anxiety, of death
Deficit-motivation, 183, 286
Depression, 163
Devotion, ontologic option of, 321, 355–356
Dialogue, 30
"Display," 140
Dominant emotional theme, 111–114, 123
Dread, neurotic, 287
and inauthentic response, 289–290, 292–293, 318–319
see also Existential anxiety

Education, authenticity of, 408
Ego, 200–201
Emancipation from the *Self*, 254–262, 322–326

Index of Subjects

Emergent man, 376–394, 395–403
　values of, 397–403
　see also Emergent society
Emergent society
　changes in, 403–411
　as open society, 411–412
Emptiness, 401–403
　anxiety of, 304–309
　see also Existential anxiety, of emptiness
　sense of, 38–39
Encounter, 28–30, 190–191, 371–372
Endgame, 306–308
Engagement, 30
Enlightenment, 278–279
Entertainment, 406–407
Estrangement, 287, 293, 310–313
Existence
　and being, 282–283
　definition of, 27
Existential-analytic thesis, 14–20, 21–30, 282–290
Existential anxiety, 22–24, 94, 287, 288, 321
　absurdity and, 306–309
　apartness and, 309–310
　autonomy and, 305–306
　blame and, 302–304
　of condemnation, 37–38, 285, 293, 300–304, 321
　contingency and, 295–298
　courage and, 288, 290
　of death, 36–37, 285, 292–300, 321
　dread and, 288–290, 292–315
　of emptiness, 38–39, 285, 287, 293, 304–309, 321
　of estrangement, 310–313
　of fate, 36–37, 285, 287, 292–300, 321
　of finiteness, 294
　forms of, 285–288
　of guilt, 37–38, 285, 287, 293, 300–304, 321
　inauthentic response and, 290, 292–293
　of isolation, 39, 285, 293, 309–313, 321
　of loneliness, 39, 285, 287, 293, 309–313, 321
　of meaninglessness, 38–39, 285, 293, 304–309, 321
　neurotic anxiety and, 24–26, 94–97
　of powerlessness, 298–300
　resistance and, 94–97
　responsibility and, 301–302
　Tillich's concepts, 285
Existential confrontations, see Confrontations
Existential crisis, 166–181
　anxiety and, 171, 172
　avoidance of reassurance in, 179
　avoidance of rewards in, 179–180
　choice and, 171–173
　concept of, 170–173
　cues to, 175–177
　focusing of associations in, 176
　freedom in, 178
　presence of therapist in, 180
　recognition of, 174–177
　reductions of resistances in, 177–178
　resistance emergence in, 176–177, 177–178
　therapeutic procedure in, 173–178
Existential givens, 15, 35–40, 285, 287, 288, 321
Existential needs, 321
　core dynamic sequence and, 286, 287, 288–290
　Fromm's observations on, 284–285
Existential neuroses, 291–293
　forms of, 292–315
　see also Existential anxiety
Existential perspective, 16, 282–283
　values of, 17–20
Experimental psychology, 249

Faith, 287, 321, 327–333
Fantasy, 398–399
Fate
　dread of, 292–300
　sense of, 36–37
　see also Existential anxiety, of fate
Fear, 405–406

INDEX OF SUBJECTS

Finiteness, 36–37, 285, 287, 294, 321
Free association, 107
Freedom, 23, 293
  see also Ontologic freedom
Fullness, emotional, 386–389

Government, 404–406
Grief, 160, 179, 353–355
Group methods, 243–244
  see also Group therapy
Group therapy, 243
  transference and, 215
Guilt
  anxiety of, see Existential anxiety, of guilt
  confusion of blame and, 303–304
  sense of, 37–38

Habits, 209
Happiness, 272
  see also Joy, existential
Hubris, 154, 161
Humanistic psychology, see Psychology, humanistic

I, 200–203
  see also *I*-process
I and the *Self*
  confusion of, 202–203, 259–260, 280, 322, 335
  distinguishing between, 213–216, 263–264, 322–323
  emancipation and, 254–262, 322–327
  false dilemma of, 260
  see also Subject–object split
Iatrogenic complications, 82–85, 362–366, 369–371
Identity, need for, 284, 285, 287, 321, 335–336
I–*Me* confusion, see *I* and the *Self*
Inhibitions, 232–233
Instincts, 209
Intensive psychotherapy, 58–60
  analytic phase of, 62, 63–64
  ontogogic phase of, 61, 62
  transcendental phase of, 61
Interpretation, see Interventions

Interventions, 207
  guides to, 31, 85–87, 115–131, 145–149, 162–163, 179–180, 236–243
  sequence, 114
  use of in psychotherapy, 115–125
Intimacy, 362
I-process, 203–208, 219, 220, 236, 402
  clinical implications of, 206
  false equation with the *Self*, see *I* and the *Self*
  identity and, 335–336
  the *Self* and, 205, 259–262
Isolation
  anxiety of, see Existential anxiety, of isolation
  threat of, 39

Joy, existential, 25, 151–152

Krapp's Last Tape, 310–311

Letting-be, 209
Limits and endings, ontological options of, 321, 330–333
Listening to the patient, 107–111, 143–145, 174–177
Living, artistry in, see Aesthetic living
Loneliness, 28–29
  anxiety of, see Existential anxiety, of loneliness
  definition of, 28–29
  response of, 353–355
  sense of, 39
Love, 287, 321, 350–357, 362–365

Magic, see Choice *and* Superstition
Man
  nature of, 142–143
  and relation to The All, 412–414
Me, 201, 202, 203, 206
  see also *Self*, the, *and I* and the *Self*
Meaningfulness, need for, 284, 285, 287, 321, 343–344
Meaninglessness, 28
  anxiety of, see Existential anxiety, of meaninglessness
  threat of, 38–39

INDEX OF SUBJECTS

Memory, 224–225
Mental illness, myth of, 54–55
Morality, see Choice
Motion picture projector analogy, 205, 279
Mourning, 347

National Training Laboratories, 243
Needs, see Existential needs
Neo-phenomenology, 10
Neuroses, see Existential neuroses
Neurosis, process of, 41–42
Non-being, 27, 135–136, 160–161, 293, 318–319
Nothingness, 28

Ontogogy, 15, 61, 62, 184, 381–382
  expanding awareness and, 235–244
  as a frame of reference, 316–319
  problems in discussion of, 186–187
  procedures, 236–244, 322–327
  state of the art of, 187–188
Ontologic freedom
  and actualization, 264–276
  conceptions of, 253–254
  nature of, 236, 247–254
  relationships and, 280
  religion and, 280
  the *Self* and, 250–251, 254–262
  state of the theory of, 279–280
  transcendence and, 277–299
Ontologic options, 321, 330–333
  of conflict, 348–350
  of devotion, 355–356
  of limits and endings, 330–333
  of participation, 340–343
  of solitude, 356–357

Participation, 270–272, 321, 340–343, 367, 371
"Peak experience," 251–252
Perception, psychology of, 220 fn.
Person, 191–194, 201–202
  and choice, see Choice
  concept of, 193–194
  "ego states" in, 211

  self-presentation of, 191
  therapeutic encounter with, 190
Powerlessness, 287, 293, 298–300
Presence, 383–386
  see also Psychotherapist, authentic presence of
Problem solving, 226–228
Psychoanalytic theory, 16
Psychodiagnostics, 73–82
  see also Tests, psychodiagnostic
Psychological mindedness, 56–57, 368
Psychology, humanistic, 8–14, 380–381
  basic postulates of, 11–13
  characteristics of, 13–14
  existentialism and, 9–10
Psychotherapist
  authentic presence of, 108–109, 180, 372
  gratifications of being a, 362–368
  guilt of, 373–374
  interventions of, see Interventions
  love for patient of, 362–365
  maturity in, 371–375
  and need to cure, 111
  pseudo-maturity in, 368–371
  "set" of, 109–110, 314–315
  silence of, 115–117
  subjective awareness of, 110–111
Psychotherapy
  analytic perspective of, 16
  concept of, 54–56
  dominant emotional theme, see Dominant emotional theme
  existential crisis in, see Existential crisis
  existential orientation in, see Intensive psychotherapy
  existential perspective, 17–20
  experience of, 51–54
  gratifications in practice of, 51–54, 362–368
  intake procedure of, 76
  and ontogogy, see Ontogogy
  patient's role in, 106–107
  phases of, 61–63
  positive products of, 266–275, 382–394

procedures of, 65–68, 85–87, 106–107, 114–131, 143–149, 155–163, 173–180
see also Ontogogy, procedures
and resistance, see Resistance
suitability for, 56–57
task of, 42–43, 288
and tragedy, see Tragedy
and transference, see Transference
writing about, 3–7

Quest for certainty, 74–75

Reality, 41
Reassurance, 162, 179
"Reducing valve," 48, 251
Reflexes, 208
Relatedness, need for, 284, 285, 287, 321, 351–352
Relationship repertoire, 144
Religion, 280, 407–408
Relinquishment, 346–347
Repetition, 123–125
Resignation, 293
Resistance, the, 88–103, 104–133, 318–319
  analysis of, 104–133
  anxiety and, 94–97
  awareness and, 97–99, 232
  chains of, 121–123
  characteristics of, 92–102
  as constraint on awareness, 232
  derived from culture, 197–199
  examples of, 90–92, 95–97
  existential meaning of, 15, 16, 42–43, 48, 63–64, 88–92, 93–103, 413–414
  exposure of in therapy, 100–101
  inadequacies in interpretations of, 125–131
  interpreting in therapy, 114–115
  layered sequence of, 95–97, 100–101
  nature of, see Resistance, existential meaning of
  threat and, 93–97, 100
  transference and, 103

ultimate meaning of, 413
unity of, 131–133
Responsibility, 23, 37–38, 196–197, 256, 334–343
  acceptance of, 338–340
  confrontation of, 287, 293, 301–302, 321
  displacing through testing, 82–83
Role and the Self, 212
Rootedness, need for, 284, 285, 287, 321, 327–328

Satori, see Enlightenment
Science, authenticity of, 408–410
Self, the, 201, 202, 203, 205, 209–216, 251
  confusion with the I, see I and the Self
  definition of, 209
  emancipation from, see Emancipation from the Self
  functioning of, 210–212
  identity and, 335–336
  image of, 212
  the I-process and, 205, 259–262
  learned descriptions of, 257–259
  ontologic freedom and, 254–262
  role and, 212
  transference and, 214–215
Self-actualization, see Actualization
Self-alienation, see Alienation
Self-as-doer, 202–203, 213
Self-as-object, 202–203, 213
Self-concept, 201
  definition of, 210
Self-consistency, 210
Self-fragmentation, 195–197
Self-perception, 249–250
Selves
  multiplicity of, 191–193, 211–212
  overlap among, 212
  "sub-selves" and, 211
  see also Self, the
Separateness, 39, 285, 287, 321
Society, see Emergent society
Solitude, 356–357
Sports, authenticity of, 407

Subject–object split, 140–142, 260–262, 275
 see also Alienation
Suchness, 272–274, 399–400
Superstition, 164, 196–197

Tests, psychodiagnostic
 existential implications of, 75–81
 disadvantages of to patient, 78–80
 disadvantages of to therapist, 76–78
 values of, 81
Therapeutic failure, 166–170, 362–365
Therapeutic procedures, see Psychotherapy, procedures of
Therapeutic relationship, 42–43, 69–87, 244
 aspects of, 139–140
 development of, 85–87
 existential-analytic goal of, 72
 models of, 70–72
 responsibility of therapist in, 244
 as a shared enterprise, 72–73
 transference in, 139–140
Therapist, see Psychotherapist
Therapy, see Psychotherapy
Thinking, 226–228, 257
Threat
 definition of, 93–94
 and the resistance, 93–97, 100
Tragedy, 25, 151–165, 173
 cathartic effect of, 160
 classical view of, 154
 guilt and, 164
 meaning of, 152
 sequence of, 154–155
 sorrow and, 163
 superstition and, 164
 therapeutic sequence in, 162–163
 the therapeutic work and, 155–165
Tragic sequence, see Tragedy, sequence of
Transcendence, 34, 209, 221–222
 enlightenment and, see Enlightenment
 Hora's conceptualization, 277–278
 ontologic freedom and, 277–279
Transference, 64, 103
 analysis of, 134–150
 definition of, 137
 dual implications of, 138
 group therapy and, 215
 incomplete resolutions of, 214
 interpretations of, 145–148
 I–Self distinction and, 214–215
 multiple, 149
 recognition of, 143–144
 resistance and, 103, 138–139
 subject–object split as a, 140–142
 therapeutic significances of, 137–138
Tropism, 208

Values, authenticity-centered, 31–33, 398–400

Wholeness of experience, 274–275
Withdrawal, 293
"World" as a construction of awareness, 97–100, 295–297
Writing, constraints upon, 3–7